Update in Ultrasound

Editor

LESLIE M. SCOUTT

RADIOLOGIC CLINICS OF NORTH AMERICA

www.radiologic.theclinics.com

Consulting Editor
FRANK H. MILLER

November 2014 • Volume 52 • Number 6

ELSEVIER

1600 John F. Kennedy Boulevard • Suite 1800 • Philadelphia, Pennsylvania, 19103-2899

http://www.theclinics.com

RADIOLOGIC CLINICS OF NORTH AMERICA Volume 52, Number 6
November 2014 ISSN 0033-8389, ISBN 13: 978-0-323-32678-0

Editor: John Vassallo (j.vassallo@elsevier.com)
Developmental Editor: Donald Mumford

Radiologic Clinics of North America (ISSN 0033-8389) is published bimonthly by Elsevier Inc., 360 Park Avenue South, New York, NY 10010-1710. Months of issue are January, March, May, July, September, and November. Periodicals postage paid at New York, NY and additional mailing offices. Subscription prices are USD 460 per year for US individuals, USD 709 per year for US institutions, USD 220 per year for US students and residents, USD 535 per year for Canadian individuals, USD 905 per year for Canadian institutions, USD 660 per year for international individuals, USD 905 per year for international institutions, and USD 315 per year for Canadian and foreign students/residents. To receive student and resident rate, orders must be accompanied by name of affiliated institution, date of term and the signature of program/residency coordinatior on institution letterhead. Orders will be billed at individual rate until proof of status is received. Foreign air speed delivery is included in all *Clinics* subscription prices. All prices are subject to change without notice. **POSTMASTER:** Send address changes to *Radiologic Clinics of North America*, Elsevier Health Sciences Division, Subscription Customer Service, 3251 Riverport Lane, Maryland Heights, MO63043. **Customer Service: Telephone: 1-800-654-2452** (U.S. and Canada); **1-314-447-8871** (outside U.S. and Canada). **Fax: 1-314-447-8029. E-mail: journalscustomerservice-usa@ elsevier.com** (for print support); **journalsonlinesupport-usa@elsevier.com** (for online support).

Reprints. For copies of 100 or more of articles in this publication, please contact the Commercial Reprints Department, Elsevier Inc., 360 Park Avenue South, New York, New York 10010-1710. Tel.: +1-212-633-3874; Fax: +1-212-633-3820; E-mail: reprints@elsevier.com.

Radiologic Clinics of North America also published in Greek Paschalidis Medical Publications, Athens, Greece.

Radiologic Clinics of North America is covered in *MEDLINE/PubMed (Index Medicus), EMBASE/Excerpta Medica, Current Contents/Life Sciences, Current Contents/Clinical Medicine, RSNA Index to Imaging Literature, BIOSIS, Science Citation Index,* and *ISI/BIOMED*.

Printed in the United States of America.

Contributors

CONSULTING EDITOR

FRANK H. MILLER, MD
Chief, Body Imaging Section and Fellowship
Program and GI Radiology; Medical Director
MRI; Professor, Department of Radiology,
Northwestern University, Feinberg School of
Medicine, Northwestern Memorial Hospital,
Chicago, Illinois

EDITOR

LESLIE M. SCOUTT, MD
Professor of Diagnostic Radiology and
Vascular Surgery; Chief, Ultrasound Section;
Medical Director, Non-Invasive Vascular
Laboratory; Associate Program Director,
Diagnostic Radiology Residency Program;
Department of Diagnostic Radiology, Yale–
New Haven Hospital, Yale University School of
Medicine, New Haven, Connecticut

AUTHORS

SMBAT AMIRBEKIAN, MD
Radiology Resident, Department of Diagnostic
Radiology, Yale University School of Medicine,
New Haven, Connecticut

ROCHELLE F. ANDREOTTI, MD
Professor of Clinical Radiology and Associate
Professor of Clinical Obstetrics and
Gynecology, Department of Radiology and
Radiological Sciences; Department of
Obstetrics and Gynecology, Vanderbilt
University Medical Center, Nashville,
Tennessee

RICHARD G. BARR, MD, PhD, FACR, FSRU
Professor of Radiology, Department of
Radiology, Northeastern Ohio Medical
University, Rootstown, Ohio; Southwoods
Imaging, Radiology Consultants Inc,
Boardman, Ohio

SHWETA BHATT, MBBS
Associate Professor, Department of Imaging
Sciences, University of Rochester, Rochester,
New York

LINDA C. CHU, MD
Assistant Professor of Radiology, The Russell
H. Morgan Department of Radiology and
Radiological Science, Johns Hopkins
University School of Medicine, Baltimore,
Maryland

STEPHANIE F. COQUIA, MD
Assistant Professor of Radiology, The Russell
H. Morgan Department of Radiology and
Radiological Science, Johns Hopkins
University School of Medicine, Baltimore,
Maryland

PAUL DiDOMENICO, MD
Mallinckrodt Institute of Radiology, Washington
University School of Medicine, St Louis, Missouri

PETER M. DOUBILET, MD, PhD
Senior Vice Chair, Department of Radiology, Brigham and Women's Hospital; Professor of Radiology, Harvard Medical School, Boston, Massachusetts

VINAY DUDDALWAR, MD, FRCR
Associate Professor of Radiology; Section Chief, Abdominal Imaging; Medical Director, Imaging, Keck Hospital of USC, USC Norris Comprehensive Cancer Center, University of Southern California, Los Angeles, California

ARTHUR C. FLEISCHER, MD
Professor of Radiology and Obstetrics and Gynecology, Department of Radiology and Radiological Sciences; Department of Obstetrics and Gynecology, Vanderbilt University Medical Center, Nashville, Tennessee

MARY C. FRATES, MD
Associate Professor of Radiology, Department of Ultrasound, Brigham and Women's Hospital, Harvard Medical School, Boston, Massachusetts

EDWARD G. GRANT, MD, FACR
Professor and Chairman, Department of Radiology, Keck Hospital of USC, USC Norris Comprehensive Cancer Center, University of Southern California, Los Angeles, California

GOWTHAMAN GUNABUSHANAM, MD
Assistant Professor, Department of Diagnostic Radiology, Yale University School of Medicine, New Haven, Connecticut

ULRIKE M. HAMPER, MD, MBA
Professor of Radiology, Urology, and Pathology, The Russell H. Morgan Department of Radiology and Radiological Science, Johns Hopkins University School of Medicine, Baltimore, Maryland

MATTHEW T. HELLER, MD
Department of Radiology, University of Pittsburgh Medical Center, Pittsburgh, Pennsylvania

REGINA J. HOOLEY, MD
Associate Professor, Department of Diagnostic Radiology, Yale University School of Medicine, New Haven, Connecticut

MINDY M. HORROW, MD, FACR
Director of Body Imaging, Einstein Medical Center; Professor of Radiology, Sidney Kimmel Medical College at Thomas Jefferson University, Philadelphia, Pennsylvania

KATHERINE A. KAPROTH-JOSLIN, MD/PhD
Fellow of Breast and Body Imaging, Department of Imaging Sciences, University of Rochester, Rochester, New York

HARSHAWN MALHI, MD
Assistant Professor of Radiology, Department of Radiology, Keck Hospital of USC, University of Southern California, Los Angeles, California

THOMAS E. McCANN, MD
Resident, Department of Diagnostic Radiology, Yale University School of Medicine, New Haven, Connecticut

WILLIAM MIDDLETON, MD
Mallinckrodt Institute of Radiology, Washington University School of Medicine, St Louis, Missouri

LAURENCE NEEDLEMAN, MD
Associate Professor of Radiology, Sidney Kimmel Medical College of Thomas Jefferson University; Director of Ultrasound, Thomas Jefferson University Hospital, Philadelphia, Pennsylvania

JULIE A. RITNER, MD
Instructor of Radiology, Department of Ultrasound, Brigham and Women's Hospital, Harvard Medical School, Boston, Massachusetts

SHUCHI K. RODGERS, MD
Clinical Assistant Professor of Radiology, Department of Radiology, Einstein Medical Center; Sidney Kimmel Medical College at Thomas Jefferson University, Philadelphia, Pennsylvania

DEBORAH J. RUBENS, MD
Professor and Associate Chair of Imaging Sciences, University of Rochester, Rochester, New York

LESLIE M. SCOUTT, MD
Professor of Diagnostic Radiology and
Vascular Surgery; Chief, Ultrasound Section;
Medical Director, Non-Invasive Vascular
Laboratory; Associate Program Director,
Diagnostic Radiology Residency Program;
Department of Diagnostic Radiology, Yale–
New Haven Hospital, Yale University School of
Medicine, New Haven, Connecticut

CHRISTOPHER P. SERENI, MD
Department of Radiology, Sidney Kimmel
Medical College at Thomas Jefferson
University, Einstein Medical Center,
Philadelphia, Pennsylvania

DANIEL SOMMERS, MD
Assistant Professor of Radiology, Department
of Radiology, University of Utah School of
Medicine, Salt Lake City, Utah

MITCHELL E. TUBLIN, MD
Department of Radiology, University of
Pittsburgh Medical Center, Pittsburgh,
Pennsylvania

THOMAS WINTER, MD
Professor of Radiology, Department of
Radiology, University of Utah School of
Medicine, Salt Lake City, Utah

Contents

Elastography is a new technique that evaluates tissue stiffness. There are two elastography methods, strain and shear wave elastography. Both techniques are being used to evaluate a wide range of applications in medical imaging. Elastography of breast masses and prostates have been shown to have high accuracy for characterizing masses and can significantly decrease the need for biopsies. Shear wave elastography has been shown to be able to detect and grade liver fibrosis and may decrease the need for liver biopsy. Evaluation of other organs is still preliminary. This article reviews the principles of elastography and its potential clinical applications.

The use of ultrasonography (US) to detect and characterize diffuse liver disease can be challenging, but remains a useful tool for the diagnosis and management of many diffuse parenchymal liver diseases such as cirrhosis, steatosis, and malignancies. Newer techniques, such as elastography, are proving useful for earlier detection of hepatic parenchymal changes. The role of US in the assessment of possible biliary ductal obstruction is well established, and Doppler US may provide additional physiologic information regarding hepatic blood flow. US plays a central role in target selection and guidance of percutaneous liver biopsies.

The clinical use of noncardiac contrast-enhanced ultrasound scan (CEUS) has been steadily gaining momentum. CEUS is a reliable and safe technique with a diverse array of applications. This article reviews the current and potential future clinical applications of CEUS. Emphasis will be placed on evaluating focal lesions with the liver and kidney. Contrast agent composition and mechanism are also briefly reviewed.

Ultrasound is a valuable diagnostic test throughout the first trimester of pregnancy. Early in this trimester, it is used to distinguish between normal intrauterine, failed intrauterine, and ectopic pregnancies. Later it can be used with maternal blood tests to screen for trisomy 21 and other forms of aneuploidy, and in some centers to assess fetal anatomy and diagnose structural anomalies. First trimester sonography is also useful for accurate assessment of gestational age. This article reviews these applications, the approach to establishing diagnoses, and ways to avoid diagnostic mistakes that can lead to serious errors in patient management and adverse pregnancy outcome.

Volume imaging in the pelvis has been well demonstrated to be an extremely useful technique, largely based on its ability to reconstruct the coronal plane of the uterus that usually cannot be visualized using traditional 2-dimensional (2D) imaging. As a result, this technique is now a part of the standard pelvic ultrasound protocol in many institutions. A variety of valuable applications of 3D sonography in the pelvis are discussed in this article.

Pelvic pain is a frequent complaint in women presenting to the emergency room or to a physician's office, and ultrasound should be considered the initial imaging modality of choice in the evaluation of women with pelvic pain. This article reviews the ultrasound imaging technique and provides a thorough differential of gynecologic and nongynecologic causes of both acute and chronic pelvic pain.

Ultrasonography is the primary imaging modality for evaluation of pelvic masses. Ultrasonography has the advantage of being inexpensive, widely available, and offering superior tissue characterization compared with computed tomography. The real-time imaging ability of ultrasonography and three-dimensional ultrasonography also has the advantage of being able to identify the organ of origin of the pelvic mass. Many pelvic masses have characteristic sonographic appearances that allow confident diagnosis and management. This article reviews the sonographic appearances and management of common pelvic masses encountered in nonpregnant women, and is organized based on anatomic location: uterus, cervix, ovaries, and fallopian tubes.

Prenatal sonography is routinely used to evaluate fetal biometry and anatomy between 16 and 20 weeks. Ventriculomegaly is easily seen on these routine views and is commonly associated with numerous intracranial anomalies. Although ventriculomegaly can be isolated, it should always prompt a detailed search to evaluate for an underlying cause. Using a systematic approach to evaluate the intracranial structures can help the clinician arrive at a correct diagnosis for many abnormalities of central nervous system.

Sonography is the ideal modality for evaluation and characterization of a scrotal mass. Extratesticular masses are usually benign, whereas intratesticular masses are generally malignant until proved otherwise. However, it is important to recognize the benign intratesticular conditions, thus possibly preventing orchiectomy when unwarranted, while appreciating the more significant findings of extratesticular masses that may warrant further intervention. This article reviews the anatomy and sonographic findings of scrotal masses. Normal anatomy, general imaging techniques, and assessment of intratesticular and extratesticular disorders will be discussed.

Sonography plays several important roles in the diagnosis and management of thyroid cancer. Ultrasound (US) is used for the detection and characterization of thyroid nodules as well as a guidance modality for fine-needle aspiration biopsy of indeterminate or suspicious nodules. US is also used to help stage thyroid cancer by identifying cervical lymph nodes suspicious for metastasis so they can be biopsied prior to subsequent neck dissection. Post-thyroidectomy, routine surveillance of the neck is performed with US to identify local recurrence and/or nodal metastatic disease so that focused and limited repeat neck dissection or alcohol ablation can be accomplished.

Palpable soft tissue masses are common and are often referred for imaging evaluation. Ultrasonography is an attractive way to image these lesions because it is inexpensive, readily available, and does not rely on ionizing radiation. Ultrasonography can easily confirm the presence of a mass, differentiate solid from cystic lesions, define the anatomic extent of the lesion, and detect vascular lesions with high sensitivity. In most cases, ultrasonography can accurately characterize the lesion, obviating biopsy and reducing unnecessary further work-up. This article reviews the capabilities of ultrasonography in evaluating superficial soft tissue lesions and the sonographic appearance of disease entities.

Ultrasonography is an excellent tool for evaluation of the renal transplant in the immediate postoperative period and for long-term follow-up. In this article, normal imaging findings and complications of renal transplantations are described. Disease processes are divided into vascular, perinephric, urologic and collecting system, and parenchymal abnormalities. Attention is paid to the time of occurrence of each complication, classic imaging findings, and potential pitfalls.

In this article, the standard ultrasonographic scanning techniques and Doppler settings necessary to produce reliable and reproducible carotid imaging are discussed. The normal carotid anatomy is reviewed, including grayscale, color Doppler, and spectral Doppler imaging appearances. The vascular abnormalities caused by atherosclerosis are examined, including plaque morphology characterization as well as waveform and velocity changes caused by stenosis, are examined. In addition, special situations are explored, such as imaging in the presence of an arrhythmia or cardiac assist devices. Imaging after carotid intervention is discussed, including the complications associated with these procedures.

Peripheral arterial disease (PAD) is an important manifestation of atherosclerosis, with an estimated age-adjusted prevalence of approximately 13% in people older than 50 years. Noninvasive vascular laboratory physiologic studies are indispensable tools in the initial evaluation and workup and postintervention follow-up. In this review, we describe a practical approach to the technique, interpretation, pitfalls, and limitations of these physiologic studies. We also provide an algorithmic approach for using these studies in the initial workup of patients with suspected PAD. Noninvasive techniques that primarily provide anatomic information have not been included in this review.

Lower extremity venous ultrasonography is an accurate method to diagnose acute deep venous thrombosis (DVT). Recurrent DVT is often a difficult diagnosis. The decision to order ultrasonography can be based on pretest risk assessment. If the ultrasonography study is negative, the report may recommend follow-up for patients whose clinical condition changes or for patients with specific risks. Lower extremity venous ultrasonography is the gold standard for diagnosis of DVT. It is accurate and objective, and because the clinical assessment of patients is limited and its potential complication, pulmonary embolism, is significant, the impact of a positive and negative test is high.

PROGRAM OBJECTIVE

The objective of the *Radiologic Clinics of North America* is to keep practicing radiologists and radiology residents up to date with current clinical practice in radiology by providing timely articles reviewing the state of the art in patient care.

TARGET AUDIENCE

Practicing radiologists, radiology residents, and other health care professionals who provide patient care utilizing radiologic findings.

LEARNING OBJECTIVES

Upon completion of this activity, participants will be able to:

1. Review ultrasound evaluation of the renal transplant, of scrotal and pelvic masses, and of diffuse liver disease.
2. Discuss the role of sonography in thyroid cancer.
3. Review an update on the lower extremity venous ultrasound.

ACCREDITATION

The Elsevier Office of Continuing Medical Education (EOCME) is accredited by the Accreditation Council for Continuing Medical Education (ACCME) to provide continuing medical education for physicians.

The EOCME designates this enduring material for a maximum of 15 *AMA PRA Category 1 Credit*(s)™. Physicians should claim only the credit commensurate with the extent of their participation in the activity.

All other health care professionals requesting continuing education credit for this enduring material will be issued a certificate of participation.

DISCLOSURE OF CONFLICTS OF INTEREST

The EOCME assesses conflict of interest with its instructors, faculty, planners, and other individuals who are in a position to control the content of CME activities. All relevant conflicts of interest that are identified are thoroughly vetted by EOCME for fair balance, scientific objectivity, and patient care recommendations. EOCME is committed to providing its learners with CME activities that promote improvements or quality in healthcare and not a specific proprietary business or a commercial interest.

The planning committee, staff, authors and editors listed below have identified no financial relationships or relationships to products or devices they or their spouse/life partner have with commercial interest related to the content of this CME activity:

Smbat Amirbekian, MD; Rochelle F. Andreotti, MD; Shweta Bhatt, MBBS; Linda C. Chu, MD; Stephanie F. Coquia, MD; Paul B. DiDomenico, MD; Peter M. Doubilet, MD, PhD; Arthur C. Fleischer, MD; Mary C. Frates, MD; Edward G. Grant, MD, FACR; Gowthaman Gunabushanam, MD; Ulrike M. Hamper, MD, MBA; Matthew T. Heller, MD; Kristen Helm; Regina J. Hooley, MD; Mindy M. Horrow, MD, FACR; Brynne Hunter; Katherine A. Kaproth-Joslin, MD/PhD; Sandy Lavery; Harshawn Malhi, MD; Thomas E. McCann, MD; Jill McNair; William Middleton, MD; Frank H. Miller, MD; Karthikeyan Subramaniam; Laurence Needleman, MD; Julie A. Ritner, MD; Shuchi K. Rodgers, MD; Deborah J. Rubens, MD; Christopher P. Sereni, MD; Daniel N. Sommers, MD; Mitchell E. Tublin, MD; John Vassallo; Thomas Winter, MD.

The planning committee, staff, authors and editors listed below have identified financial relationships or relationships to products or devices they or their spouse/life partner have with commercial interest related to the content of this CME activity:

Richard G. Barr, MD, PhD, FACR, FSRU is on speakers bureau, is a consultant/advisor for, and has research grant from Philips Ultrasound and Siemens Ultrasound; is on speakers bureau and has research grant from SuperSonic Imagine; is a consultant/advisor for Toshiba America Medical Systems; and has a research grant from Esaote.
Vinay A. Duddalwar, MD, FRCR has a research grant from GE Healthcare.
Leslie M. Scoutt, MD is on speakers bureau for Philips Healthcare.

UNAPPROVED/OFF-LABEL USE DISCLOSURE

The EOCME requires CME faculty to disclose to the participants:

1. When products or procedures being discussed are off-label, unlabelled, experimental, and/or investigational (not US Food and Drug Administration [FDA] approved); and
2. Any limitations on the information presented, such as data that are preliminary or that represent ongoing research, interim analyses, and/or unsupported opinions. Faculty may discuss information about pharmaceutical agents that is outside of FDA-approved labelling. This information is intended solely for CME and is not intended to promote off-label use of these medications. If you have any questions, contact the medical affairs department of the manufacturer for the most recent prescribing information.

TO ENROLL

To enroll in the *Radiologic Clinics of North America* Continuing Medical Education program, call customer service at 1-800-654-2452 or sign up online at http://www.theclinics.com/home/cme. The CME program is available to subscribers for an additional annual fee of USD $315.

METHOD OF PARTICIPATION

In order to claim credit, participants must complete the following:

1. Complete enrolment as indicated above.
2. Read the activity.
3. Complete the CME Test and Evaluation. Participants must achieve a score of 70% on the test. All CME Tests and Evaluations must be completed online.

CME INQUIRIES/SPECIAL NEEDS

For all CME inquiries or special needs, please contact elsevierCME@elsevier.com.

RADIOLOGIC CLINICS OF NORTH AMERICA

NOW AVAILABLE FOR YOUR iPhone and iPad

Preface
Update in Ultrasound

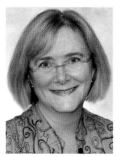

Leslie M. Scoutt, MD
Editor

Ultrasound has been an integral part of diagnostic imaging for many years, is readily accessible, is without known adverse bioeffects, and is relatively inexpensive. As such, ultrasound has been actively embraced by diagnostic radiologists as well as by many other medical subspecialties. Hence, ultrasound plays an integral role in the diagnostic evaluation of patients of all ages and is often used in screening, follow-up of therapy and chronic illness as well as in the evaluation of the acutely ill patient. Ultrasound has a broad range of clinical applicability, ranging from pediatrics, women's imaging, urology, and endocrinology, to vascular, abdominal, and musculoskeletal pathology. Ultrasound can be used to confirm diagnosis and to guide recommendations for further imaging or intervention. Recently, advances in technology, such as 3-dimensional imaging, elastography, and intravenous ultrasound contrast, have resulted in a renaissance in ultrasound imaging.

This volume introduces many of these new technologies, describing principles and theory, current clinical applications as well as how to introduce such new technology into clinical practice. In addition, guidelines for the evaluation of the first trimester of pregnancy, thyroid nodules, adnexal masses, and lower extremity venous pathology have been recently revised and current guidelines and controversies are presented here. Last, a series of articles are offered that review many common or emerging areas where ultrasound is particularly clinically useful, such as MSK, OB, GYN, abdominal, and vascular pathology.

I am honored to have been asked to serve as editor for this volume. I wish to thank the many authors, all experts in the field, for their excellent contributions, which provide state-of-the-art information on a wide variety of topics. In addition, I wish to acknowledge their forbearance with my editorial efforts. I sincerely appreciate the hard work of the Elsevier staff and I especially wish to thank Donald Mumford and John Vassallo for their administrative and editorial assistance. Thanks to all of our wonderful sonographers, who obtain such outstanding images on a daily basis. Last, thanks to our readers for their commitment, interest, and enthusiasm in ultrasound and for stretching the limits of this modality to provide optimal care for their patients.

Leslie M. Scoutt, MD
Diagnostic Radiology and Vascular Surgery
Ultrasound Section
Non-Invasive Vascular Laboratory
Diagnostic Radiology Residency Program
Yale University School of Medicine
Yale–New Haven Hospital
PO Box 208042
New Haven, CT, 06529-8042, USA

E-mail address:
leslie.scoutt@yale.edu

Radiol Clin N Am 52 (2014) xv
http://dx.doi.org/10.1016/j.rcl.2014.08.003

Elastography in Clinical Practice

Richard G. Barr, MD, PhD, FACR, FSRU[a,b,*]

KEYWORDS

- Elastography - Ultrasound - Breast mass - Breast cancer - Prostate cancer - Liver fibrosis
- Thyroid mass

KEY POINTS

- Both strain and shear wave elastography have high sensitivity and specificity in characterizing breast lesions as benign or malignant.
- Shear wave point quantification and 2-dimensional shear wave elastography can be used to assess liver fibrosis and as a noninvasive method of monitoring disease progression or treatment response.
- Shear wave elastography has a high negative predictive value for assessing malignancy in the peripheral zone of the prostate.
- Strain elastography can be performed anywhere a good B-mode image can be obtained.

INTRODUCTION

With the recent Food and Drug Administration approval for quantification using ultrasound elastography, these techniques are rapidly gaining acceptance for many clinical applications. Multiple vendors have some form of elastography available on their systems. In this article, the principles of the 2 major types of ultrasound elastography are briefly reviewed, highlighting their advantages and disadvantages. The clinical applications that are becoming widely accepted as the standard of care are discussed. Emphasis is placed on how to incorporate these techniques into your practice. A brief review of other potential applications that are not yet mature enough for routine clinical use is provided.

PRINCIPLES

There are 2 types of ultrasound elastography presently available, strain elastography (SE) and shear wave elastography (SWE).[1,2] Although these both measure tissue stiffness, there are differences in the techniques and how they are used in clinical practice.

SE is a qualitative (not quantitative) technique. The images obtained demonstrate the relative stiffness of the tissues within the field of view (FOV). However, the absolute stiffness of the tissue is not known; other factors, such as relative stiffness compared with normal tissue or change in size compared with B-mode, must be used to obtain clinically useful information.[2,3] SE images are obtained by comparing the frame-to-frame changes of tissues when a vibratory or compression/release force is applied to the tissue. Soft tissues deform more, whereas hard tissues deform less (Fig. 1). The amount of compression/release force to obtain optimal SE images varies by vendor. In some cases, only the patients' breathing and/or heartbeat are required to generate optimal elastograms, whereas, in others,

Disclosures: Philips Ultrasound – equipment grant, research grant, speaker's bureau, advisory panel; Siemens Ultrasound – equipment grant, research grant, speaker's bureau, advisory panel; SuperSonic Imagine – equipment grant, speaker's bureau; Esaote – equipment grant; Toshiba America Medical Systems – advisory panel.
[a] Department of Radiology, Northeastern Ohio Medical University, 4209 Ohio 44, Rootstown, OH 44272, USA;
[b] Southwoods Imaging, Radiology Consultants Inc, 7623 Market Street, Boardman, OH 44512, USA
* Southwoods Imaging, Radiology Consultants Inc, 7623 Market Street, Boardman, Ohio 44512.
E-mail address: rgbarr@zoominternet.net

radiologic.theclinics.com

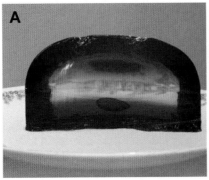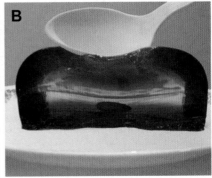

Fig. 1. SE is based on how a tissue deforms when a force is applied to it. Soft tissues will deform more than stiff tissues. A simple example is if we have an almond in gelatin (*A*) and then apply a force with a spoon (*B*), the gelatin deforms significantly; however, the almond does not change shape. Therefore, the gelatin is soft, whereas the almond is hard. In SE, the system compares the frame-to-frame changes when a force is applied. The relative stiffness of the tissues is determined by how much they deform.

compression and release using the transducer are required. With practice, the optimal scanning technique can be learned and be reproducible. Some vendors have a bar, or quality measure, on the monitor that provide real-time feedback on the appropriateness of the amount of compression/release being applied.[2]

The results are provided in an image that can be displayed in gray scale or in a variety of color maps. The data provided are the same regardless of which color map is used, and the map choice is often dictated by the user's experience. It is important to remember that because SE is a relative measure of stiffness, the FOV should contain a range of tissues with varying stiffness to allow for an appropriate dynamic range in the scale for adequate interpretation.[2]

SWE is a technique that provides a quantitative measure of stiffness that is expressed in meters per second (the shear wave speed) or in kilopascals (Young's Modulus).[1,2] Most systems allow for either to be displayed, and they are easily converted from one to the other. In SWE, a push pulse, often referred to as acoustic radiation force impulse (ARFI), is used to generate shear waves within the tissues, which is similar to dropping a stone into a pond (the push pulse) and generating waves on the water (shear waves). Note that the shear waves are generated perpendicular to the push pulse. Conventional B-mode imaging is used to monitor the shear waves generated through the tissue and calculate the shear wave speed (**Fig. 2**).

In this technique, either a single measurement over a small FOV can be obtained (*point quantification* SWE) or color mapping of a large FOV of individual pixel shear wave speeds is depicted (*2-dimensional [2D] SWE*). The color map used

to display the data is usually red as hard and blue as soft. The color scale can be adjusted to allow better depiction of the range of shear wave speeds within the FOV, and careful attention to the scale is advised if interpretation based on color is used.

A limitation of SWE is that the push pulse is attenuated as it traverses tissue and ultimately reaches a point where it is too weak to generate shear waves. In this case, the area/tissue where adequate shear waves are not obtained is not color coded (black) on 2D SWE or a value of x.xx or 0.00 is obtained with point quantification SWE.[1,2]

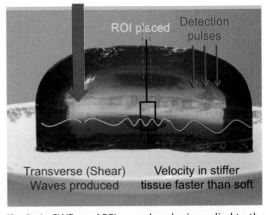

Fig. 2. In SWE, an ARFI or push pulse is applied to the tissue. This strong acoustic pulse generates shear waves perpendicular to the applied push pulse. The shear wave speed can be measured by using B-mode imaging to detect the shear wave displacements at different positions from the pulse push. The shear wave speed varies with the stiffness of the tissue, slower for softer lesions and faster for stiffer lesions. ROI, region of interest.

In SWE, the absolute stiffness value can be used for lesion characterization or the ratio of the lesion stiffness to normal tissue stiffness can be used.

Another elastography technique is available whereby ARFI is used to generate tissue deformation and the deformation is used to calculate a strain image. This method is a qualitative strain method and not an SWE method. This technique is called Virtual Touch Imaging (VTI, Siemens Ultrasound, Mountain View, CA).

One factor that is critical in obtaining accurate elastograms using either the SE or SWE techniques is the amount of precompression or preload used when obtaining the elastogram.[2] This precompression is the amount of pressure exerted on the tissues when the scan is taken. As tissues are compressed with the transducer (ie, using a heavy hand), the tissues become stiffer. In general, softer tissues are affected more than stiffer tissues; therefore, both the relative values in SE as well as the absolute values of SWE can be affected enough to lead to inaccurate tissue assessment. A method of applying minimal precompression has been described and found to be highly reproducible.[4]

BREAST ELASTOGRAPHY

Both SE and SWE have been shown to have high sensitivity and specificity for characterization of breast masses as benign or malignant.[5–13] Breast elastography has been recommended for breast lesion characterization in the guidelines of both the European Federation of Societies for Ultrasound in Medicine and Biology (EFSUMB) and the World Federation for Ultrasound in Medicine and Biology (WFUMB).[14,15] Previous work in vitro has demonstrated that breast cancers are significantly stiffer than benign breast lesions with little overlap, suggesting elastography would be an excellent method for breast lesion characterization.[16] Careful attention to technique is important for both types of elastography and are descripted in detail elsewhere.[2,17]

There have been several methods for reporting, analyzing, and interpretation of SE in breast lesion characterization. These methods include the ratio of elastogram to B-mode length (E/B ratio),[5,6] a 5-point color scale (Tsukuba score),[18] and the lesion-to-fat ratio or strain ratio.[19] All of these methods depend on obtaining adequate strain images with minimal precompression and an FOV containing a wide range of tissue stiffness (fat, fibroglandular tissue, lesion, and pectoralis muscle). A detailed description of how to obtain optimal SE images is provided elsewhere.[2]

In early work on breast elastography, it was noticed that breast malignancies appear larger on the elastogram than the corresponding B-mode image, whereas benign lesions appear smaller.[20] This phenomenon seems to be unique to breast lesions and can be used to characterize a lesion as benign or malignant. In a single-site pilot study using an E/B ratio of 1.0 or more as malignant and less than 1.0 as benign, Barr[5] reported a sensitivity of 100% and a specificity of 99% in characterizing breast lesions as benign or malignant. In a larger multicenter, international study evaluating 651 biopsy-proven lesions, a sensitivity of 99% and a specificity of 85% was obtained.[6] Additional studies have had similar results.[7] Fig. 3 demonstrates an example of a benign and malignant breast lesion.

To use this technique, the lesion must be accurately measured on both the B-mode image and the elastogram. Early work suggests that the E/B ratio may be reflective of tumor grade, with low-grade malignancies (ductal carcinoma in situ or mucinous cancers) having an E/B ratio of at or near 1.0, whereas higher-grade tumors have ratios of up to 3.0 or greater.[21] Some investigators have suggested using an E/B ratio of 1.2 to increase specificity but at the expense of decreased sensitivity.

The 5-point color scale has been proposed for interpretation of many SE applications (Fig. 4).[18,22–25] In this scale, a tissue that is entirely soft is given a score of 1; a tissue with mixed soft and stiff components is given a score of 2; a stiff lesion that is smaller than the appearance on B-mode imaging is given a score of 3; if the lesion is stiff and the same size as on B-mode, it is given a score of 4; if the lesion is stiff and larger than on B-mode, it is given a score of 5. Using this scale, Ueno[9] determined a cutoff between 3 and 4 had a sensitivity of 86% and a specificity of 90% in characterizing breast lesions as benign or malignant.[18] Multiple studies have reported similar results. Fig. 5 is an example of this technique.

In order to semiquantitate the SE results, Itoh and colleagues[18] suggested using the ratio of lesion stiffness to the stiffness of fat, the lesion-to-fat ratio, or the strain ratio. In order to use this method, the lesion and fat need to be within the same image. A region of interest (ROI) is placed within the lesion and a second within fat. Most ultrasound systems allow for the calculation of the relative stiffness of the tissues. Note that precompression can significantly affect the results, as fat stiffness increases faster than lesion stiffness.[4] Using this technique, Itoh and colleagues[18] found a sensitivity of 77% and a

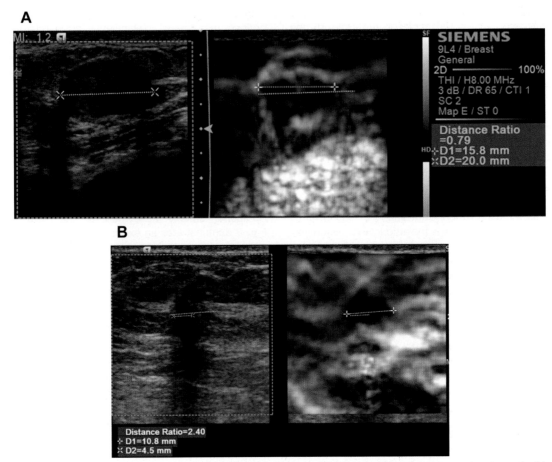

Fig. 3. Examples of a benign (*A*) and malignant (*B*) lesion on SE. (*A*) A 43 year old who presented with a palpable breast mass. The B-mode image is on the left and measures 20.0 mm. The image on the right is the SE image. The lesion measures 15.8 mm on SE, giving a ratio of elastogram to B-mode length (E/B) of 0.79 suggesting a benign lesion. The lesion was a benign fibroadenoma on biopsy. (*B*) A 63-year-old woman had a suspicious lesion noted on screening mammography. On B-mode ultrasound (*left image*), there is a taller-than-wide BI-RADS category 4C lesion with a diameter of 4.5 mm. On the SE image (*right*), the lesion measures 10.8 mm, giving an E/B ratio of 2.4 suggestive of a malignant lesion. The lesion was an invasive ductal cancer.

specificity of 77% in breast lesion characterization.[19] Several other studies have been published with a wider range of accuracy, most likely because of the variability in the techniques and effects of precompression. An example of this technique is presented in **Fig. 6**.

Using shear wave imaging, an absolute value of lesion stiffness can be obtained and used to characterize a breast lesion as benign or malignant.[2,8,26,27] The cutoff values in various studies have varied between 60 and 80 kPa (4.5–5.2 m/s), with sensitivities ranging from 63% to 97% and

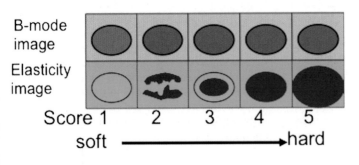

Score 1   2   3   4   5
soft ⟶ hard

Fig. 4. The 5-point color scale for lesion classification with SE. A score of 1 is given to a lesion that is entirely soft; a score of 2 is given if the lesion has both soft and stiff components; a score of 3 corresponds to a stiff lesion that is smaller than identified on B-mode; a score of 4 is given if the lesion is stiff and same size as the B-mode image; if the lesion is stiff and larger than the B-mode image, it is given a score of 5.

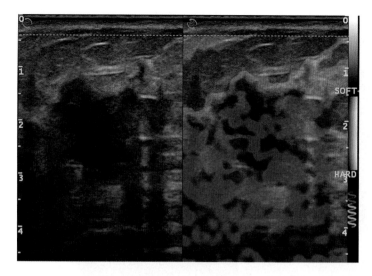

Fig. 5. A 55-year-old woman presented with a new lesion on screening mammography. On B-mode imaging (*left*) the lesion has angular borders and is taller than wide BI-RADS category 4C lesion. On the color-coded SE image (*red* is soft and *blue* is hard), the lesion is mostly blue with occasional green that corresponds to a score of 4 consistent with a malignant lesion. On image-guided core biopsy, the lesion was an invasive ductal cancer.

specificities ranging from 83% to 100%. Some breast cancers do not allow for the generation of measureable shear waves for accurate assessment of the cancer stiffness. When this occurs, the cancer is not color coded or has a low-quality map.[28] There may be a ring of high velocity surrounding the lesion. Breast cancers tend to have increased heterogeneity on SWE. Examples of benign and malignant lesions are presented in **Fig. 7**.

In a large multicenter study,[8] the evaluation of SWE signal homogeneity and lesion-to-fat ratios were the best differentiators of benign and malignant. The addition of SWE improved the characterization of breast lesions compared with using Breast Imaging-Reporting and Data System (BI-RADS) alone, with a sensitivity and specificity of 93% and 59% for BI-RADS and 92% and 76% with the addition of SWE. The investigators comment that the major value of the addition of SWE is in BI-RADS 3 and 4a lesions whereby the SWE results are used to upgrade or downgrade the lesion.

In a study comparing SE and SWE in the same patient population, both demonstrated high sensitivity (98% and 93% respectively) and specificity (95% and 89% respectively) of breast lesion characterization as benign or malignant when a quality map is used with SWE to aid in lesion characterization.[29]

With some vendors, SE a bull's-eye artifact is identified in benign simple and complicated

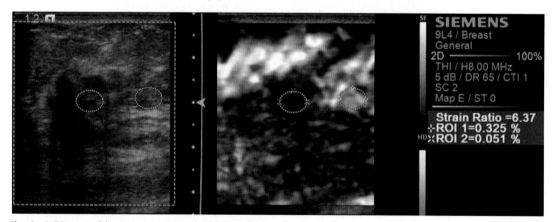

Fig. 6. A 75-year-old woman presented with an abnormal screening mammogram. To calculate the lesion-to-fat ratio, or strain ratio, a region of interest (ROI) (*yellow circles*) is placed in the lesion and a second ROI is placed in fat. The ratio of the relative lesion stiffness can then be calculated. In this example, the same patient in **Fig. 5** has a strain ratio of 6.37, that is, the lesion is 6.37 times stiffer than fat. This ratio (>4.5) is suggestive of a malignancy consistent with this invasive ductal carcinoma.

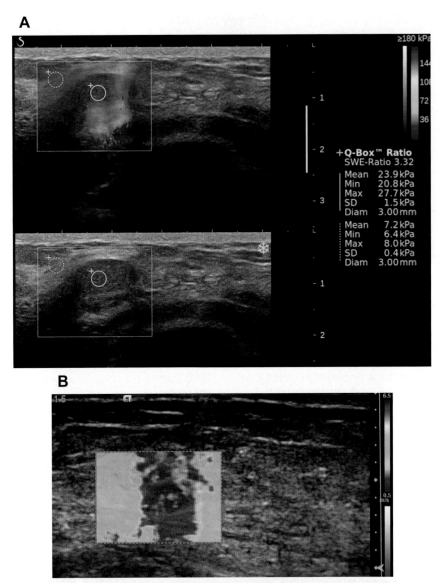

Fig. 7. Examples of a benign (A) and malignant (B) lesion on SWE. (A) A 43-year-old woman presented with a palpable mass. The SWE image is the upper image and the B-mode image is the lower image. The lesion has a maximum kilopascal of 27.7 (3.0 m/s) (*yellow circles*) consistent with a benign lesion. This lesion was a benign fibroadenoma on biopsy. (B) A 68-year-old woman presented with an abnormal screening mammogram. The velocity map of an SWE study is presented here. The lesion is color coded red with a shear wave velocity (Vs) of 6.8 m/s (135 kPa) consistent with a malignant lesion. The lesion was an invasive ductal cancer on biopsy.

cysts.[30] This artifact is characterized by a white central signal within a black outer signal and a bright spot posterior to the lesion (**Fig. 8**). This artifact has been used to decrease the number of biopsies performed in breast lesions.[30]

LIVER
Focal Liver Lesions

Focal liver lesions have been evaluated with both SE and SWE techniques. Because SE is qualitative, a lesion can be compared with normal liver to determine its relative stiffness. However, this technique is limited in that the background liver may have variable stiffness depending on the degree of fibrosis. Another confounding factor is that both benign and malignant lesions can be soft or hard compared with normal liver. Using SWE, a true measurement of stiffness is obtained. However, because of the wide variability of a given pathologic conditions stiffness, characterization of a lesion as benign or malignant is

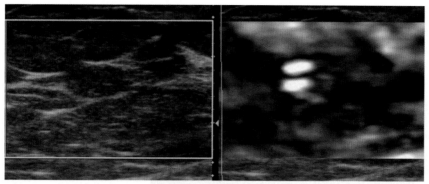

Fig. 8. The bull's-eye artifact is identified with Siemens (Mountain View, CA) and Philips (Bothell, WA) SE imaging. The artifact has been shown to be highly specific for benign simple and complicated cysts. In this example of a 45-year-old woman who presented with a palpable mass, the bull's-eye artifact is identified at the site of the palpable abnormality. On B-mode imaging, the lesion is an isoechoic, complicated cyst that would not have been identified without the use of elastography.

problematic. In a series by Yu and Wilson,[31] hemangioma had a range of shear wave velocity (Vs) of 0.87 to 4.01 m/s with an average of 0.71 m/s, whereas hepatocellular carcinomas had a range of 0.77 to 4.34 m/s with an average of 1.01 m/s. Although the overall difference in Vs of malignant 2.57 ± 1.01 m/s and benign lesions 1.73 ± 0.8 was statistically significant ($P<.01$), the large overlap between benign and malignant makes the technique unreliable for focal liver mass characterization in any given case. **Fig. 9** is a selected SWE of a patient with multiple metastatic lesions from colorectal carcinoma demonstrating the variability of metastatic lesions in the same patient. At this time, the use of elastography is not recommended for characterization of focal liver lesions. Elastography can be used to improve visualization of a lesion for biopsy (**Fig. 10**) and may be useful in following lesions after treatment.

Liver Fibrosis Assessment

Diffuse liver disease, most commonly caused by hepatitis C and hepatitis B infection, is a major worldwide health concern. Appropriate diagnosis and staging is required for adequate treatment and follow-up. The need for a noninvasive method of assessing treatment is needed, especially with the development of new antiviral medications for the treatment of hepatitis C. Liver biopsy has been the gold standard but only assesses a

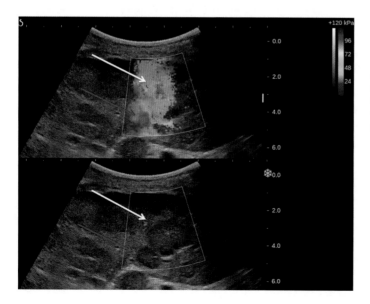

Fig. 9. Shear wave elastogram of the liver in a patient with diffuse colorectal metastatic disease. Note that 2 selected metastatic lesions (*arrows*) are of markedly different stiffness, one very stiff and one soft. The variability of lesion stiffness even in the same patient limits the use of liver lesion characterization in focal liver lesions.

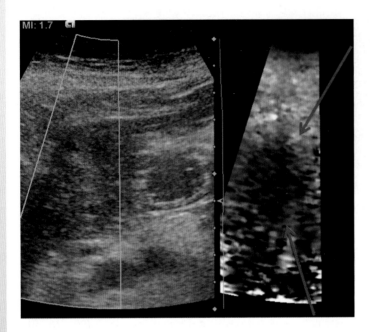

Fig. 10. VTI imaging of a patient with a liver metastasis from ovarian cancer. The lesion has increased conspicuity on elastography (*red arrows*).

minimal amount of tissue and is invasive with possible serious complications.[32–34]

There are several classification methods for liver fibrosis based on the histologic grading of liver biopsy specimens. The most widely used is the Metavir score.[35] This scale ranges from 0 to 4, with 0 representing normal, F1 as minimal fibrosis, F2 as moderate fibrosis, F3 as severe fibrosis, and F4 as cirrhosis. With increasing fibrosis, the stiffness of the liver increases. There are several SWE methods that can be used to assess liver stiffness (LS). These methods include Fibroscan[36–50] as well as SWE point quantification[51–57] and 2D SWE.[14,58,59] Fibroscan is a nonimaging method that uses a mechanical push to generate shear waves that are measured with B-mode ultrasound. The point quantification and 2D methods use ARFI push pulses to generate shear waves. The shear wave speed is estimated using B-mode imaging techniques to monitor the shear waves. Fibroscan cannot be used in the presence of ascites and does not provide imaging of the liver. SWE can be used if ascites is present and all systems provide B-mode and color Doppler for liver imaging.

Technique is critical to obtain accurate measurements of LS regardless of which methodology is used. Measurements should be taken in the right lobe of the liver with patients in the left lateral oblique or decubitus position with their arm above the head. This positioning allows for a wider window between the ribs. Measurements in the left lobe of the liver have been found to be more variable and less accurate and, therefore,

not recommended for liver fibrosis assessment. The ROI used for measurements should not contain large blood vessels. Patients should suspend respiration in a neutral position. Taking a breath in or out can change stiffness measurements secondary to changes in hepatic venous pressure. A window with an excellent B-mode image should be used. The probe should be perpendicular to the liver capsule. The ROI box should be placed at least 1.5 cm to 2.0 cm below the liver capsule. Measurements taken closer to the liver capsule are less accurate and suffer from artifacts.

Multiple measurements should be taken and averaged. The literature suggests a minimum of 10 measurements should be obtained and a mean value used. The interquartile measurement or the interquartile/mean measurements are useful quality measures to confirm that the results are accurate. Quality indicators have been recommended, including an interquartile range less than 30% and a success rate of greater than 60%.[60] With increasingly defined protocols to limit variability, the number of measurements may be decreased as long as the quality measures remain high.

TRANSIENT ELASTOGRAPHY

In patients with chronic hepatitis C, LS values obtained using transient elastography (TE) greater than 6.8 to 7.6 kPa signify a high probability of significant fibrosis (F = >2) on biopsy. The cutoff values for predicting cirrhosis (F = 4) range between 11.0 and 13.6 kPa.[39,40] Although TE is less accurate in distinguishing between contiguous stages of fibrosis, it can differentiate absence and mild fibrosis from significant fibrosis and cirrhosis. A meta-analysis in recurrent hepatitis C posttransplantation demonstrated 98% sensitivity and 84% specificity of TE for predicting cirrhosis.[41] The use of TE in chronic hepatitis C has been endorsed in the recommendations for the management of viral hepatitis by the European Association for the Study of the Liver.[61]

Studies performed in patients with nonalcoholic fatty liver disease (NAFLD) and nonalcoholic steatohepatitis (NASH) have found steatosis does not seem to affect LS measurements.[38,44,45] TE has been used to assess many other diffuse liver diseases with similar good results.[47] TE has been evaluated for predicting complications of cirrhosis, such as portal hypertension and mortality. The area under the receiver operating characteristic curves (AUROCs) for predicting clinically significant portal hypertension (hepatic venous pressure gradient of >12 mm Hg) were 0.94 to 0.99 for cutoffs ranging from 13.6 to 21.0 kPa.[48,49] Measurements of splenic stiffness have also been evaluated and showed better correlation with portal pressure (r = 0.89) in patients with cirrhosis than LS.[62] In a large prospective study of patients with chronic hepatitis C, TE was more accurate than liver biopsy in predicting prognosis. Patients with TE greater than 9.5 kPa had a significantly reduced 5-year survival.[50]

Recommendations for routine clinical use of TE have been published by the EFSUMB.[14]

Shear Wave Speed Measurement

With increasing fibrosis, the liver becomes stiffer, which can be monitored using SWE.[63,64] **Fig. 11**

shows the results from a 27 year old with chronic hepatitis C. The stiffness average of 4.77 kPa is consistent with the patient's liver biopsy result of mild fibrosis. **Fig. 12** is the image from a patient with marked cirrhosis demonstrating a markedly elevated stiffness of 66 kPa.

How this new technology can be best used in clinical practice is under extensive investigation.[63] The use of this technique may be able to decrease the number of liver biopsies performed for evaluation of chronic liver disease. Potential uses of this technique include liver cirrhosis suspected but not obvious on B-mode ultrasound, evaluation of patients with chronic hepatitis C, follow-up of patients to detect progression of liver disease, and to determine when to initiate treatment.

SWE can be performed in a small ROI, point quantification SWE (pSWE), or with a color-coded map of the shear wave speed (in either meters per second or kilopascals) over a larger ROI, 2D SWE. Interobserver variability with pSWE has been shown to be good with an intraclass correlation coefficient of 0.87.[51,52] Interoperator reproducibility has also been reported to be good using 2D SWE.[58]

Cutoff values of 1.21 to 1.34 m/s have been shown to predict significant fibrosis (F = >2) with an AUROC of 0.85 to 0.89.[53,65] For diagnosis of cirrhosis, SWE cutoff values range from 1.55 to 2.0 m/s with AUROCs of 0.89 to 0.93.[53,54,65] In a recent meta-analysis of 518 patients with chronic liver disease,[55] the AUROC was 0.87 for predicting significant fibrosis (F = >2), 0.91 for severe fibrosis (F = >3), and 0.93 for cirrhosis. The values for 2D SWE are similar to pSWE with AUROCs of 0.95 to 0.98 for F = >2, 0.96 for F = >3, and 0.97 to 0.98 for F = 4.[56,57]

The accuracy of SWE for the assessment of liver fibrosis is similar to TE.[53,66] Preliminary findings using SWE show promising results

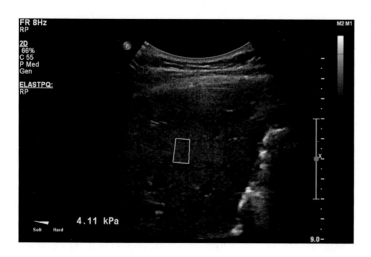

Fig. 11. Point SWE of a 28 year old with chronic hepatitis C infection. The stiffness value of 4.11 kPa is consistent with the patient's mild fibrosis on liver biopsy. The white rectangle is the FOV where the measurement is taken.

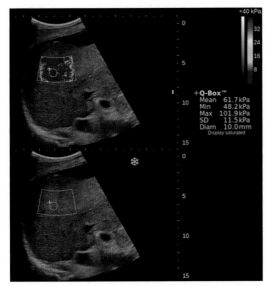

+Q-Box™
Mean   61.7 kPa
Min   48.2 kPa
Max   101.9 kPa
SD   11.5 kPa
Diam   10.0 mm
Display saturated

Fig. 12. In this 64-year-old man with advanced alcohol-induced cirrhosis, the 2D shear wave elastogram confirms a markedly stiff liver with a max kilopascal value of 102 (5.8 m/s). The white circle in the FOV is where the measurement of stiffness is taken.

in patients with NAFLD and NASH[67,68] and posttransplantation.[69]

The EFSUMB[14] and WFUMB[70] have guidelines for the use of SWE in assessment of liver fibrosis, particularly in hepatitis C. At this time, the cutoff values for the various manufactures are different; the appropriate cutoff values for the system should be used when assessing the degree of liver fibrosis.

THYROID ELASTOGRAPHY

Thyroid nodules are a common finding. Fine-needle aspiration is the most widely used method of lesion characterization. B-mode imaging and color Doppler have been used to characterize lesions, and guidelines have been published elsewhere.[71]

Both SE and SWE have been used to characterize thyroid lesions as benign or malignant. Preliminary results are mixed, with some investigators obtaining good results, whereas others are less encouraging. Asteria and colleagues[72] used a 4-point color scale in SE and found a sensitivity and specificity for thyroid cancer of 94% and 81%, respectively. Ragu and colleagues,[73] using a 5-point color-scale with SE, found a sensitivity of 97% and a specificity of 100%. Bojunga and colleagues[24] performed a meta-analysis of SE and found a mean sensitivity of 92% and mean specificity of 90%. Sebag and colleagues,[74] using SWE and a cutoff of 65 kPa, found a sensitivity of

85% and a specificity of 94%. An example of both SE and SWE of a thyroid lesion is presented in **Fig. 13.**

PROSTATE ELASTOGRAPHY

Prostate cancer (PC) is the most common malignancy in American men (excluding skin cancers) and is second only to lung cancer as a cause of cancer-related death.[75] Serum prostate-specific antigen (PSA) has been used as a screening test for PC, with PSA levels greater than 4.0 ng/mL considered abnormal. In addition to adenocarcinoma, a variety of benign diseases of the prostate, such as acute prostatitis and benign prostatic hypertrophy, as well as prostatic instrumentation will elevate PSA levels; false-positive PSA results are common. About 20% of PC will present with a PSA less than 4.0 ng/mL. A commonly used screening protocol for PC combines serum PSA measurement with digital rectal examination (DRE). The positive predictive value (PPV) of this combination is quoted as 61%, an improvement over DRE alone (PPV 31%) or PSA alone (PPV 42%). Transrectal ultrasound–guided sextant prostate biopsies are then used to evaluate those patients identified as abnormal by this screening protocol. Only 25% of these patients will have at least one positive biopsy, whereas the biopsy technique will fail to detect tumors in at least 25% of patients proven subsequently to have PC.[76]

Multi-parametric MRI is increasingly being used for tumor detection and localization. However, although its sensitivity is high, its specificity is low, particularly for the detection of small lesions with Gleason scores less than 6. Contrast-enhanced ultrasound is also being evaluated for detection and characterization of PC. Reports of the use of both SE and SWE to detect PC have been published.

STRAIN ELASTOGRAPHY

When using SE, the FOV should cover the entire prostate gland and surrounding tissue. A strain ratio between normal and abnormal tissue can be used for semiquantitative analysis. Minimal amounts of pressure should be used in performing the examination. Studies using SE have demonstrated a sensitivity and specificity of 55% to 70%, PPV of 57% to 85%, and a negative predictive value (NPV) of 72% to 87%. There is controversy regarding the inability to differentiate PC from chronic prostatitis. SE has been reported to improve biopsy guidance; a well-designed study did not confirm these results.[77–80]

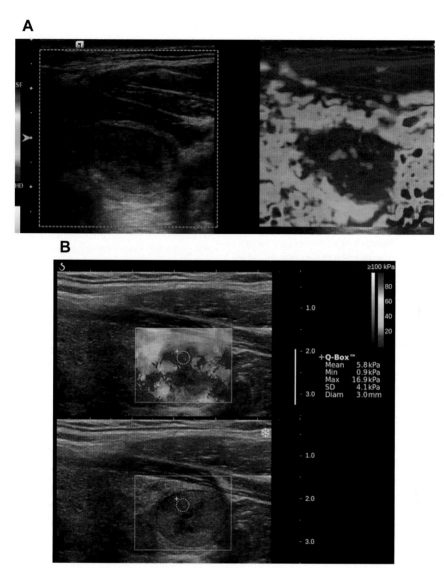

Fig. 13. The SE (*A*) of a 53-year-old man with a thyroid nodule demonstrates that the lesion is stiffer (*blue*) than the surrounding normal thyroid tissue. The 2D SWE (*B*) can estimate the stiffness of the nodule that in, this case, is a maximum kilopascal of 16.9 (2.4 m/s) (*circles*).

SHEAR WAVE ELASTOGRAPHY

A small single-center prospective study of 53 patients using SWE found excellent results in lesion detection and characterization in the peripheral zone.[76] The kilopascal value of cancers ranged from 30 to 110, with a mean value of 58.0 ± 20.7, whereas benign lesions had kilopascal values ranging from 9 to 107, with a mean value of 21.5 ± 11.5. Correas and colleagues[81,82] have obtained similar results. Based on the ROC curve, a value of 37 kPa was used as the cutoff between benign and malignant. This cutoff produced a sensitivity of 96.0%, specificity of 96.0%, PPV of 69.0%, and NPV of 99.6%.[76] Most false positives were secondary to calcifications noted on B mode in benign tissue. Nodules identified on B-mode imaging had a 12% positive biopsy rate. Using SWE to characterize B-mode–detected nodules, a sensitivity of 100%, specificity of 96%, PPV of 75%, and NPV of 100% were observed.[76] To obtain 100% sensitivity at the sextant level, a cutoff value of 30 kPa was required. Using this technique, a 140% increase in the positive biopsy rate could have been obtained.[76]

Correas and colleagues[82] found that the Vs ratio of the lesion to background prostate tissue was more discriminatory, as it takes into account the increased stiffness of the peripheral zone from calcification and chronic prostatitis. The ratio between the nodule and the adjacent peripheral gland for benign and malignant was 1.5 ± 0.9 and 4.0 ± 1.9, respectively (P<.002).

Fig. 14 is a benign prostate gland in a 74-year-old black man who presented with a PSA of 12.3 ng/mL. His PSA was 8.0 ng/mL 5 years earlier. DRE was unremarkable, and the sextant biopsy was negative. B-mode ultrasound was negative with a prostate volume of 26 mL. On SWE, the peripheral zone is blue throughout, corresponding to a low (<20 kPa) shear wave velocity.

Fig. 15 is a selected image from a 54-year-old white patient with a hypoechoic nodule in the peripheral zone. The nodule has a low kilopascal value of less than 20, consistent with a benign cause. However, there is an area of high kilopascal value of 75 (red) suggestive of a malignancy. On image-guided biopsy, the hypoechoic nodule was benign, whereas the area of high stiffness was a Gleason grade 7 PC. This finding highlights the clinical strength of elastic imaging. Malignant lesions can be differentiated from benign prostatic hyperplasia or prostatitis, as their stiffness often differs by a factor of 3 and can reach a factor of 10 in extreme cases. Elastography can also be used to guide a prostate biopsy. SWE can also be used to evaluate for extracapsular extension of tumor.

SWE is a very promising technique for the detection and biopsy guidance of PC. Of particular interest is its high NPV that may reduce the need for invasive procedures, such as biopsies. Using the sextant biopsy technique, only 25% to 30% of patients have a positive biopsy. The use of SWE could have deceased the biopsy rate by 53%. Also, by assuming lesions with calcifications noted on B mode are benign, the biopsy rate could have been decreased by 69%.

FUTURE POTENTIAL APPLICATIONS

Many other organs are presently under investigation with elastography, but there is no consensus on their routine clinical use.

Musculoskeletal Applications

Musculoskeletal applications with assessment of tendons, ligaments, and muscle are possible with both SE and SWE techniques. As these structures are anisotropic, the direction of probe placement in elastography is important. These structures are generally very stiff when normal and become soft when pathologic as opposed to other organs. Limited work has demonstrated that the elastographic abnormalities are similar in size to that of MRI. Tendonitis or tendon tears can be monitored noninvasively with this technique to document healing.[83] Fig. 16 compares the results of MRI and SE of a patient with Achilles tendonitis. Fig. 17 demonstrates the ability to monitor healing of lateral epicondylitis.

Gynecologic Applications

Both SE and SWE are available on endo-cavity probes and can be used to assess the stiffness of ovarian and uterine masses. At this time, there are no studies available to assess the use of these techniques in characterizing ovarian or uterine masses as benign or malignant. An interesting application being investigated is cervical ripening. The cervix is usually relatively stiff but softens

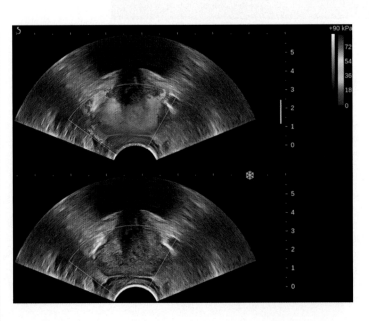

Fig. 14. A 74-year-old black man presented with an elevated PSA of 12.3 ng/mL increased from 8.0 ng/mL. Patient had undergone 2 prior sextant biopsies that were both negative. In this 2D SWE, the prostate gland has low kilopascal values throughout (<20 kPa, <2.6 m/s). With an NPV of greater than 99%, 2D SWE can influence management in this patient to monitor and not repeat a biopsy.

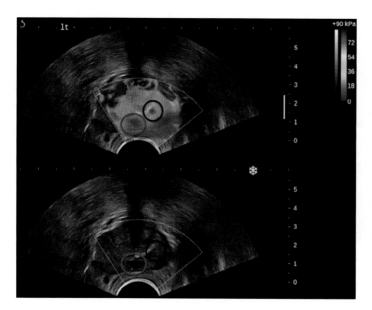

Fig. 15. This patient presented with an elevated PSA. On B-mode ultrasound, a hypoechoic nodule was identified (*red circle*). On 2D SWE, the nodule identified on B mode was found to have a low stiffness (<20 kPa); however, an area with a kilopascal value of 75 (5.0 m/s) was identified suspicious for a neoplasm (*black circle*). On biopsy, the nodule identified on B mode with low kilopascal was benign, whereas the lesion not identified on B mode with a high kilopascal was a Gleason grade 7 prostate adenocarcinoma. This finding highlights the clinical advantage of SWE in detection and characterization of prostate lesions.

during the delivery process. Elastography can be used to assess cervical stiffness to identify patients in danger of preterm delivery.

Testicular Applications

Ultrasound including color Doppler is the imaging modality of choice for evaluating scrotal abnormalities. A study evaluating testicular lesions identified on B-mode ultrasound found that benign and pseudonodules masses of the testes were very soft. Using the 5-point color scale, they were classified as a score of 1. Malignant lesions were stiff and had scores of 4 or 5. An 87% sensitivity, 98% specificity, 93% PPV, and a 96% NPV were found in differentiating intratesticular malignant from benign lesions.[84]

Pancreatic Applications

Pancreatic masses have been evaluated using elastography using both an endoscopic and

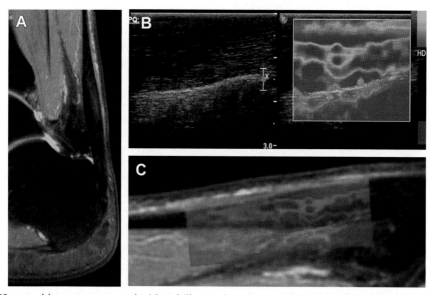

Fig. 16. A 42-year-old runner presented with Achilles tendon pain. An MRI (*A*) confirms tendonitis. The SE image performed at the same setting as the MRI (*B*) also confirms an abnormal soft area of the tendon representing tendonitis. When the SE image and the MRI are fused (*C*), the abnormalities identified on the two examinations are identical.

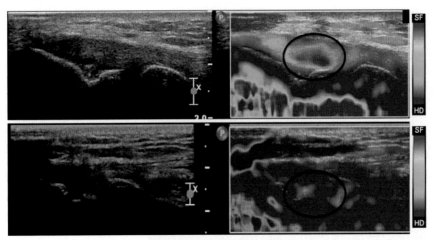

Fig. 17. The ultrasound and SE image of a 58 year old presenting with elbow pain. The upper image is on initial presentation. On the SE image, the tendon is abnormally soft (*black circle*) representing lateral epicondylitis. The lower image is the same patient after a month of treatment. Note that the tendonitis has resolved and the SE image now appears normal. Being a noninvasive, easily performed examination, SE (or SWE) can be used to monitor treatment of tendons or muscles.

transabdominal approach. The pancreas is of uniform intermediate stiffness; but with advancing age, it may become heterogeneous.

Preliminary studies using an endoscopic approach suggest that a homogeneous green pattern (red as soft and blue as hard) can be used to exclude malignancy. However, the clinical usefulness of this technique in distinguishing benign from malignant pathologies is limited. Inflammatory lesions of the pancreas can be hard or soft depending on the stage of the inflammation. Neoplasms can have necrotic areas that appear soft in contrast to the viable tumor that is hard. Itokawa and colleagues[85] found the strain ratio (strain of lesion compared with strain of normal pancreas) was 23.7 ± 12.7 for mass-forming pancreatitis and 39.1 ± 20.5 for pancreatic cancer.

In differentiating benign and malignant focal pancreatic masses, qualitative and semiquantitative strain techniques have been reported, both showing high overall accuracy. Two meta-analyses published have indicated endoscopic ultrasound elastography has a high sensitivity but lower specificity in the differentiation of focal pancreatic masses.[86,87]

SWE may be able to distinguish serous from mucinous malignancies. Serous fluid has low viscosity and does not propagate shear waves. A value of x.xx or 0 is obtained indicating shear waves were not identified in the fluid. However, mucinous cystic lesions have high viscosity that does propagate shear waves. In cystic lesions containing mucin, a shear wave velocity will be obtained. Preliminary results using this technique seem promising. In a study by D'Onofrio and

colleagues[88,89] that included 14 mucinous cystadenomas, 4 pseudocysts, 3 intraductal papillary-mucinous neoplasms, and 2 serous cystadenomas were studied. The values obtained ranged from x.xx/0 to 4.85 m/s in mucinous cystadenomas, from x.xx/0 to 3.11 m/s in pseudocysts, and from x.xx/0 to 4.57 m/s in intraductal papillary-mucinous neoplasms. In serous cystadenomas, all values measured were x.xx/0 m/s. Diagnostic accuracy in benign and nonbenign differentiation of pancreatic cystic lesions was 78%.

SUMMARY

Ultrasound elastography is a rapidly growing technique for many clinical applications. There is enough clinical evidence that this technique can be used to improve the characterization of breast masses, to detect PC, and to assess liver fibrosis, all of which should decrease the need for invasive biopsies. Preliminary work suggests that in other organs, such as focal liver lesions, there may be significant overlap of the stiffness of benign and malignant lesions that will limit this technique in clinical practice.

REFERENCES

1. Bamber J, Cosgrove D, Dietrich CF, et al. EFSUMB guidelines and recommendations on the clinical use of ultrasound elastography. Part 1: basic principles and technology. Ultraschall Med 2013; 34(2):169–84.
2. Barr RG. Sonographic breast elastography: a primer. J Ultrasound Med 2012;31(5):773–83.

3. Barr RG. US elastography: applications in tumors. In: Luna A, Vilanova JC, Hygino da Cruz LC, et al, editors. Functional imaging in oncology. New York: Springer-Verlag Berlin Heidelberg; 2014. p. 459–86. http://dx.doi.org/10.1007/978-3-642-40412-2_21.

4. Barr RG, Zhang Z. Effects of precompression on elasticity imaging of the breast: development of a clinically useful semiquantitative method of precompression assessment. J Ultrasound Med 2012; 31(6):895–902.

5. Barr RG. Real-time ultrasound elasticity of the breast: initial clinical results. Ultrasound Q 2010; 26(2):61–6.

6. Barr RG, Destounis S, Lackey LB 2nd, et al. Evaluation of breast lesions using sonographic elasticity imaging: a multicenter trial. J Ultrasound Med 2012;31(2):281–7.

7. Destounis S, Arieno A, Morgan R, et al. Clinical experience with elasticity imaging in a community-based breast center. J Ultrasound Med 2013;32(2):297–302.

8. Berg WA, Cosgrove DO, Dore CJ, et al. Shear-wave elastography improves the specificity of breast US: the BE1 multinational study of 939 masses. Radiology 2012;262(2):435–49.

9. Ueno EI. Diagnosis of breast cancer by elasticity imaging. Eizo Joho Medical 2004;36:2–6.

10. Tozaki M, Isobe S, Sakamoto M. Combination of elastography and tissue quantification using the acoustic radiation force impulse (ARFI) technology for differential diagnosis of breast masses. Jpn J Radiol 2012;30(8):659–70.

11. Raza S, Odulate A, Ong EM, et al. Using real-time tissue elastography for breast lesion evaluation: our initial experience. J Ultrasound Med 2010; 29(4):551–63.

12. Lee SH, Chang JM, Kim WH, et al. Differentiation of benign from malignant solid breast masses: comparison of two-dimensional and three-dimensional shear-wave elastography. Eur Radiol 2013;23(4): 1015–26.

13. Evans A, Whelehan P, Thomson K, et al. Invasive breast cancer: relationship between shear-wave elastographic findings and histologic prognostic factors. Radiology 2012;263(3):673–7.

14. Cosgrove D, Piscaglia F, Bamber J, et al. EFSUMB guidelines and recommendations on the clinical use of ultrasound elastography. Part 2: clinical applications. Ultraschall Med 2013;34(3): 238–53.

15. Barr RG. WFUMB guidelines for breast elastography. Ultrasound Med Biol, in press.

16. Krouskop TA, Wheeler TM, Kallel F, et al. Elastic moduli of breast and prostate tissues under compression. Ultrason Imaging 1998;20(4):260–74.

17. Barr RG. Breast elastography. New York: Thieme Publishers; 2014.

18. Itoh A, Ueno E, Tohno E, et al. Breast disease: clinical application of US elastography for diagnosis. Radiology 2006;239(2):341–50.

19. Ueno E, Umemoto T, Bando H, et al. New quantitative method in breast elastography: fat lesion ratio (FLR). In: Paper presented at: Radiological Society of North America 93rd Scientific Assembly and Annual Meeting. Chicago, IL, November 25–30, 2007.

20. Hall TJ, Zhu Y, Spalding CS. In vivo real-time free-hand palpation imaging. Ultrasound Med Biol 2003;29(3):427–35.

21. Grajo JR, Barr RG. Strain elastography in the prediction of breast cancer tumor grade. J Ultrasound Med 2014;33:129–34.

22. Friedrich-Rust M, Sperber A, Holzer K, et al. Real-time elastography and contrast-enhanced ultrasound for the assessment of thyroid nodules. Exp Clin Endocrinol Diabetes 2010;118(9):602–9.

23. Cantisani V, D'Andrea V, Biancari F, et al. Prospective evaluation of multiparametric ultrasound and quantitative elastosonography in the differential diagnosis of benign and malignant thyroid nodules: preliminary experience. Eur J Radiol 2012;81(10):2678–83.

24. Bojunga J, Herrmann E, Meyer G, et al. Real-time elastography for the differentiation of benign and malignant thyroid nodules: a meta-analysis. Thyroid 2010;20(10):1145–50.

25. Brock M, von Bodman C, Sommerer F, et al. Comparison of real-time elastography with grey-scale ultrasonography for detection of organ-confined prostate cancer and extra capsular extension: a prospective analysis using whole mount sections after radical prostatectomy. BJU Int 2011;108(8 Pt 2):E217–22.

26. Athanasiou A, Tardivon A, Tanter M, et al. Breast lesions: quantitative elastography with supersonic shear imaging–preliminary results. Radiology 2010;256(1):297–303.

27. Evans A, Whelehan P, Thomson K, et al. Quantitative shear wave ultrasound elastography: initial experience in solid breast masses. Breast Cancer Res 2010;12(6):R104.

28. Barr RG. Shear wave imaging of the breast: still on the learning curve. J Ultrasound Med 2012;31(3): 347–50.

29. Barr RG. Comparison of strain and shear wave without or with a quality measure in evaluation of breast masses. J Ultrasound Med 2013;32(suppl): S12,1540665.

30. Barr RG, Lackey AE. The utility of the "bull's-eye" artifact on breast elasticity imaging in reducing breast lesion biopsy rate. Ultrasound Q 2011; 27(3):151–5.

31. Yu H, Wilson SR. Differentiation of benign from malignant liver masses with Acoustic Radiation Force Impulse technique. Ultrasound Q 2011; 27(4):217–23.

32. Seeff LB, Everson GT, Morgan TR, et al. Complication rate of percutaneous liver biopsies among persons with advanced chronic liver disease in the HALT-C trial. Clin Gastroenterol Hepatol 2010; 8(10):877–83.

33. Seeff LB, Hoofnagle JH. National Institutes of Health Consensus Development Conference: management of hepatitis C: 2002. Hepatology 2002; 36(5 Suppl 1):S1–2.

34. Stotland BR, Lichtenstein GR. Liver biopsy complications and routine ultrasound. Am J Gastroenterol 1996;91(7):1295–6.

35. Bedossa P, Poynard T. An algorithm for the grading of activity in chronic hepatitis C. The METAVIR Cooperative Study Group. Hepatology 1996; 24(2):289–93.

36. Castera L, Foucher J, Bernard PH, et al. Pitfalls of liver stiffness measurement: a 5-year prospective study of 13,369 examinations. Hepatology 2010; 51(3):828–35.

37. Fraquelli M, Rigamonti C, Casazza G, et al. Reproducibility of transient elastography in the evaluation of liver fibrosis in patients with chronic liver disease. Gut 2007;56(7):968–73.

38. Myers RP, Pomier-Layrargues G, Kirsch R, et al. Feasibility and diagnostic performance of the FibroScan XL probe for liver stiffness measurement in overweight and obese patients. Hepatology 2012;55(1):199–208.

39. Talwalkar JA, Kurtz DM, Schoenleber SJ, et al. Ultrasound-based transient elastography for the detection of hepatic fibrosis: systematic review and meta-analysis. Clin Gastroenterol Hepatol 2007;5(10):1214–20.

40. Friedrich-Rust M, Ong MF, Martens S, et al. Performance of transient elastography for the staging of liver fibrosis: a meta-analysis. Gastroenterology 2008;134(4):960–74.

41. Adebajo CO, Talwalkar JA, Poterucha JJ, et al. Ultrasound-based transient elastography for the detection of hepatic fibrosis in patients with recurrent hepatitis C virus after liver transplantation: a systematic review and meta-analysis. Liver Transpl 2012;18(3):323–31.

42. Chon YE, Choi EH, Song KJ, et al. Performance of transient elastography for the staging of liver fibrosis in patients with chronic hepatitis B: a meta-analysis. PLoS One 2012;7(9):e44930.

43. Chan HL, Wong GL, Choi PC, et al. Alanine aminotransferase-based algorithms of liver stiffness measurement by transient elastography (Fibroscan) for liver fibrosis in chronic hepatitis B. J Viral Hepat 2009;16(1):36–44.

44. de Ledinghen V, Wong VW, Vergniol J, et al. Diagnosis of liver fibrosis and cirrhosis using liver stiffness measurement: comparison between M and XL probe of FibroScan(R). J Hepatol 2012;56(4):833–9.

45. Friedrich-Rust M, Hadji-Hosseini H, Kriener S, et al. Transient elastography with a new probe for obese patients for non-invasive staging of non-alcoholic steatohepatitis. Eur Radiol 2010;20(10): 2390–6.

46. Wong VW, Vergniol J, Wong GL, et al. Diagnosis of fibrosis and cirrhosis using liver stiffness measurement in nonalcoholic fatty liver disease. Hepatology 2010;51(2):454–62.

47. Wong GL, Wong VW, Choi PC, et al. Assessment of fibrosis by transient elastography compared with liver biopsy and morphometry in chronic liver diseases. Clin Gastroenterol Hepatol 2008;6(9): 1027–35.

48. Bureau C, Metivier S, Peron JM, et al. Transient elastography accurately predicts presence of significant portal hypertension in patients with chronic liver disease. Aliment Pharmacol Ther 2008;27(12): 1261–8.

49. Vizzutti F, Arena U, Romanelli RG, et al. Liver stiffness measurement predicts severe portal hypertension in patients with HCV-related cirrhosis. Hepatology 2007;45(5):1290–7.

50. Vergniol J, Foucher J, Terrebonne E, et al. Noninvasive tests for fibrosis and liver stiffness predict 5-year outcomes of patients with chronic hepatitis C. Gastroenterology 2011;140(7):1970–9, 1979. e1–3.

51. Piscaglia F, Salvatore V, Di Donato R, et al. Accuracy of VirtualTouch Acoustic Radiation Force Impulse (ARFI) imaging for the diagnosis of cirrhosis during liver ultrasonography. Ultraschall Med 2011;32(2):167–75.

52. D'Onofrio M, Gallotti A, Mucelli RP. Tissue quantification with acoustic radiation force impulse imaging: measurement repeatability and normal values in the healthy liver. AJR Am J Roentgenol 2010; 195(1):132–6.

53. Friedrich-Rust M, Wunder K, Kriener S, et al. Liver fibrosis in viral hepatitis: noninvasive assessment with acoustic radiation force impulse imaging versus transient elastography. Radiology 2009; 252(2):595–604.

54. Sporea I, Bota S, Peck-Radosavljevic M, et al. Acoustic radiation force impulse elastography for fibrosis evaluation in patients with chronic hepatitis C: an international multicenter study. Eur J Radiol 2012;81(12):4112–8.

55. Friedrich-Rust M, Nierhoff J, Lupsor M, et al. Performance of acoustic radiation force impulse imaging for the staging of liver fibrosis: a pooled meta-analysis. J Viral Hepat 2012;19(2):e212–9.

56. Bavu E, Gennisson JL, Couade M, et al. Noninvasive in vivo liver fibrosis evaluation using supersonic shear imaging: a clinical study on 113 hepatitis C virus patients. Ultrasound Med Biol 2011;37(9):1361–73.

57. Ferraioli G, Tinelli C, Dal Bello B, et al. Accuracy of real-time shear wave elastography for assessing liver fibrosis in chronic hepatitis C: a pilot study. Hepatology 2012;56(6):2125–33.

58. Ferraioli G, Tinelli C, Zicchetti M, et al. Reproducibility of real-time shear wave elastography in the evaluation of liver elasticity. Eur J Radiol 2012; 81(11):3102–6.

59. Friedrich-Rust M, Ong MF, Herrmann E, et al. Real-time elastography for noninvasive assessment of liver fibrosis in chronic viral hepatitis. AJR Am J Roentgenol 2007;188(3):758–64.

60. Bota S, Sporea I, Sirli R, et al. Factors that influence the correlation of acoustic radiation force impulse (ARFI), elastography with liver fibrosis. Med Ultrason 2011;13(2):135–40.

61. European Association for the Study of the Liver. EASL Clinical Practice Guidelines: management of hepatitis C virus infection. J Hepatol 2011; 55(2):245–64.

62. Colecchia A, Montrone L, Scaioli E, et al. Measurement of spleen stiffness to evaluate portal hypertension and the presence of esophageal varices in patients with HCV-related cirrhosis. Gastroenterology 2012;143(3):646–54.

63. Ferraioli G, Lissandrin R, Zicchetti M, et al. Diffuse liver diseases. In: Calliada F, Canepari M, Ferraiolo G, et al, editors. Sono-elastography main clinical applications. 1st edition. Pavia (IT): Edizioni Medico Scientifiche; 2012. p. 13–30.

64. Yu H, Wilson SR. New noninvasive ultrasound techniques: can they predict liver cirrhosis? Ultrasound Q 2012;28(1):5–11.

65. Sporea I, Sirli R, Bota S, et al. Is ARFI elastography reliable for predicting fibrosis severity in chronic HCV hepatitis? World J Radiol 2011;3(7):188–93.

66. Rizzo L, Calvaruso V, Cacopardo B, et al. Comparison of transient elastography and acoustic radiation force impulse for non-invasive staging of liver fibrosis in patients with chronic hepatitis C. Am J Gastroenterol 2011;106(12):2112–20.

67. Yoneda M, Suzuki K, Kato S, et al. Nonalcoholic fatty liver disease: US-based acoustic radiation force impulse elastography. Radiology 2010; 256(2):640–7.

68. Friedrich-Rust M, Romen D, Vermehren J, et al. Acoustic radiation force impulse-imaging and transient elastography for non-invasive assessment of liver fibrosis and steatosis in NAFLD. Eur J Radiol 2012;81(3):e325–31.

69. Crespo G, Fernandez-Varo G, Marino Z, et al. ARFI, FibroScan, ELF, and their combinations in the assessment of liver fibrosis: a prospective study. J Hepatol 2012;57(2):281–7.

70. Ferraioli G, Filice C, Castera L, et al. WFUMB guidelines and recommendations on the clinical use of ultrasound elastography: liver. UMB, in press.

71. American Thyroid Association (ATA) Guidelines Taskforce on Thyroid N, Differentiated Thyroid C, Cooper DS, et al. Revised American Thyroid Association management guidelines for patients with thyroid nodules and differentiated thyroid cancer. Thyroid 2009;19(11):1167–214.

72. Asteria C, Giovanardi A, Pizzocaro A, et al. US-elastography in the differential diagnosis of benign and malignant thyroid nodules. Thyroid 2008;18(5): 523–31.

73. Rago T, Santini F, Scutari M, et al. Elastography: new developments in ultrasound for predicting malignancy in thyroid nodules. J Clin Endocrinol Metab 2007;92(8):2917–22.

74. Sebag F, Vaillant-Lombard J, Berbis J, et al. Shear wave elastography: a new ultrasound imaging mode for the differential diagnosis of benign and malignant thyroid nodules. J Clin Endocrinol Metab 2010;95(12):5281–8.

75. American Cancer Society. Cancer facts & figures. Atlanta (GA): American Cancer Society; 2010.

76. Barr RG, Memo R, Schaub CR. Shear wave ultrasound elastography of the prostate: initial results. Ultrasound Q 2012;28(1):13–20.

77. Aigner F, Pallwein L, Junker D, et al. Value of real-time elastography targeted biopsy for prostate cancer detection in men with prostate specific antigen 1.25 ng/ml or greater and 4.00 ng/ml or less. J Urol 2010;184(3):913–7.

78. Kapoor A, Mahajan G, Sidhu BS, et al. Real-time elastography in the detection of prostate cancer in patients with raised PSA level. Ultrasound Med Biol 2011;37(9):1374–81.

79. Zhu Y, Chen Y, Qi T, et al. Prostate cancer detection with real-time elastography using a bi-plane transducer: comparison with step section radical prostatectomy pathology. World J Urol 2014;32: 329–33.

80. Sparchez Z. Real-time ultrasound prostate elastography. An increasing role in prostate cancer detection? Med Ultrason 2011;13(1):3–4.

81. Correas JM, Khairoune A, Tissier AM. Transrectal quantitative shear wave elastography: application to prostate cancer a feasibility study. Vienna (Austria): European Congress of Radiology; 2011.

82. Correas JM, Khairoune A, Tissier AM, et al. Quantitative ShearWave Elastography of the prostate: correlation to sextant and targeted biopsies. Vienna (Austria): European Congress of Radiology; 2012.

83. Barr RG. Elastography in evaluation of musculoskeletal abnormalities. Appl Radiol 2012;41(12 Suppl):S53–5.

84. Goddi A, Sacchi A, Magistretti G, et al. Real-time tissue elastography for testicular lesion assessment. Eur Radiol 2012;22(4):721–30.

85. Itokawa F, Itoi T, Sofuni A, et al. EUS elastography combined with the strain ratio of tissue elasticity for diagnosis of solid pancreatic masses. J Gastroenterol 2011;46(6):843–53.

86. Mei M, Ni J, Liu D, et al. EUS elastography for diagnosis of solid pancreatic masses: a meta-analysis. Gastrointest Endosc 2013;77(4): 578–89.

87. Pei Q, Zou X, Zhang X, et al. Diagnostic value of EUS elastography in differentiation of benign and malignant solid pancreatic masses: a meta-analysis. Pancreatology 2012;12(5):402–8.

88. D'Onofrio M, Gallotti A, Mucelli RP. Pancreatic mucinous cystadenoma at ultrasound acoustic radiation force impulse (ARFI) imaging. Pancreas 2010;39(5):684–5.

89. D'Onofrio M, Gallotti A, Salvia R, et al. Acoustic radiation force impulse (ARFI) ultrasound imaging of pancreatic cystic lesions. Eur J Radiol 2011;80(2): 241–4.

The Role of Ultrasonography in the Evaluation of Diffuse Liver Disease

Matthew T. Heller, MD*, Mitchell E. Tublin, MD

KEYWORDS

• Ultrasound • Sonography • Diffuse • Liver disease • Hepatic disease

KEY POINTS

- Coarsening and heterogeneity of hepatic echotexture, altered echogenicity, and surface nodularity are key ultrasonography (US) findings that suggest diffuse liver disease.
- Identification of vascular displacement, altered flow, or thrombosis during color and Doppler US interrogation are critical ancillary features that support a diagnosis of diffuse liver disease by US.
- Even in the absence of a specific diagnosis, US findings interpreted in the proper clinical context often facilitate the next step in the patient's evaluation.

INTRODUCTION

Ultrasonography (US) is frequently the initial modality for evaluating patients with hepatic dysfunction or suspected diffuse disease. Availability, low cost, and lack of ionizing radiation contribute to its popularity. Rapid acquisition of structural and physiologic data has made US an indispensable tool in assessing diffuse liver disease.

Gray-scale findings that suggest diffuse liver disease include surface nodularity, heterogeneous echotexture, and altered parenchymal echogenicity. Doppler US findings of vessel distortion, thrombosis, neovascularity, the arterial buffer response, and variceal formation are important ancillary findings. In addition, assessment of the biliary system and perihepatic spaces are helpful in detecting diffuse hepatic abnormality.

Ultrasound elastography has evolved over the past 30 years as a noninvasive method of assessing liver fibrosis.[1] Although elastography platforms differ by method of excitation and measurement, they all have shown utility for evaluation of numerous diffuse liver diseases. Newly developed applications, such as real-time tissue elastography, virtual touch quantification, and color map integration are promising developments that are anticipated to enable elastography to play a prognostic role in diffuse liver disease.[2] Similarly, it is possible that perfusion data afforded by dynamic contrast-enhanced US will be an additional area of growth once microbubble contrast agents gain approval in the United States.

Despite its popularity, the utility of US may be limited by a relatively small field of view, operator dependence, and artifacts. Several diffuse hepatic processes are not detectable during initial US examinations early in the course of the disease. Furthermore, the abnormalities that are eventually detected by US may be nonspecific, requiring further evaluation with contrast-enhanced

The authors have no relevant disclosures.
Department of Radiology, University of Pittsburgh Medical Center, 200 Lothrop Street, Suite 3950 PST, Pittsburgh, PA 15213, USA
* Corresponding author.
E-mail address: hellmt@upmc.edu

radiologic.theclinics.com

computed tomography (CT), magnetic resonance (MR) imaging, or biopsy.

NORMAL ANATOMY AND IMAGING TECHNIQUE
Hepatic Parenchyma

Hepatic US is performed with standard curvilinear and high-resolution linear probes. The curvilinear probe (2–6 MHz) allows acoustic penetration of deeper parenchyma while a high-resolution probe (7–12 MHz) may be used to depict greater surface detail. Optimization of the gain, time-gain compensation, and tissue harmonics by an experienced sonologist, and second-look sonography by informed radiologists are requisites for achieving diagnostic examinations.

Normal liver parenchyma has a homogeneous echotexture (**Fig. 1**); the assessment is subjective but the liver should not appear granular or coarsened if speckle reduction and compound imaging parameters are optimized. Hepatic echogenicity is subjectively compared with that of adjacent solid viscera such as the kidneys and spleen; normal hepatic echogenicity is marginally higher than that of the kidney but less than that of the spleen. The spleen provides a more reliable comparison because numerous intrinsic kidney diseases can alter their echogenicity. Normal relative hepatic echogenicity is summarized in **Box 1**.

Hepatic Vasculature

Normal hepatic vessels have smooth walls and anechoic lumens. Intrahepatic arteries are difficult to resolve on gray scale alone, but parallel the portal veins. Normal spectral Doppler interrogation shows a low-resistance waveform with continuously hepatopetal diastolic flow. Normal portal veins have thin echogenic walls and monophasic waveforms with mild respiratory variation. Alterations of portal mural echogenicity should be

---

> **Box 1**
> **Normal relative hepatic echogenicity**
>
> - Liver > kidneys
> - Liver < spleen
> - Liver < portal tracts
> - Liver < diaphragm muscle

---

considered abnormal. Normal hepatic veins and the inferior vena cava (IVC) lack discernible walls. The normal hepatic venous waveform is triphasic, owing to 2 hepatofugal peaks and 1 hepatopetal peak reflecting primarily right atrial pressure.

Miscellaneous

The normal common bile duct measures up to 6 mm in normal individuals, but radiology dogma suggest that the diameter of the duct can increase with age.[3] The central intrahepatic ducts should normally measure 3 mm or less. The diameter of the common bile duct may vary following cholecystectomy.

The normal perihepatic spaces should contain a variable amount of homogeneous fat; any ascites, fluid collection, or soft-tissue lesion should be considered abnormal.

Imaging Protocol

Scanning typically commences with the use of a curved linear-array probe at 3 to 6 MHz. With the patient in a supine position, the left hepatic lobe is insonated via a subcostal approach; an intercostal window in the left lateral decubitus position is usually required for evaluation of the right lobe. Repositioning and breathing instructions may be used for problematic anatomic regions such as the subcostal surface, the tip of the lateral segment, and the subdiaphragmatic regions.

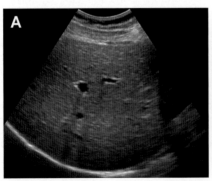 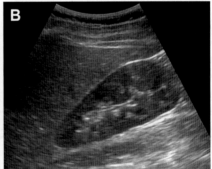

Fig. 1. Normal liver ultrasonogram. (*A*) Transverse ultrasonography (US) shows homogeneous echotexture. (*B*) Sagittal image demonstrates that the liver echogenicity is slightly higher than that of the right kidney.

Vascular landmarks are identified so that images are acquired according to the Couinaud classification. Color and spectral Doppler are used to evaluate vessel patency and altered flow dynamics. High-resolution probes should be used to evaluate the surface and parenchyma of the left lobe. The biliary system and perihepatic spaces should also be evaluated. A right intercostal window is generally used for elastography; the intercostal approach prevents excessive compression of the liver by the probe, and the right lobe is less affected by cardiac motion than the left. Measurements are taken during a breath-hold in a fasting patient after a region of interest is determined.

A typical scan protocol is summarized in **Table 1**.

IMAGING FINDINGS AND PATHOLOGY
Diagnostic Criteria

Hepatitis
Numerous features can cause acute hepatitis; common entities include acetaminophen toxicity, alcohol poisoning, and viruses. Although US findings are variable, a more common manifestation is hepatomegaly.[4] Findings include right lobe extension inferior to the kidney in the setting of a normal-sized left lobe; some investigators consider a height exceeding 15.5 cm in the midclavicular line to be a reliable measurement.[5] Increased periportal echogenicity, the so-called starry sky sign, has been thought in the past to be due to background diffuse parenchymal edema and hypoechogenicity, although the appearance may also be due to periportal edema (**Fig. 2**).[6] Unfortunately, the rarity and poor sensitivity in addition to the specificity of this sign preclude clinical utility.[5,7] Marked circumferential gallbladder wall edema/thickening (normally $\leq$3 mm) is variably observed and has been associated with hepatitis A virus.[8]

The prolonged inflammation of chronic hepatitis results in a variable degree of hepatic steatosis and fibrosis. Therefore, the US findings consist of parenchymal heterogeneity, increased echogenicity, and decreased penetration; surface nodularity ensues as cirrhosis develops.

Steatosis
Diffuse hepatic steatosis is the end product of numerous pathologic processes that cause chronic hepatocellular injury. The differential diagnosis for diffuse hepatic steatosis is summarized in **Box 2**.

Hepatic steatosis manifests as increased hepatic echogenicity relative to the right kidney or spleen.[9] Impaired acoustic penetration results in poor visualization of the posterior segment and diaphragm. Finally, vascular landmarks are suboptimally resolved; in particular, the echogenicity of the portal walls becomes less apparent (**Fig. 3**).[10] Prior investigations have shown that these 3 US findings strongly correlate with biopsy results.[9,11] Diffuse hepatic steatosis can result in hepatomegaly, but does not cause changes of size in particular hepatic segments.

Nonalcoholic fatty liver disease (NAFLD) is a spectrum of hepatic disorders that includes diffuse steatosis, nonalcoholic steatohepatitis (NASH), fibrosis, and cirrhosis. NAFLD is one of the most common causes of chronic liver disease in the United States, with an estimated prevalence of 20% to 30% of the population; NAFLD is strongly associated with obesity and type 2 diabetes

---

Table 1
Summary of hepatic ultrasonography protocol

Probes	Gray Scale	Color Doppler	Spectral Doppler	Elastography
Curved linear array (2–6 MHz)	Entire liver (left lateral decubitus for right lobe) Couinaud segments (transverse, sagittal) Bile duct caliber Perihepatic spaces	Major arteries, hepatic veins, portal veins, splenic vein, IVC, aorta Any focal lesion or segmental abnormality	Waveforms for arteries, hepatic veins, portal veins, splenic vein, IVC, ± aorta Interrogate thrombosis for waveforms	ROI on right lobe via intercostal window Measure at breath-hold in fasting patient
High-resolution linear (7–12 MHz)	Ventral or dorsal margin of lateral segment			
Small sector	Regions of anatomic difficulty			

Abbreviations: IVC, inferior vena cava; ROI, region of interest.

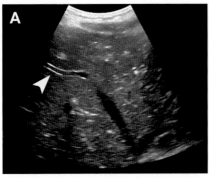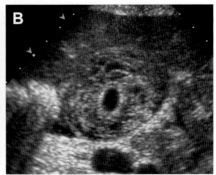

Fig. 2. Acute hepatitis. (*A*) Transverse US of the right lobe shows increased echogenicity of the portal venous walls (*arrowhead*) caused by parenchymal edema. (*B*) Transverse image shows extensive gallbladder wall edema.

mellitus. The spectrum of NAFLD is characterized by progressive fat deposition, abnormal liver function, inflammation, and fibrosis.[12] The current role of US is to detect and grade the degree of hepatic steatosis. Elastography has also been investigated for longitudinal monitoring of NASH patients.[13]

Box 2
Differential diagnosis of diffuse hepatic steatosis

Common

Chronic alcohol ingestion

Obesity/hyperlipidemia

Nonalcoholic fatty liver disease/Nonalcoholic steatohepatitis

Hepatitis B/C

Medication-Related

Various chemotherapy agents

Steroids

Amiodarone

Valproic acid

Storage Diseases

Glycogen storage diseases

α1-Antitrypsin deficiency

Hemochromatosis

Wilson disease

Other

Cystic fibrosis

Total parenteral nutrition

Radiation

Pregnancy

Aminoacidopathy

Cirrhosis

Cirrhosis is characterized by extensive bridging fibrosis and innumerable regenerative nodules that replace the normal liver parenchyma. Cirrhosis is regarded as the final common pathway for numerous causes of chronic liver injury. Common causes of cirrhosis are summarized in **Box 3**.

US findings include a coarsened echotexture, parenchymal heterogeneity, regenerative nodules, and surface nodularity.[14] However, liver morphology may be normal in the early stages. As cirrhosis progresses, a characteristic lobar atrophy-hypertrophy complex manifests as a relatively increased size of the caudate and lateral segment with corresponding volume loss of the right lobe, especially in the posterior segment (**Fig. 4**). Use of the ratio ($\geq$0.65) of the transverse diameter of the caudate to the right lobe has yielded a sensitivity of 84%, specificity of 100%, and accuracy of 94% in one investigation.[15] A highly sensitive finding for cirrhosis is reduction of the transverse diameter (<30 mm) of the medial segment (segment 4) of the left lobe.[16]

Although these findings lack high sensitivity and specificity, ancillary findings of portal hypertension may facilitate the diagnosis; common findings include hepatofugal portal venous flow, portosystemic collaterals, ascites, and splenomegaly.[5] Advanced portal hypertension can result in venous stasis and development of bland thrombus. Alterations of the normal hepatic venous waveform have been shown to correlate with the presence and severity of cirrhosis.[17] As cirrhosis progresses, the normally triphasic waveform becomes biphasic and then monophasic, owing to diminished venous compliance secondary to the parenchymal fibrosis.[18] In addition, enlargement and tortuosity of hepatic arteries, the so-called corkscrew appearance, can be shown with color Doppler analysis (**Fig. 5**); hyperdynamic arterial flow manifests as aliasing and increased velocities

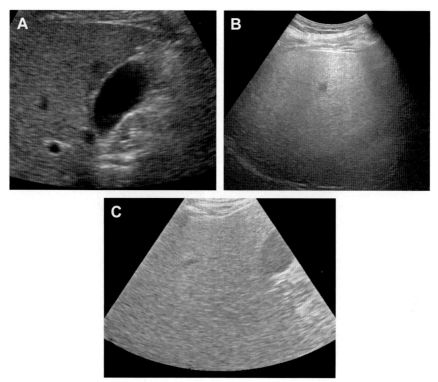

Fig. 3. Steatosis. Transverse US shows (*A*) mild, (*B*) moderate, and (*C*) severe diffuse steatosis. Note the increasing parenchymal echogenicity and loss of vascular and diaphragmatic definition as steatosis progresses.

Box 3
Etiology of cirrhosis
Toxins
Alcohol
Drugs (methotrexate)
Infection
Hepatitis B/C virus
Schistosomiasis
Autoimmune
Cryptogenic/autoimmune hepatitis
Primary biliary cirrhosis
Sclerosing cholangitis
Metabolic
Hemochromatosis
Wilson disease
α1-Antitrypsin deficiency
Other
Venous congestion
Postgastric bypass

because of relatively decreased portal venous flow.[19]

Elastography has proved to be useful in patients who require assessment of liver fibrosis (**Fig. 6**). Allowing for inherent variability between investigations, methodology, and underlying etiology, elasticity measurements of 7 kPa and greater, and from 12.5 to 15 kPa have been regarded as indicating advanced fibrosis and cirrhosis, respectively.[2,20] A meta-analysis of investigations studying transient elastography have shown sensitivities and specificities of 0.87 and 0.91 for the diagnosis of cirrhosis and 0.91 and 0.85 for the diagnosis of fibrosis, respectively.[21] Finally, although not currently available for routine use in the United States, dynamic contrast-enhanced US has potential applications in cirrhosis; it has been shown that measurement of diminished mean hepatic venous transit time of liver blood flow with contrast-enhanced US is similar to that measured by perfusion CT.[22]

Malignancy

Although typically presenting as a discrete mass, hepatocellular carcinoma (HCC) can be infiltrating and indistinguishable from other diffuse processes (**Fig. 7**). The gray-scale features of infiltrating HCC are variable and nonspecific; therefore, any mass

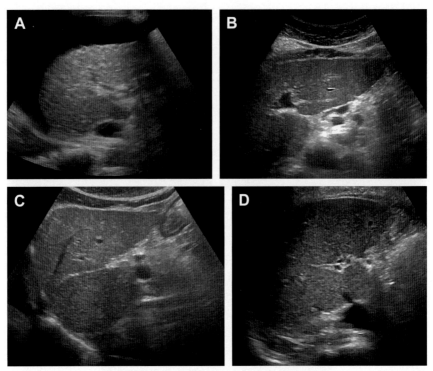

Fig. 4. Cirrhosis. (*A*) Sagittal US reveals surface nodularity, ascites, and parenchymal coarsening. Sagittal images show (*B*) hypertrophy of the lateral segment, (*C*) caudate hypertrophy, and (*D*) right lobe atrophy.

in a patient should undergo further evaluation to exclude HCC. Correlation to serum α-fetoprotein levels, MR imaging, and biopsy are usually required for diagnosis. Metastatic lesions, such as breast carcinoma, can spread along the hepatic sinusoids, resulting in diffuse infiltration of tumor (**Fig. 8**).

Budd-Chiari

Although Budd-Chiari syndrome is not a primary condition of the liver parenchyma, it results in diffuse parenchymal changes. The clinical presentation of Budd-Chiari depends on the extension and acuity of venous outflow obstruction and may include abdominal discomfort, jaundice,

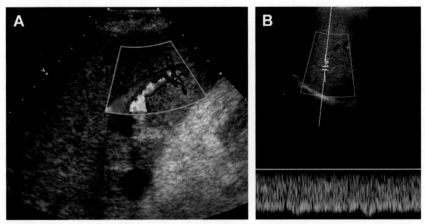

Fig. 5. Cirrhosis: vascular changes. (*A*) Color Doppler shows hepatofugal flow in the left portal vein and compensatory hypertrophy of the adjacent hepatic artery. Note coarsening of the hepatic echotexture. (*B*) Spectral Doppler shows blunting of the hepatic venous waveform caused by cirrhosis.

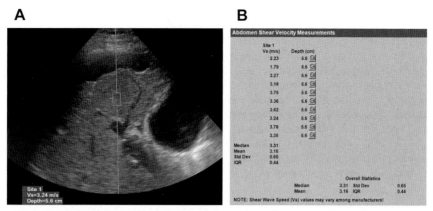

Fig. 6. Cirrhosis: elastography. (*A*) Transverse US shows the region of interest in the right lobe, providing a velocity measurement. (*B*) The elastography data consist of an average of 10 velocity measurements, which are converted to kilopascals. Findings confirmed fibrosis in this case. IQR, interquartile range. (*Courtesy of* Dr Myra Feldman.)

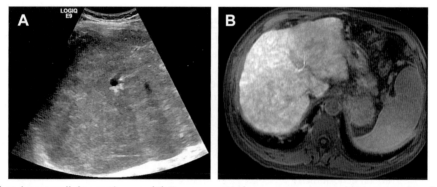

Fig. 7. Diffuse hepatocellular carcinoma. (*A*) Transverse US shows coarsening and heterogeneity of the parenchyma. (*B*) Postcontrast magnetic resonance (MR) imaging during the hepatobiliary phase reveals innumerable nodules that do not take up contrast material. Biopsy proved diffuse hepatocellular carcinoma.

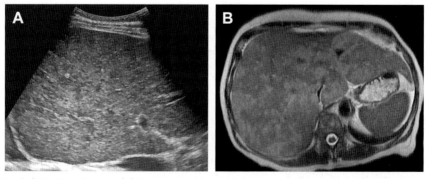

Fig. 8. Metastatic breast carcinoma. (*A*) Transverse US reveals heterogeneity and coarsening of the echotexture. (*B*) Transverse T2-weighted MR image shows extensive abnormal signal throughout the liver. Biopsy proved diffuse, infiltrative tumor.

encephalopathy, and fulminant hepatic failure. Budd-Chiari syndrome is multifactorial in etiology, but the underlying mechanism is hepatic venous outflow obstruction and increased sinusoidal pressure. Acutely, US reveals venous occlusion, hepatomegaly, and parenchymal heterogeneity. In the chronic form, there is fibrosis and atrophy of the periphery, caudate hypertrophy, and development of regenerative nodules and intrahepatic venous collaterals.

Salient US features of some of the more common diffuse hepatic diseases are summarized in **Table 2**.

DIFFERENTIAL DIAGNOSIS

The differential diagnosis for the US findings of diffusely abnormal hepatic parenchyma is broad, and summarized in **Box 4**.

PEARLS, PITFALLS, AND VARIANTS
Hepatitis

In chronic active hepatitis, increased caliber of the hepatic arteries can be mistaken for biliary ductal dilatation on gray scale; application of color Doppler helps to avoid this pitfall.

Steatosis

Diagnosis of advanced diffuse hepatic steatosis by US is usually straightforward because of the profoundly increased parenchymal echogenicity. However, a potential pitfall exists when mild to moderate hepatic steatosis coexists with chronic renal diseases. Because numerous chronic renal diseases can result in increased echogenicity of the renal cortex, the steatotic liver may appear to be isoechoic to the diseased kidney, resulting in

---

Table 2
Summary of ultrasonography findings for more common diffuse hepatic diseases

Pathologic Entity	Gray Scale	Color Doppler	Spectral Doppler
Hepatitis, acute	Hepatomegaly Hypoechoic parenchyma ↑ Periportal echoes	Normal	Normal
Hepatitis, chronic	Parenchymal heterogeneity ↑ Echogenicity ↓ Penetrability ↑ Caliber of hepatic arteries in chronic active hepatitis	↑ Caliber of hepatic arteries in chronic active hepatitis	Normal
Steatosis, NAFLD	↑ Echogenicity ↓ Penetrability ↓ Portal echogenicity Parenchymal heterogeneity	Normal	Normal
Cirrhosis	Coarsened echotexture Hypertrophy of caudate and lateral segment Volume loss in right lobe and medial segment Surface nodularity	Hepatofugal portal flow if advanced cirrhosis and portal hypertension present ↑ Arterial caliber and flow (arterial buffer response) compensating for ↓ portal venous flow	Hepatofugal portal flow if advanced Loss of hepatic vein and IVC phasicity
Malignancy	Coarsened, heterogeneous echotexture Focal satellite lesions Surface nodularity (pseudocirrhosis) Biliary obstruction	Displacement, narrowing, occlusion	Blunted waveforms due to compression Occlusion Arterial neovascularity in malignant thrombus
Budd-Chiari	Acute: hepatomegaly, heterogeneity due to congestion Chronic: peripheral atrophy, central hypertrophy, regenerative nodules	Hepatic venous occlusion Development of small intrahepatic venous collaterals	Hepatic venous occlusion Slow flow in small collaterals

Abbreviations: IVC, inferior vena cava; NAFLD, nonalcoholic fatty liver disease; ↑, increase; ↓, decrease.

Box 4
Differential diagnosis of diffusely abnormal liver ultrasonography

- Inflammatory/metabolic:

  Alcoholic cirrhosis

  Steatosis

  Drug toxicity (acetaminophen)

- Neoplastic:

  Primary liver neoplasms (hepatocellular carcinoma, adenomatosis)

  Metastatic neoplasms (colon, neuroendocrine, pancreatic, biliary, renal, melanoma, breast)

- Vascular:

  Budd-Chiari

- Autoimmune:

  Primary sclerosing cholangitis

  Primary biliary cirrhosis

  Sarcoidosis

- Infectious:

  Viral hepatitis

  Multifocal pyogenic abscesses

a false-negative result if only this criterion is used. Instead, it has been suggested that the relative echogenicity of the right kidney and liver be compared with the relative echogenicity of the left kidney and spleen. If the echogenicity of the kidneys is equal, a greater echogenicity difference between the right kidney and liver compared with that between the left kidney and spleen indicates that the hepatic parenchymal echogenicity is abnormally elevated.[5]

Steatosis may also affect all segments of the liver without being uniform in distribution. Variants of diffuse steatosis include formation of multiple nodules, lobar or segmental deposition with sparing, or perivascular infiltration. In these cases, the US findings of echogenic regions or "lesions" that do not displace or occlude the hepatic vessels may suggest the diagnosis of atypical diffuse steatosis; however, MR imaging with opposed-phase imaging may be needed for corroboration. Focal fatty infiltration and sparing are commonly observed in segments 4 and 5 near the gallbladder fossa, but can also occur in the other segments.

Cirrhosis

Parenchymal coarsening and heterogeneity are nonspecific findings caused by various pathologic conditions such as cirrhosis, steatosis, infiltrative malignancy, diffuse miliary metastases, or granulomatous diseases (Fig. 9). Surface nodularity is a more specific sign of cirrhosis, and is more apparent in the setting of ascites or with use of high-frequency probes (Fig. 10). However, because lower-frequency curved linear-array probes are generally used for screening, nodularity may be more readily identified along the posterior surfaces of the liver.[23] Regardless of its optimal anatomic depiction, surface nodularity is not always attributable to cirrhosis. Pseudocirrhosis can result from diffuse parenchymal distortion and scarring arising from various metastases and treatment; common causes include breast carcinoma and neuroendocrine tumors (Fig. 11).[23] In addition, extrahepatic lesions, such as pseudomyxoma peritonei and ovarian carcinoma metastases, may result in extensive irregularity and scalloping of the liver surfaces.

Malignancy

Infiltrating hepatic malignancies that are nearly isoechoic to normal background liver cause only subtle parenchymal changes, and may evade detection during US examinations (Fig. 12). Therefore, application of color and spectral Doppler is critical for detection; absent, distorted, displaced, or thrombosed vessels should raise concern for neoplastic involvement and additional imaging or biopsy. Mass effect may be subtle on gray scale but more apparent as a blunted, monophasic waveform. Although cirrhosis also results in venous blunting, it affects all hepatic veins and is associated with the typical lobar atrophy-hypertrophy complex. An additional helpful gray-scale finding of infiltrating tumor is the multiple refractive edge shadows that occur at the interfaces between background liver and tumor (Fig. 13).

Cirrhosis can also result in bland thrombosis of the portal veins. However, approximately one-third of patients with hepatocellular carcinoma have been shown to have portal venous thrombus on US.[24] Although US is highly sensitive for detecting portal venous thrombus, the specificity is not as high. Findings that increase the specificity for tumor thrombus include expansion of the portal vein and the demonstration of an arterial waveform within the thrombus[25]; reliance on color Doppler flow alone may be complicated by the presence of a small amount of residual flow in nonocclusive portal venous thrombus.

Infiltrating malignancies and numerous nonmalignant etiologic factors can cause Budd-Chiari syndrome and result in loss of normal vascular

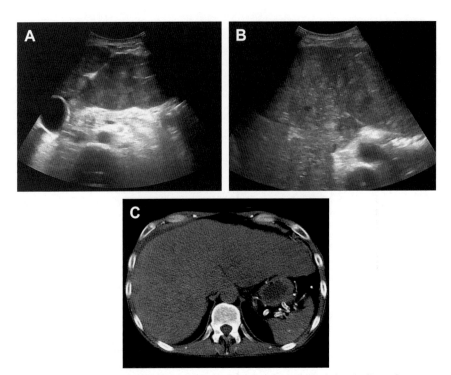

Fig. 9. Sarcoidosis. Transverse US images of the (*A*) left and (*B*) right hepatic lobes indicate heterogeneity of the echotexture and surface nodularity, seen best on the posterior surface in image *A*. (*C*) Noncontrast computed tomography (CT) corroborates the US findings. Biopsy proved sarcoidosis.

landmarks. With nonmalignant causes, the hepatic veins are occluded but can typically still be identified on gray scale, whereas infiltrative malignancies are more likely to displace or invade and obscure the vessels. Infiltrating malignancies are also more likely when portal vein occlusion is present. In addition, the presence of characteristic peripheral atrophy, caudate hypertrophy, and intrahepatic venous collaterals are consistent with chronic Budd-Chiari syndrome.

WHAT THE REFERRING CLINICIAN NEEDS TO KNOW

The primary goal is to provide data to determine the next step in evaluation (**Box 5**). First, limitations resulting in suboptimal evaluation should be stated in the context of any required additional imaging. Next, because hepatic function relates to structure, any focal or diffuse morphologic and parenchymal changes are reported regardless of subtlety. Ancillary findings of vascular deformation, biliary ductal dilatation, and abnormalities of the perihepatic spaces should be described. Finally, a specific diagnosis is offered if US and clinical criteria are met; if not, a concise differential diagnosis is integrated with recommendations for further characterization. Considerations for CT, MR imaging, or image-guided biopsy are placed within the context of patient age, comorbidities, and prior imaging. Diagnostic yield of biopsies can often be optimized if the US report indicates the segment or lobe in which the diffuse abnormality is most pronounced.

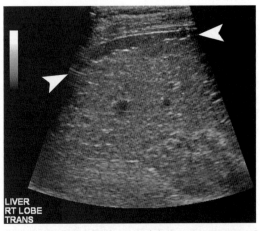

Fig. 10. Cirrhosis: surface nodularity. Transverse US obtained with a high-resolution probe reveals subtle surface nodularity (*arrowheads*) that was not apparent with a standard curvilinear probe (not shown). There is a small volume of ascites.

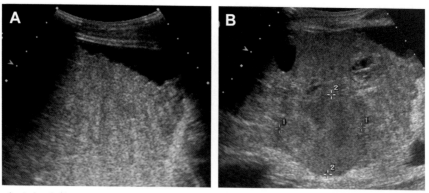

Fig. 11. Pseudocirrhosis: breast cancer. Transverse US images show (*A*) ascites and surface nodularity, and (*B*) a solid mass (*calipers*).

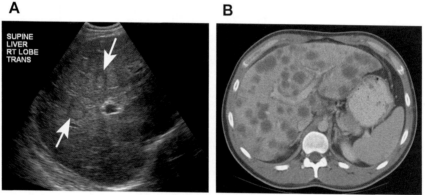

Fig. 12. Diffuse colon cancer metastases. (*A*) Transverse US shows parenchymal heterogeneity and subtle lesions (*arrows*). (*B*) Postcontrast CT shows multifocal tumor that was underestimated by US.

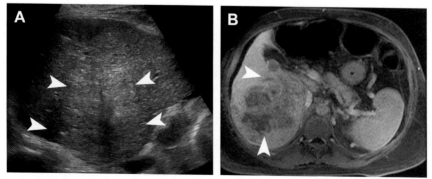

Fig. 13. Refractive edge shadows. (*A*) Transverse US shows heterogeneity of the right hepatic lobe and subtle refractive edge shadows (*arrowheads*) attributable to an ill-defined mass. (*B*) Postcontrast T1-weighted MR image corroborates the infiltrative mass in the right lobe (*arrowheads*).

Box 5
Summary of what the referring clinician needs to know and do

- List significant limitations requiring further evaluation
- Determine focal versus diffuse hepatic disease
- Describe hepatic vessel involvement
- Provide specific diagnosis or recommendation for further evaluation
- Describe target or anatomic landmarks to guide biopsy

SUMMARY

US is commonly used to evaluate patients presenting with abnormal liver function tests, right upper quadrant symptoms, or suspected diffuse hepatic disease. Detection and characterization of diffuse disease can be challenging; altered hepatic parenchymal echogenicity, echotexture, and contour are essential, but nonspecific findings should prompt further evaluation with CT, MR imaging, or biopsy. In addition, deformation of vascular landmarks, altered flow, biliary ductal dilatation, and abnormalities in the perihepatic spaces are ancillary findings that often herald the presence of diffuse hepatic abnormality. In the future, further refinement of elastography and ultrasound contrast agents may improve the specificity of the ultrasound diagnosis of diffuse liver disease.

REFERENCES

1. Parker KJ, Doyley MM, Rubens DJ. Imaging the elastic properties of tissue: the 20 year perspective. Phys Med Biol 2011;56:R1–29.
2. Kudo M, Shiina T, Moriyasu F, et al. JSUM ultrasound elastography practice guidelines: liver. J Med Ultrasonics 2013;40:325–57.
3. Horrow MM, Horrow JC, Niakosari A, et al. Is age associated with size of adult extrahepatic bile duct: sonographic study. Radiology 2001;221:411–4.
4. Zwiebel WJ. Sonographic diagnosis of diffuse liver disease. Semin Ultrasound CT MR 1995;16:8–15.
5. Tchelepi H, Ralls PW, Radin R, et al. Sonography of diffuse liver disease. J Ultrasound Med 2002;21:1023–32 [quiz: 1033–4].
6. Needleman L, Kurtz AB, Rifkin MD, et al. Sonography of diffuse benign liver disease: accuracy of pattern recognition and grading. AJR Am J Roentgenol 1986;146:1011–5.
7. Giorgio A, Amoroso P, Fico P, et al. Ultrasound evaluation of uncomplicated and complicated acute viral hepatitis. J Clin Ultrasound 1986;14:675–9.
8. Juttner HU, Ralls PW, Quinn MF, et al. Thickening of the gallbladder wall in acute hepatitis: ultrasound demonstration. Radiology 1982;142:465–6.
9. Joy D, Thava VR, Scott BB. Diagnosis of fatty liver disease: is biopsy necessary? Eur J Gastroenterol Hepatol 2003;15:539–43.
10. Hamer OW, Aguirre DA, Casola G, et al. Fatty liver: imaging patterns and pitfalls. Radiographics 2006;26:1637–53.
11. Sanford NL, Walsh P, Matis C, et al. Is ultrasonography useful in the assessment of diffuse parenchymal liver disease? Gastroenterology 1985;89:186–91.
12. Reid AE. Nonalcoholic steatohepatitis. Gastroenterology 2001;121:710–23.
13. Foucher J, Chanteloup E, Vergniol J, et al. Diagnosis of cirrhosis by transient elastography (FibroScan): a prospective study. Gut 2006;55:403–8.
14. Brown JJ, Naylor MJ, Yagan N. Imaging of hepatic cirrhosis. Radiology 1997;202:1–16.
15. Harbin WP, Robert NJ, Ferrucci JT Jr. Diagnosis of cirrhosis based on regional changes in hepatic morphology: a radiological and pathological analysis. Radiology 1980;135:273–83.
16. Lafortune M, Matricardi L, Denys A, et al. Segment 4 (the quadrate lobe): a barometer of cirrhotic liver disease at US. Radiology 1998;206:157–60.
17. Bolondi L, Li Bassi S, Gaiani S, et al. Liver cirrhosis: changes of Doppler waveform of hepatic veins. Radiology 1991;178:513–6.
18. Arda K, Ofelli M, Calikoglu U, et al. Hepatic vein Doppler waveform changes in early stage (Child-Pugh A) chronic parenchymal liver disease. J Clin Ultrasound 1997;25:15–9.
19. Gulberg V, Haag K, Rossle M, et al. Hepatic arterial buffer response in patients with advanced cirrhosis. Hepatology 2002;35:630–4.
20. Sandrin L, Fourquet B, Hasquenoph JM, et al. Transient elastography: a new noninvasive method for assessment of hepatic fibrosis. Ultrasound Med Biol 2003;29:1705–13.
21. Talwalkar JA, Kurtz DM, Schoenleber SJ, et al. Ultrasound-based transient elastography for the detection of hepatic fibrosis: systematic review and meta-analysis. Clin Gastroenterol Hepatol 2007;5:1214–20.
22. Blomley MJ, Lim AK, Harvey CJ, et al. Liver microbubble transit time compared with histology and Child-Pugh score in diffuse liver disease: a cross sectional study. Gut 2003;52:1188–93.
23. Filly RA, Reddy SG, Nalbandian AB, et al. Sonographic evaluation of liver nodularity: inspection of

deep versus superficial surfaces of the liver. J Clin Ultrasound 2002;30:399–407.

24. Connolly GC, Chen R, Hyrien O, et al. Incidence, risk factors and consequences of portal vein and systemic thromboses in hepatocellular carcinoma. Thromb Res 2008;122:299–306.

25. Dodd GD 3rd, Memel DS, Baron RL, et al. Portal vein thrombosis in patients with cirrhosis: does sonographic detection of intrathrombus flow allow differentiation of benign and malignant thrombus? AJR Am J Roentgenol 1995;165: 573–7.

Contrast-Enhanced Ultrasound of the Liver and Kidney

Harshawn Malhi, MD[a],*, Edward G. Grant, MD[b],
Vinay Duddalwar, MD, FRCR[c]

KEYWORDS

- Contrast ultrasound scan • Imaging • Mass • Lesion • Renal • Liver • Microbubble

KEY POINTS

- Contrast-enhanced ultrasound scan is a safe and effective imaging technique with a growing number of clinical applications.
- Targeted contrast-enhanced ultrasound scan can greatly aid in the characterization and diagnosis of perfusion defects and focal lesions of several visceral organs, including the liver and kidney.

INTRODUCTION

Over the last decade, the clinical applications of noncardiac contrast-enhanced ultrasound (CEUS) have been steadily increasing. The development of new second-generation contrast agents has allowed superior visualization of the microcirculation, once a domain restricted to angiography, contrast-enhanced computed tomography (CECT), and contrast-enhanced magnetic resonance imaging (CEMR). Ultrasound (US) contrast agents possess a good safety profile and, given their lack of nephrotoxicity, are indispensable in patients with critical renal function who may have contraindications to undergoing CECT or CEMR imaging. In addition, CEUS allows for real-time dynamic imaging of lesions and organs. This article provides a survey of the current clinical applications and potential future uses of CEUS in the liver and kidney.

CONTRAST AGENTS

US contrast agents, commonly referred to as *microbubbles*, are composed of tiny bubbles of a perfluorocarbon or nitrogen gas contained within a stabilizing shell made from a lipid or protein. The composition of the shell determines how long the agent remains in the circulation. These microbubbles avoid filtration in the lungs and heart because of their equivalent size to red blood cells. The highly echogenic microbubble gas core provides useful contrast from the background tissue.[1]

LIVER

In the evaluation of focal liver masses, magnetic resonance imaging (MRI) signal, computed tomography (CT) attenuation, and echogenicity on conventional US taken alone are often nonspecific imaging characteristics. The distinguishing feature

Disclosure: Nothing to disclose (H. Malhi); General Electric research grant, General Electric company medical advisory board, Nuance Communications, Inc (E.G. Grant); General Electric research grant (V. Duddalwar).
[a] Department of Radiology, Keck Hospital of USC, University of Southern California, 1500 San Pablo Street, Los Angeles, CA 90033, USA; [b] Department of Radiology, Keck Hospital of USC, USC Norris Comprehensive Cancer Center, University of Southern California, 1500 San Pablo Street, Los Angeles, CA 90033, USA; [c] Abdominal Imaging, Imaging, Keck Hospital of USC, USC Norris Comprehensive Cancer Center, University of Southern California, 1500 San Pablo Street, Los Angeles, CA 90033, USA
* Corresponding author.
E-mail address: harshawn.malhi@usc.edu

0033-8389/14/$ – see front matter © 2014 Elsevier Inc. All rights reserved.

radiologic.theclinics.com

of many lesions remains their vascularity and hemodynamic parameters. CEUS has become increasingly accepted as an equally effective and sustainable alternative to multiphase CEMR or CECT while saving cost and avoiding potential nephrotoxicity and harmful radiation to the patient. The established recommended indications for CEUS in the liver include evaluation of lesions or a suspected lesion in a patient with a history of chronic liver disease or known malignancy, workup for incidental findings on routine US or inconclusive MRI/CT or biopsy results, and characterization of portal vein thrombosis (**Box 1**).

Hemangioma

Cavernous hemangiomas are the most common benign tumors of the liver, occurring in approximately 4% of the population. Most hemangiomas are small and asymptomatic, usually discovered incidentally, although large lesions can occasionally present with acute abdominal pain caused by hemorrhage or thrombosis.

The typical appearance of a hemangioma on conventional US is a well-circumscribed or lobulated mass that is homogeneously hyperechoic. This lesion may have posterior acoustic enhancement. Of note, echogenicity is relative to the background tissue; thus, in the setting of hepatic steatosis, a hemangioma may appear hypoechoic or isoechoic relative to the echogenic fatty liver parenchyma.[2]

On CEUS, hemangiomas will typically have peripheral globular-nodular enhancement in the arterial phase. This is followed by centripetal progression of the enhancement until the entire lesion is enhancing and hyperechoic compared with the background liver parenchyma (**Fig. 1**). This enhancement usually persists in the portal venous and more delayed phases.[1] Small flash hemangiomas typically show diffuse and immediate arterial enhancement, which will often persist on the later phases.[3]

Box 1
Uses of contrast US in the liver

1. Incidental findings on routine US

2. Lesion(s) or suspected lesion(s) detected with US in patients with a known history of a malignancy, as an alternative to CT or MRI

3. Need for a contrast study when CT and MRI contrast are contraindicated

4. Inconclusive MRI/CT

5. Inconclusive cytology/histology results

Focal Nodular Hyperplasia

Focal nodular hyperplasia (FNH) is the second most common benign liver mass and histologically represents developmental hyperplastic lesions containing a mix of abnormally arranged nonneoplastic hepatocytes, Kupffer cells, biliary ducts, and components of portal triads.[4] Similar to hemangioma, FNH is usually discovered incidentally and is asymptomatic.

Sonographically, FNH can be subtle and difficult to detect in large part because histologically FNH is essentially hyperplastic normal liver tissue. When seen, FNH typically becomes apparent because of displacement of the normal surrounding vasculature and subtle contour abnormalities rather than an inherent difference in the echogenicity of the lesion compared with the surrounding liver parenchyma. The linear or stellar central scar seen in FNH is usually hypoechoic although occasionally hyperechoic.[5]

After contrast administration, FNHs will enhance (predominately within the central scar) and a large feeding vessel can often be seen on the arterial phase. This is followed by a centrifugal filling direction in the portal venous phase (in contrast to the centripetal filling seen in hemangiomas). Enhancement is sustained in the portal venous phase with equal or greater enhancement than the background liver tissue (**Fig. 2**). Occasionally, an unenhanced scar may be seen in both the arterial and portal venous phases.

Adenoma

Adenomas consist of normal to slightly atypical hepatocytes that occasionally contain bile ducts, Kupffer cells, calcification, and fat, thus, making their appearance highly variable on all imaging modalities. They are associated with women using oral contraceptives and, although typically asymptomatic, can present with severe pain in the setting of hemorrhage or infarction. The risk of rupture, hemoperitoneum, and shock makes the management of these lesions more complicated than, for instance, hemangiomas. Thus, small adenomas are often managed conservatively, whereas large or growing adenomas are considered for resection.

The gray-scale US appearance of adenomas is extremely variable. With regard to their vascularity, adenomas may have well-defined intralesion blood vessels (usually venous) and can, therefore, be difficult to distinguish from FNH based on their nonspecific conventional US and Doppler appearance.[6]

CEUS can aid in distinguishing between adenomas and FNHs. Adenomas will typically be hypervascular on the arterial phase just as FNH,

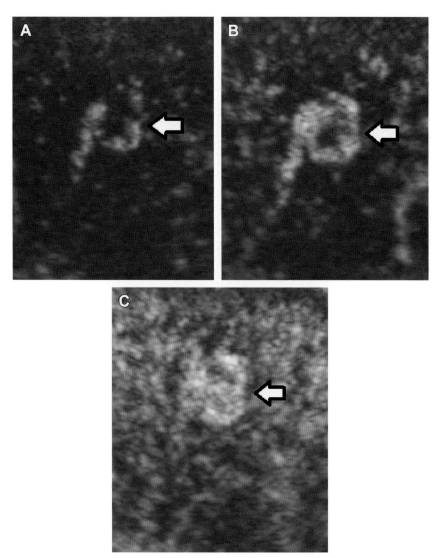

Fig. 1. A 42-year-old man with a hepatic hemangioma. Three sequential CEUS images of a liver mass (*arrows*). (*A*) Early peripheral nodular enhancement. (*B*) Progressive centripetal contrast enhancement. (*C*) Near-complete enhancement of the hemangioma.

although usually to a lesser extent.[7] The distinguishing factor, however, is the centripetal filling pattern seen on the subsequent phases with adenomas. This is in contrast to the centrifugal filling pattern of FNH (**Fig. 3**).

Hepatocellular Carcinoma

Hepatocellular carcinoma (HCC) commonly occurs in the setting of chronic liver disease and cirrhosis (alcoholic and viral) and is the most common primary visceral malignancy in the world, accounting for 80% to 90% of all primary liver malignancies.[5] Of note, the liver does not necessarily have to have a cirrhotic appearance on imaging to be predisposed to increased risk of HCC, as in the setting of hepatitis B virus. Although usually solitary tumors, HCCs may be multifocal or infiltrative in nature.

Sonographically, HCC is variable in appearance. When larger in size, HCCs often have mixed echogenicity because of tumor necrosis and hypervascularity, whereas smaller lesions are usually solid and appear hypoechoic. HCCs may also be hyperechoic if fatty metamorphosis or sinusoidal dilation is present. Small hyperechoic HCCs can, therefore, simulate hemangiomas, hypervascular metastases, or lipomas. On color Doppler, HCCs usually show hypervascularity and tumor shunting.

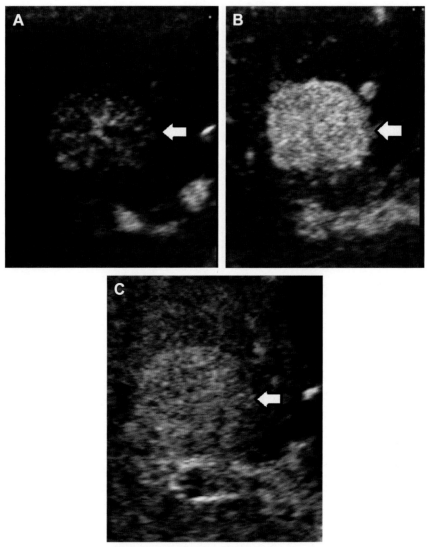

Fig. 2. A 21-year-old woman with FNH. Three sequential CEUS images of a liver lesion (*arrows*). (*A*) Early hypervascular enhancement within the central scar. (*B*) Progressive centrifugal direction of contrast enhancement. (*C*) Sustained mild enhancement on the portal venous phase.

On CEUS, HCCs show classic and characteristic arterial enhancement owing to arterial neovascularity. This is followed by decreased portal venous flow (washout), findings similar to those seen on 4-phase CEMRIs and CECTs (Fig. 4). Of note, several atypical variations of enhancement patterns of HCCs have been described, including arterial-phase hypovascularity with delayed or no enhancement and arterial enhancement without washout.[8]

HCC tumor thrombus within the portal and hepatic veins can be diagnosed with CEUS. The enhancement patterns should be similar to those of the tumor from which it originated and will have a different appearance than a normally enhancing vessel (ie, an arterial tumor blush rather than discrete vessels), secondary to malignant neovascularity (Fig. 5).[9] A marked wash out in the portal and late phases may occur in metastatic portal vein thrombosis. A bland thrombus, however, will show no arterial enhancement (Fig. 6).

Fibrolamellar HCC is a histologic subtype of HCC often seen in younger individuals and is not associated with chronic liver disease. These tumors are usually solitary and well encapsulated. Similar to HCC, fibrolamellar HCC can have a variable sonographic appearance. Common findings include punctate calcifications and a hyperechoic central scar. On CEUS, fibrolamellar HCC will

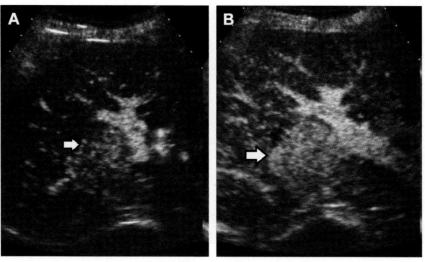

Fig. 3. A 63-year-old woman with a hepatic adenoma. Two sequential CEUS images of a liver lesion (*arrows*). (*A*) Hypervascular early central enhancement on the arterial phase, typically less intense than FNH. (*B*) Centripetal filling pattern seen on more delayed phase.

typically show heterogeneous arterial enhancement secondary to necrosis with washout during the portal venous phase.[10]

Cholangiocarcinoma

Cholangiocarcinomas are the second most common primary hepatic tumor after HCC. Histologically, cholangiocarcinomas are usually adenocarcinomas arising from the bile duct epithelium and are highly malignant, occurring primarily in the sixth and seventh decades of life. They can arise peripherally or centrally in the liver, with the hilar variant known as a *Klatskin tumor*. Given their biliary origin, both variants may cause more proximal biliary ductal dilation secondary to luminal obstruction.

Sonographically, cholangiocarcinomas usually appear as mixed echogenicity masses with associated biliary ductal dilatation. On CEUS, most cholangiocarcinomas show peripheral irregular rimlike enhancement with heterogeneous central hypoenhancement during the arterial phase followed by characteristic wash out on portal and late phases.[10]

Cystadenoma/Cystadenocarcinoma

Biliary cystadenomas and cystadenocarcinomas are rare cystic tumors that likely arise from ectopic

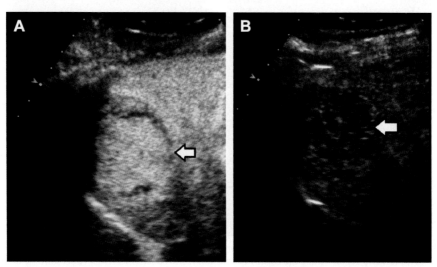

Fig. 4. A 61-year-old woman with HCC. Two sequential CEUS images. (*A*) Intense early arterial enhancement (*arrow*). (*B*) Contrast washout of HCC (*arrow*) on later phase (approximately 4-minute delay).

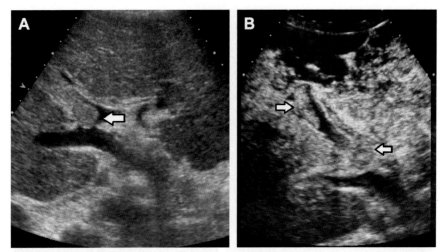

Fig. 5. A 59-year-old man with infiltrating HCC and secondary malignant portal vein thrombus. (*A*) Thrombus within the left and possibly main portal vein (*arrow*); unclear if bland or malignant on unenhanced gray-scale image. (*B*) CEUS images show enhancement of the malignant thrombus (*arrows*) in left portal vein.

nests of primitive biliary tissue. Unfortunately, on imaging, benign cystadenomas cannot be reliably differentiated from malignant cystadenocarcinomas. Sonographically, they appear as large, well-defined multiloculated anechoic masses with highly echogenic septa. Nodular components may be present. Because they are largely avascular, minimal enhancement is seen with CEUS; however, abnormal enhancing vessels may be seen peripherally or within the septa.[11]

Metastasis

Metastatic lesions to the liver most commonly originate from primary tumors of the gallbladder, colon, stomach, pancreas, breast, and lung. Metastases are the most common liver tumor in the United States, up to 20 times more common than HCC.[5]

Patients with metastatic liver disease usually present with multifocal disease and less commonly with a solitary lesion or as an infiltrative process. Sonographically, they may be hypoechoic, isoechoic, or hyperechoic depending on vascularity, hemorrhage, and mucin content. The so-called target appearance of a hepatic parenchymal mass with a hypoechoic halo is a common sonographic pattern for liver metastases. Many metastatic lesions are similar in echogenicity to the background liver, making their detection

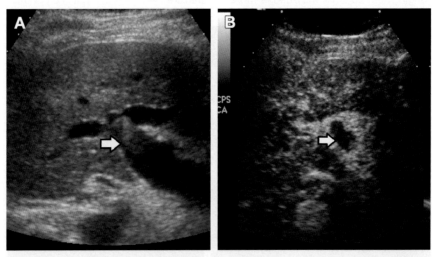

Fig. 6. A 62-year-old woman with HCC, portal hypertension, and new portal vein thrombus. (*A*) Gray-scale image shows subtle echogenicity within the bifurcation of the main portal vein (*arrow*), representing a nonocclusive thrombus, either bland or malignant. (*B*) Corresponding CEUS image in the portal venous phase shows no enhancement (*arrow*), consistent with bland thrombus.

difficult or impossible. CEUS can help combat this problem by improving the conspicuity of metastasis. After contrast administration, the appearance of metastatic disease on the arterial phase is variable depending on the vascularity of the lesion. During the arterial phase, hypovascular metastases (ie, gastrointestinal tumors, ovarian, pancreatic) are hypoenhancing, whereas hypervascular metastases (ie, neuroendocrine tumors, melanoma, renal) are hyperenhancing. The portal venous phase is often more useful in detecting and characterizing metastases, as they almost always washout (**Fig. 7**). When detected initially on US, the diagnosis can be confirmed with biopsy.[12]

Infection

Hepatic abscesses (whether pyogenic, parasitic, or fungal in etiology) may have a rimlike enhancement pattern, which may persist or fade to background on the delayed phases. If the abscess center is liquefied, it will not enhance and will appear as a persistent hypoechoic defect on delayed phases. Occasionally, enhancing septae may be seen within the central defect.[3]

Postprocedure Monitoring (Local Ablative and Transarterial Chemoembolization Treatment)

Percutaneous ablation and trans-arterial chemoembolization have become viable alternatives for the management of selected patients with liver malignancies. It is essential to follow up with these treated lesions to exclude residual or nontreated disease, and to assess for recurrence and CEUS is a useful modality with the ultimate goal being complete devascularization of the mass. Live scanning through the entire treated lesion is necessary to detect focal areas of persistently enhancing tissue within or surrounding the treated lesion. For hypovascular malignancies, the completeness of treatment can be assessed by comparing the pretreatment lesion appearance with that of the posttreatment necrotic region (**Fig. 8**). For this reason, obtaining a pretreatment CEUS of the lesion to be ablated or embolized is of high utility. Of note, normal peripheral uniform enhancement can be seen in the postablative setting for up to 30 days, and careful consideration should be made before misinterpreting this hyperemic halo as residual disease. A treated lesion with nodular or irregular enhancement should raise the suspicion for residual disease (**Fig. 9**). If residual malignancy is suspected, the patient may be referred for retreatment of the tumor.[3]

RENAL

The use of CEUS in evaluating renal pathology is maturing and evolving. Current uses include evaluation of the general vascular perfusion of the kidney and its most publicized use—the evaluation of focal renal masses (**Box 2**).[1,13]

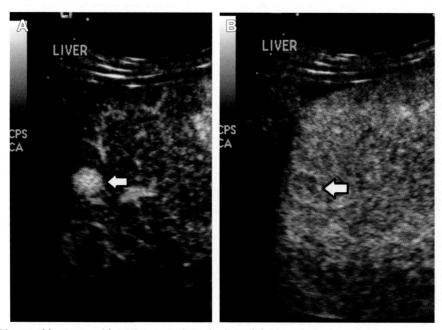

Fig. 7. A 66-year-old woman with RCC metastasis to the liver. (*A*) Arterial phase contrast-enhanced image shows rapid enhancement (11 seconds) of a small liver mass (*arrow*). (*B*) Rapid early washout (*arrow*) is also present (19 seconds).

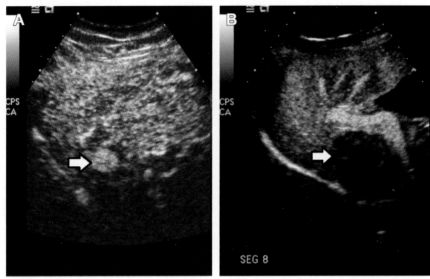

Fig. 8. A 64-year-old man with HCC. CEUS images of the HCC before and after radiofrequency ablation (RFA). (*A*) Arterially enhancing HCC (*arrow*) within the right hepatic lobe. (*B*) No residual arterial enhancement and a large devascularized defect (*arrow*) after RFA.

Normal Appearance

In the arterial phase, the renal cortex enhances rapidly. This phase is followed by successive perfusion of the medulla and then a more homogenous appearance corresponding to the nephrographic phase as seen on CECT or CEMRI. As contrast is reduced within the circulation, enhancement gradually fades. Although there is thought to be a fair amount of potential in the

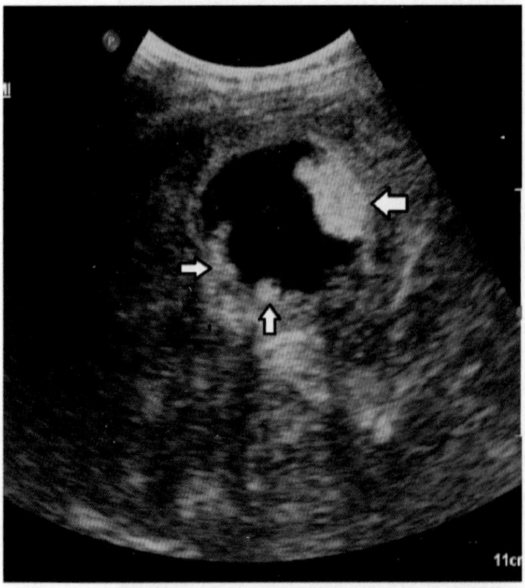

Fig. 9. A 75-year-old woman with HCC after radiofrequency ablation treatment. Partially treated HCC with 3 regions (*arrows*) of residual peripheral mural nodular enhancement.

evaluation of renal perfusion and blood flow quantification, this has not yet translated into routine clinical use (**Fig. 10**).[14,15]

Renal Cell Carcinoma

Renal cell carcinomas (RCCs) are the eighth most common malignancy affecting adults and the most common malignant renal neoplasm. On conventional US, these masses are typically heterogeneously hypoechoic or isoechoic, although small masses (<2 cm) may be echogenic. On CEUS, RCCs typically are heterogeneously hypervascular with early washout on the delayed phase. A pseudocapsule may be present (**Fig. 11**).[16]

Complex Renal Cysts

Complex cystic masses have variable malignant potential depending on the existence of certain

---

Box 2
Uses of contrast US in the kidney

1. Characterization of renal masses
   a. Evaluation and characterization of renal pseudotumors versus true mass lesions
   b. Characterization of complex mass lesions
   c. Characterization of renal cysts
2. Renal ischemia and perfusion
3. Abdominal/renal trauma
4. Guidance of renal biopsy and ablative procedures

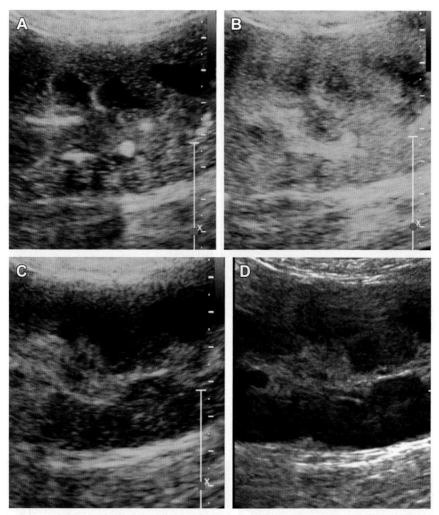

Fig. 10. Appearance of renal cortex and medulla after ultrasound contrast injection. (*A*) Early arterial phase after contrast injection: normal renal cortex enhances early with renal pyramids well seen as relative areas hypoperfusion at this stage. (*B*) Nephrographic phase equivalent: there is a more homogenous appearance to the entire kidney. (*C*) Late phase: appearance of the kidney is similar to normal gray-scale US images. (*D*) Gray-scale image of normal kidney.

characteristics such as septations and wall thickness, the presence or absence of mural nodules, and septal enhancement. The role of CEUS in delineating these features has been studied with good results. CEUS can also be used to classify cysts through Bosniak grading.[16–18] The presence of contrast-enhanced septations and nodular protuberances can help differentiate a benign cyst from an indeterminate or neoplastic cyst (**Fig. 12**).

Angiomyolipoma

Angiomyolipomas (AMLs) are benign mesenchymal tumors of the kidney that are usually asymptomatic, but larger (>4 cm) lesions can hemorrhage. On conventional US, AMLs are commonly

hyperechoic. On CEUS, AMLs tends to enhance peripherally and enhance less than the normal cortex centrally.[16]

Oncocytoma

Oncocytoma is the most common benign solid renal tumor but unfortunately, it shares many of the imaging features also found in RCC. Conventional US may show a well-defined, homogeneous, and hypoechoic to isoechoic solid mass, with or without an echogenic central scar. CEUS features of oncocytoma include early enhancement, enhancement greater than adjacent cortex and rapid washout (**Fig. 13**). The well described avascular scar depicted on CT and MR has also been reported.[19]

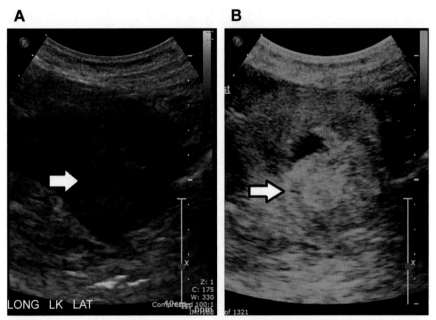

Fig. 11. A 65-year-old woman with a left-sided renal mass. (*A*) Gray-scale image shows a solid left renal mass (*arrow*). (*B*) Early phase CEUS image shows very early enhancement centrally (*arrow*). Surgical pathology showed RCC.

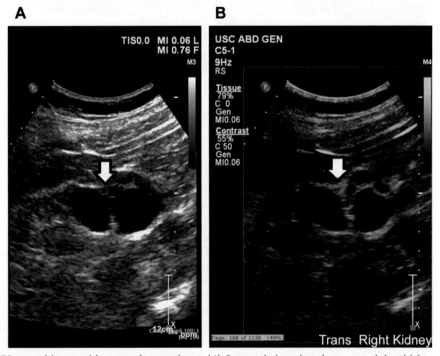

Fig. 12. A 56-year-old man with a complex renal cyst. (*A*) Gray-scale imaging shows a nodular thickened complex septation along the margin of the larger cyst (*arrow*). (*B*) After contrast injection, there is marked enhancement of the septation (*arrow*). This classifies the cyst as a Bosniak III lesion. On resection, this was a cystic clear cell renal carcinoma.

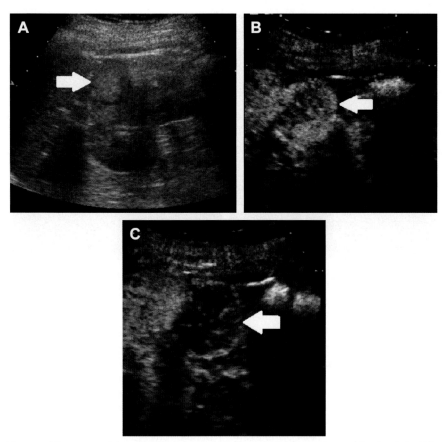

Fig. 13. A 64-year-old woman with a right renal mass. (*A*) Hyperechoic mass (*arrow*) in the right kidney, which is well marginated. (*B*) After contrast injection, there is early enhancement of most of the mass (*arrow*) with a non-enhancing area in the center. (*C*) Delayed images show early washout from most of the mass (*arrow*). Surgical pathology showed an oncocytoma.

Pseudotumor

A renal pseudotumor is a mass that simulates a tumor on imaging but is composed of nonneoplastic tissue. CEUS can aid in differentiating a true mass from a pseudotumor. Examples include a congenital hypertrophied column of Bertin and a postprocedural surgical bed mass as those seen in patients undergoing minimally invasive treatment of renal tumors (ie, laparoscopic/robotic-assisted nephron-sparing surgery, cryoablation, and radiofrequency ablation). There is an established role of CEUS in the evaluation of renal masses during and after minimally invasive treatments to monitor completeness of therapy and for the detection of disease recurrence. Specifically, postoperative renal pseudotumors should not have any internal enhancement, as they often represent surgical gelatin sponge material or hematoma and usually resolve or decrease in size over time (**Fig. 14**).[20–22]

Metastasis

Metastasis to the kidney is uncommon. The main diagnostic dilemma is to distinguish a renal metastasis from a primary renal tumor. Renal metastases do not have a characteristic enhancement pattern on CEUS but tend to be hypovascular compared with normal cortical enhancement (**Fig. 15**).

Ischemia/Infarction

Renal ischemia/infarction results from reduced or a complete lack of perfusion to the kidney. Underlying etiologies include thromboembolism (most common), aortic or renal artery dissection, vasculitis, and iatrogenic. CEUS aids in evaluating the presence and extent of renal parenchymal ischemia and, therefore, can be used in the evaluation of suspected infarction. Renal infarcts will appear as wedge-shaped areas of nonperfusion.

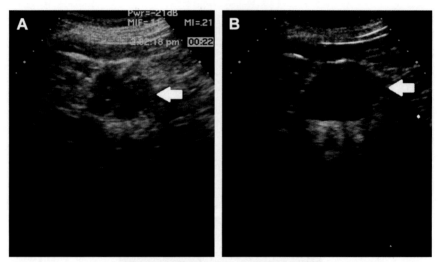

Fig. 14. A 60-year-old man after resection of a left RCC. (A) Postoperative gray-scale US shows a complex septated mass (arrow) measuring 4.6 cm within the surgical bed. Differential of tumor recurrence versus postoperative pseudotumor was given. (B) CEUS of the mass (arrow) shows no enhancement, findings consistent with benign pseudotumor.

In addition, CEUS can help detect a nonperfused or hypoperfused organ such as a failing transplanted kidney.[23,24]

Infection

An abnormal finding on conventional US is seen in only around 20% of patients with bacterial pyelonephritis. When positive findings of pyelonephritis are discovered on sonography, they may include renal enlargement, hydronephrosis, increased renal cortical echogenicity, and abscess formation. Gas identified in the renal parenchyma aids in diagnosing emphysematous pyelonephritis. CEUS can assist in differentiating focal pyelonephritis from mass lesions and aids in delineating abscesses, either parenchymal or perinephric (Fig. 16).[23]

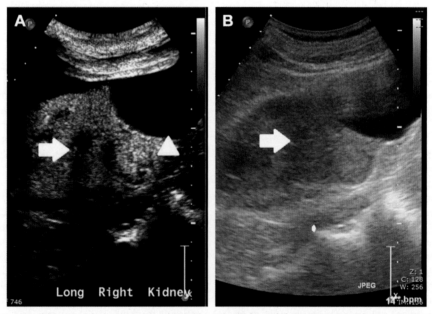

Fig. 15. A 78-year-old man with metastatic melanoma to the kidney. (A) CEUS image shows a poorly defined relatively hypovascular focal lesion (arrow). Incidental note is made of a Bosniak I simple cyst (arrowhead). (B) Corresponding gray-scale images unable to reliably identify the focal lesion.

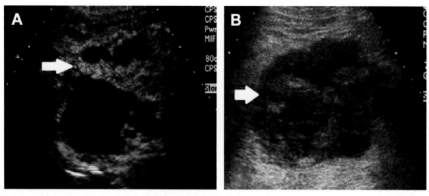

Fig. 16. A 59-year-old man after renal transplant with fevers and leukocytosis and a peritransplant fluid collection found to represent abscess. (*A*) CEUS image shows enhancing septations and loculations (*arrow*), features suggestive of a complex fluid collection such as an abscess. (*B*) Gray-scale image alone does not show septations as readily (*arrow* indicates general area).

CEUS is a safe and effective imaging technique with a growing number of clinical applications. Targeted CEUS can greatly aid in the characterization and diagnosis of perfusion defects and focal lesions of several visceral organs, including the liver and kidney.

REFERENCES

1. Wilson SR, Burns PN. Microbubble enhanced ultrasound imaging: what role? Radiology 2010;257:24–39.
2. Marsh JI, Gibney RG, Li DK. Hepatic hemangioma in the presence of fatty infiltration: an atypical sonographic appearance. Gastrointest Radiol 1989;14:262–4.
3. Claudon M, Cosgrove D, Albrecht T, et al. Guidelines and good clinical practice recommendations for contrast enhanced ultrasound (CEUS) - Update 2008. Ultraschall Med 2008;29:28–44.
4. Wanless IR, Mawdsley C, Adams R. On the pathogenesis of focal nodular hyperplasia of the liver. Hepatology 1985;5:1194–200.
5. Rumack C, Wilson S, Charboneau J, et al. The liver, diagnostic ultrasound. 4th edition. Philadelphia: Elsevier Mosby; 2011. p. 78–145.
6. Golli M, Van Nhieu JT, Mathieu D, et al. Hepatocellular adenoma: color Doppler and pathologic correlations. Radiology 1994;190:741–4.
7. Kim TK, Jank HJ, Burns PN, et al. Focal nodular hyperplasia and hepatic adenoma: differentiation with low mechanical index contrast-enhanced sonography. AJR Am J Roentgenol 2008;190:58–66.
8. Jang HG, Kim TK, Burns PN, et al. Enhancement patterns of hepatocellular carcinoma at contrast-enhanced US: comparison with histologic differentiation. Radiology 2007;244:898–906.
9. Claudon M, Dietrich C, Choi B, et al. Guidelines and good clinical practice recommendations for contrast enhanced ultrasound (CEUS) - Update 2012. A WFUSMB-EFSUMB initiative in cooperation with representatives of AFSUMB, AIUM, ASUM, FLAUS and ICUS. Ultrasound Med Biol 2013;39:187–210.
10. Zhi-Hui F, Min-Hua C, Ying D, et al. Evaluation of primary malignancies of the liver using contrast-enhanced sonography: correlation with pathology. AJR Am J Roentgenol 2006;186:1512–9.
11. Xu H, Lu M, Liu L, et al. Imaging features of intrahepatic biliary cystadenoma and cystadenocarcinoma on B-mode and contrast-enhanced ultrasound. Ultraschall Med 2012;33:241–9.
12. Larsen L. Role of contrast enhanced ultrasonography in the assessment of hepatic metastases: a review. World J Hepatol 2010;27:8–15.
13. Cokkinos DD, Antypa EG, Skilakaki M, et al. Contrast enhanced ultrasound of the kidneys: what is it capable of? Biomed Res Int 2013;2013:595873.
14. Wei K, Le E, Bin JP, et al. Quantification of renal blood flow with contrast-enhanced ultrasound. J Am Coll Cardiol 2001;37:1135–40.
15. Kishimoto N, Mori Y, Nishiue T, et al. Renal blood flow measurement with contrast-enhanced harmonic ultrasonography: evaluation of dopamine-induced changes in renal cortical perfusion in humans. Clin Nephrol 2003;59:423–8.
16. Barr RG, Peterson C, Hindi A. Evaluation of indeterminate renal masses with contrast-enhanced US: a diagnostic performance study. Radiology 2013;271:133–42.
17. Nicolau C, Bunesch L, Sebastia C. Renal complex cysts in adults: contrast-enhanced ultrasound. Abdom Imaging 2011;36:742–52.
18. Quaia E, Bertolotto M, Cioffi V, et al. Comparison of contrast-enhanced sonography with unenhanced sonography and contrast-enhanced CT in the diagnosis of malignancy in complex cystic renal masses. AJR Am J Roentgenol 2008;191:239–49.
19. Wu Y, Du L, Li F, et al. Renal oncocytoma: contrast-enhanced sonographic features. J Ultrasound Med 2013;32:441–8.

20. McArthur C, Baxter G. Current and potential renal applications of contrast-enhanced ultrasound. Clin Radiol 2012;67:909–22.

21. Chen Y, Huang J, Xia L, et al. Monitoring laparoscopic radiofrequency renal lesions in real time using contrast-enhanced ultrasonography: an open-label, randomized, comparative pilot trial. J Endourol 2013; 27:697–704.

22. Meloni MF, Bertolotto M, Alberzoni C, et al. Follow-up after percutaneous radiofrequency ablation of renal cell carcinoma: contrast-enhanced sonography versus contrast-enhanced CT or MRI. Am J Roentgenol 2008;191:1233–8.

23. Correas JM, Claudon M, Tranquart F, et al. The kidney: imaging with microbubble contrast agents. Ultrasound Q 2006;22:53–66.

24. Bertolotto M, Martegani A, Aiani L, et al. Value of contrast-enhanced ultrasonography for detecting renal infarcts proven by contrast enhanced CT. A feasibility study. Eur Radiol 2008;18:376–83.

Ultrasound Evaluation of the First Trimester

Peter M. Doubilet, MD, PhD

KEYWORDS

- Ultrasound • Pregnancy • First trimester • Ectopic pregnancy • Fetal anatomy

KEY POINTS

- In a woman with a positive pregnancy test, any intrauterine saclike fluid collection seen on ultrasound is highly likely to be a gestational sac.
- Sonographic criteria for definite pregnancy failure (ie, miscarriage) include nonvisualization of cardiac activity in an embryo whose crown-rump length is at least 7 mm, or nonvisualization of an embryo in a gestational sac whose mean sac diameter is at least 25 mm.
- Diagnosis of ectopic pregnancy should be based on visualization of an extraovarian mass in a woman with a positive pregnancy test; the concept of a pseudogestational sac is not helpful and may be misleading.
- A variety of fetal anatomic structures and fetal anomalies can be identified in the first trimester via transvaginal sonography.

INTRODUCTION

The first trimester of pregnancy is a 3-month span of remarkable growth and development. The embryo, microscopic in size near the beginning of this period, transforms into a fetus approximately 80 mm in length with identifiable features and internal organs by the end. (Note: by convention, the term *embryo* is used until 8–10 weeks' gestation and *fetus* is used thereafter.)

Ultrasound has undergone major advances since its first use in pregnancy approximately 50 years ago.[1] As the technology progressed from bistable to gray scale and static to real-time, and since transvaginal, Doppler, and 3-dimensional sonography were introduced, the applications of ultrasound in pregnancy have exploded.[2] This article reviews the use of ultrasound in the first trimester.

NORMAL SONOGRAPHIC APPEARANCE OF FIRST TRIMESTER PREGNANCY

During the first 3 weeks after conception, the gestational sac of the developing pregnancy is generally too small to be seen on ultrasound. Because conception occurs approximately 2 weeks after a woman's last menstrual period (LMP) and gestational age corresponds to time since LMP, this means that the pregnancy is not generally visible on ultrasound before a gestational age of 5 weeks.[3]

When the gestational sac is first identifiable on transvaginal ultrasound at approximately 5 weeks' gestation, it appears as a round or oval intrauterine fluid collection 2 to 3 mm in diameter (**Fig. 1**). It is located in the central echogenic portion of the uterus, which corresponds to the decidualized endometrium (also termed *decidua*). In some cases, this fluid collection is surrounded partly by 2 echogenic rings, which are thought to represent 2 layers of decidua: the decidua parietalis and capsularis. The double-ringed appearance has been termed the *double sac sign* of early intrauterine pregnancy.[4] In other cases, the gestational sac is eccentrically located on one side of a thin white line that corresponds to the collapsed uterine cavity. This appearance has been termed the *intradecidual sign*.[5] In many cases, however, the early gestational sac appears as a small, featureless,

Department of Radiology, Brigham and Women's Hospital, 75 Francis Street, Boston, MA 02116, USA
E-mail address: pdoubilet@partners.org

Radiol Clin N Am 52 (2014) 1191–1199
http://dx.doi.org/10.1016/j.rcl.2014.07.004
0033-8389/14/$ – see front matter

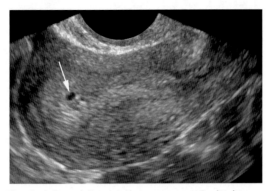

Fig. 1. A 5-week intrauterine pregnancy. Sagittal transvaginal view of the uterus shows a 5-week gestational sac, which appears as a fluid collection (*arrow*) with rounded edges, 3 mm in maximum diameter, located in the central echogenic portion of the uterus. Follow-up scan 7 weeks later showed a normal-appearing 12-week pregnancy, including a fetus with cardiac activity.

saclike structure without either of these signs.[6] Thus, the absence of a double sac sign or intradecidual sign does not exclude an intrauterine pregnancy. In fact, any saclike structure in the mid-uterus in a woman with a positive pregnancy test result is highly likely to represent an intrauterine pregnancy.[6]

At approximately 5.5 weeks' gestation, the gestational sac has grown to approximately 6 mm in diameter and a small thin-walled circular structure, the yolk sac, is seen within it (**Fig. 2**).[3] The embryo itself is first visible on transvaginal ultrasound at approximately 6 weeks' gestation (**Fig. 3**), at which time the gestational sac is 10 mm in diameter.[7] At that point, the embryo appears as a small structure at the edge of the yolk sac, 1 to 2 mm in length, and usually demonstrates

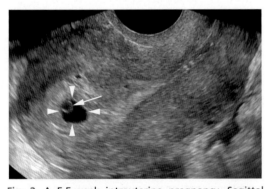

Fig. 2. A 5.5-week intrauterine pregnancy. Sagittal transvaginal view of the uterus shows a 5.5-week gestational sac, which appears as an intrauterine fluid collection (*arrowheads*) containing a yolk sac (*arrow*) and no visible embryo. Follow-up scan 4 weeks later showed a normal-appearing 9.5-week pregnancy, including a fetus with cardiac activity.

the flickering motion of cardiac activity. The embryonic length, termed the *crown-rump length* (CRL), grows progressively to 5 mm at 6.5 weeks, 10 mm at 7.0 weeks, and approximately 80 mm by the end of the first trimester.[8,9]

For the first 1 to 2 weeks after it appears on ultrasound, the embryo is a featureless structure without identifiable body parts. By 8 weeks' gestation, the head can be seen separate from the body and the limb buds are visible. At that point, the relative sizes of the body parts differ considerably from those of the newborn: the head is bigger in relation to the body and the limbs are very short. From then until the end of the first trimester, the body proportions become progressively more similar to those of a neonate.

At 8 to 10 weeks, a round hypoechoic structure can be seen within the fetal head (**Fig. 4**), which represents the developing rhombencephalon (or hindbrain), an anatomic structure in the brain that comprises the medulla, pons, and cerebellum.[10]

At approximately 10 to 13 weeks, an echogenic structure is seen protruding from the anterior abdominal wall (**Fig. 5**).[11] This sonographic finding, termed *physiologic bowel herniation*, corresponds to a stage in the normal embryologic development of the gestational tract in which the intestine temporarily extends into the base of the umbilical cord.

Beginning at approximately 10 weeks' gestation, a hypoechoic space can be seen in the posterior fetal neck. Termed the *nuchal translucency*, it is located just internal to the posterior skin surface and measures approximately1 to 2 mm in diameter in the normal fetus (**Fig. 6**).[12]

By approximately 12 weeks' gestation, many internal fetal anatomic structures can be imaged, especially with transvaginal sonography.[13] Among the structures that can be seen are the choroid plexus (**Fig. 7**) and other brain components; face; cardiac chambers and outflow tracts; stomach; bladder; spine; and extremities.

DIAGNOSIS OF FIRST TRIMESTER ABNORMALITIES
Early Pregnancy Failure ("Miscarriage")

The sonographic appearance of a normal intrauterine pregnancy follows a predictable pattern during the 5- to 7-week period. Any substantial deviation from this pattern raises concern that the pregnancy has already, or will soon, fail ("miscarry"). An important aspect of ultrasound in early pregnancy is distinguishing between the abnormal sonographic findings that are definitive for pregnancy failure and those that are suspicious but not definitive, requiring follow-up testing to establish a definitive diagnosis.

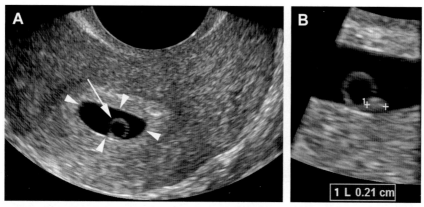

Fig. 3. A 6-week intrauterine pregnancy. (*A*) Sagittal transvaginal view of the uterus shows a gestational sac (*arrowheads*) containing a yolk sac (*arrow*). (*B*) Close-up view shows an embryo (*calipers*) measuring 0.21 cm (2.1 mm) in length. Cardiac activity was visible on real-time scanning.

The criteria for definitive pregnancy failure must be set to avoid false-positive diagnoses, because an erroneous diagnosis of miscarriage can have a disastrous consequence: intervention, such as uterine evacuation, that will disrupt a normal intrauterine pregnancy. The generally accepted criteria for diagnosing definite pregnancy failure have become more stringent since 2011 because of evidence that criteria previously in use could occasionally lead to false-positive diagnoses.[14] Current criteria for definitive pregnancy failure on transvaginal ultrasound are the following[15]:

- Nonvisualization of cardiac activity in an embryo whose CRL is at least 7 mm.

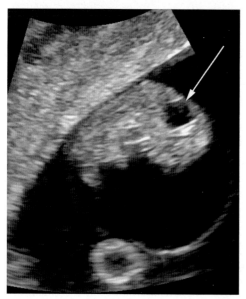

Fig. 4. Rhombencephalon. An intracranial cystic space (*arrow*) is present in a 8-week fetus, corresponding to the developing hindbrain (rhombencephalon).

- Nonvisualization of an embryo in a gestational sac whose mean sac diameter is at least 25 mm.
- Nonvisualization of an embryo at least 2 weeks after a scan that showed a gestational sac without a yolk sac.
- Nonvisualization of an embryo at least 11 days after a scan that showed a gestational sac with a yolk sac.

Failure to visualize cardiac activity in an embryo whose CRL is less than 7 mm or failure to visualize an embryo in a gestational sac whose mean sac diameter is 16 to 24 mm is suspicious but not definitive for pregnancy failure.

After miscarriage of a first trimester pregnancy, a woman may experience passage of blood and/or tissue. When this occurs, ultrasound is often used to determine whether all pregnancy-related tissue has passed or whether there are retained products of conception (RPOC). If ultrasound shows material within the uterus, the sonologist must attempt to determine whether it represents blood or RPOC. Published studies addressing RPOC after first trimester miscarriage (as opposed to those involving RPOC in postpartum women) have found that the presence of a discrete mass in the mid-uterus indicates a high likelihood of RPOC, especially if there is flow in the mass on color Doppler.[16,17] Absence of color flow, however, has a low negative predictive value, because RPOC may be avascular.[16] Another useful point is that expectant management of miscarriage is more likely to be successful when no flow is seen on color Doppler.[18]

Ectopic Pregnancy

Ectopic pregnancies, which most commonly are located in the isthmic or ampullary portions of

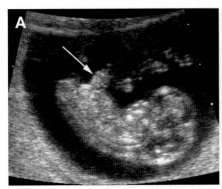
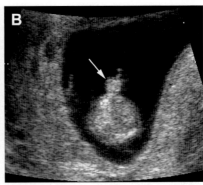

Fig. 5. Physiologic bowel herniation. Sagittal (*A*) and transverse (*B*) views of a 10-week fetus show a soft tissue mass (*arrows*) protruding from the anterior abdominal wall. The protruding mass measured 4 mm in maximum diameter, and was no longer present on a subsequent 18-week scan.

the fallopian tube, constitute approximately 2% of all pregnancies in the United States.[19] Ectopic pregnancy is clinically suspected when a woman with a positive pregnancy test presents with symptoms of bleeding and/or pain. In such a patient, ultrasound is the primary diagnostic test to establish the diagnosis. The sonogram should be performed both transabdominally and transvaginally; the former to assess for a mass or fluid high in the pelvis and the latter to obtain a detailed view of the uterus and adnexa.

If the sonogram shows an intrauterine pregnancy, ectopic pregnancy is highly unlikely (although examination of the adnexa for signs for ectopic pregnancy is still essential, as discussed later). In this case, a key role of ultrasound is to distinguish a normal intrauterine pregnancy from a failed intrauterine pregnancy.

In the absence of an intrauterine pregnancy, the likelihood of an ectopic pregnancy depends on the extraovarian adnexal findings.[20] If there is an adnexal mass containing an embryo with, or even without, cardiac activity, or a mass containing a yolk sac, then the diagnosis of ectopic pregnancy is established with certainty (100% positive predictive value). If an adnexal mass separate from the ovary is seen, then ectopic pregnancy is highly likely—more than 90% in the clinical context of a symptomatic woman with a positive pregnancy test and no sonographic evidence of an intrauterine pregnancy. Ectopic pregnancy should be suspected whether the extraovarian mass appears as a fluid collection surrounded by a thick echogenic wall (**Fig. 8**), an appearance termed a *tubal*

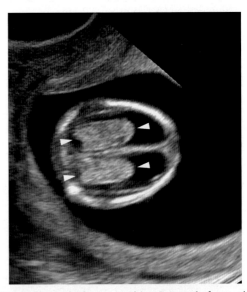

Fig. 7. Choroid plexus. In this 12.4-week fetus, the choroid plexus is seen as echogenic structures (*arrowheads*) in the lateral ventricles of the brain. At this stage of pregnancy, the choroid plexus constitutes a much larger fraction of the intracranial space than it does later in pregnancy and at birth.

Fig. 6. Nuchal translucency. Sagittal view of a 12.7-week fetus shows a hypoechoic space (*calipers*) measuring 0.19 cm (1.9 mm) in thickness in the posterior neck. The amnion (*arrow*) is seen behind the fetus.

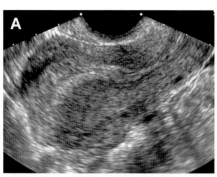
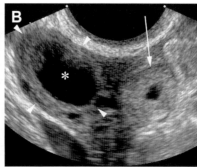

Fig. 8. Ectopic pregnancy appearing as a tubal ring. (*A*) Sagittal view of the uterus shows no evidence of an intrauterine pregnancy. (*B*) Transverse view of the right adnexa shows a structure (*arrow*) consisting of a hypoechoic central region and a thick echogenic rim, an appearance termed a *tubal ring*. The right ovary (*arrowheads*), containing a cyst (*asterisk*), is seen adjacent to the tubal ring.

ring,[20–22] or has a more amorphous appearance (**Fig. 9**). The likelihood of ectopic pregnancy is also high if a large amount of free pelvic fluid is present. If the sonogram shows neither an intrauterine pregnancy nor an extraovarian mass, a situation termed *pregnancy of unknown location*,[23] then follow-up testing with human chorionic gonadotropin (hCG) measurement and sonography is necessary to determine whether the woman has a normal intrauterine pregnancy, failed intrauterine pregnancy, or ectopic pregnancy.[24]

To apply these diagnostic criteria, an intraovarian mass must be distinguished from an extraovarian mass. The former is likely to be a corpus luteum, which is a normal feature of pregnancy and can have a highly variable sonographic appearance: simple cyst, thick-walled cyst, complex cyst, or homogeneous "solid" appearance.[25] When uncertainty exists about whether an adnexal mass is intraovarian or contiguous with the ovary, the distinction can often be made when observing what happens when pressure is applied to the adnexa by the transvaginal transducer or through palpation of the anterior abdominal wall. If the mass moves separately from the ovary, then it is extraovarian and the likely diagnosis is ectopic pregnancy. If the mass moves together with the ovary, it is likely to be a corpus luteum.[26]

It is important to avoid errors in diagnosing ectopic pregnancy that can occur from misapplying concepts that originated in the early days of sonography: hCG "discriminatory level" and "pseudogestational sac." The former refers to an hCG measurement above which a normal intrauterine pregnancy can be excluded if no intrauterine pregnancy is seen on ultrasound, a value first reported to be 6500 mIU/mL,[27] and more recently to be 1000 to 2000 mIU/mL.[3,28] It is now evident, however, that nonvisualization of an intrauterine gestational sac when the hCG measurement is more than 2000, or even more than 3000 mIU/mL, does not rule out a normal intrauterine pregnancy,[29] and that treatment should not be initiated based on a single hCG measurement in a hemodynamically stable woman with a pregnancy of uncertain location.[15]

The concept of the pseudogestational sac arose more than 30 years ago, before the use of transvaginal ultrasound. At that time, in some cases it was not possible to distinguish between 2 types of intrauterine fluid collection in a woman with a positive pregnancy test: (1) fluid within an intrauterine

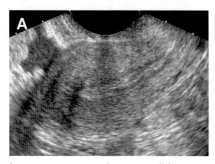
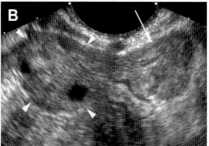

Fig. 9. Ectopic pregnancy appearing as a solid extraovarian mass. (*A*) Sagittal view of the uterus shows no evidence of an intrauterine pregnancy. (*B*) Transverse view of the left adnexa shows a solid mass (*arrow*) adjacent to the left ovary (*arrowheads*).

gestational sac; and (2) intrauterine blood or secretions in a woman with ectopic pregnancy. With modern equipment, these fluid collections are clearly distinguishable in almost all cases: intrauterine gestational sacs are round or oval in shape, whereas intrauterine fluid in women with ectopic pregnancies are generally irregular shaped with pointed edges and/or filled with debris.[30]

Although most ectopic pregnancies are implanted in the isthmic or ampullary portions of the fallopian tube, pregnancies can implant in other abnormal sites. An interstitial (or cornual) ectopic pregnancy appears on ultrasound as a gestational sac that is located in a very superolateral location (within the isthmic portion of the tube as it courses through the myometrium to the endometrial cavity), with little or no hypoechoic myometrium surrounding part of it.[31] A cervical ectopic pregnancy appears as a well-formed gestational sac located in the cervix, although it must be distinguished from a miscarriage-in-progress, which typically is seen as a flattened, irregular sac. Cesarean scar implantation, another abnormally located pregnancy that is not technically an ectopic pregnancy, appears as a gestational sac located low in the uterus, just above the cervix, extending anteriorly to (or close to) the serosal surface of the uterus.[32] For each of these entities, care must be taken to avoid false-positive and false-negative diagnoses. When the diagnosis is in doubt, 3-dimensional sonography with multiplanar reconstruction can be helpful in some cases.[33] When the location of the pregnancy remains uncertain and the patient is hemodynamically stable, follow-up scanning may be necessary to establish the diagnosis.

Thickened Nuchal Translucency

The relationship between thickening of the first trimester nuchal translucency and aneuploidy has been recognized for more than 20 years. In a 1992 study evaluating 51 fetuses with a nuchal translucency measuring 3 mm or greater at 10 to 14 weeks' gestation, 18 (35%) had chromosomal abnormalities, most often trisomy 21.[12] The rate of aneuploidy when the nuchal translucency was 2 mm or less was only 1%.

Since that time, the use of nuchal translucency as a screening tool for aneuploidy has been studied extensively. Instead of using a single cutoff value of 3 mm at 10 to 14 weeks, it became clear that the 95th percentile for nuchal translucency increases over this gestational age range.[34] Furthermore, instead of using the nuchal translucency alone to screen for aneuploidy, screening has been found to be more accurate using the nuchal translucency in conjunction with maternal serum

tests: pregnancy-associated plasma protein A (PAPP-A) and hCG. The combination of these 3 measurements detects 87% of cases of trisomy 21 at 11 weeks, 85% at 12 weeks, and 82% at 13 weeks, at a 5% false-positive rate.[35]

Because the nuchal translucency is a very small structure, even minor errors can have substantial effects on false-positive and false-negative diagnoses, which in turn can lead to unnecessary invasive tests (chorionic villous sampling or amniocentesis) or missed diagnoses of aneuploidy. In view of this, careful technique and ongoing quality assessment are important.[36] Nuchal translucency certification is offered by several groups to document compliance with training and quality assessment.

A fetus with thickening of the nuchal translucency is also at elevated risk for abnormalities other than aneuploidy (**Fig. 10**). Even if the chromosomes are normal, a fetus with a thickened nuchal translucency at 10 to 14 weeks is at increased risk of intrauterine demise and structural abnormalities, especially cardiac anomalies.[37] In a large study of chromosomally normal fetuses, the prevalence of cardiac anomalies increased progressively with increasing nuchal translucency, from 4.9 per 1000 when the nuchal translucency was below the median for gestational age, to 126.7 per 1000 when the nuchal translucency measured 5.5 mm or greater.[38]

Fetal Structural Anomalies

During the 1980s, when transabdominal sonography was the predominant ultrasound technique, published reports of first trimester diagnosis of

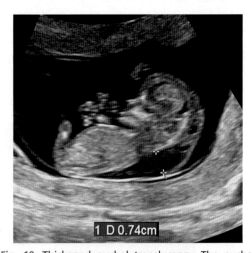

Fig. 10. Thickened nuchal translucency. The nuchal translucency (*calipers*) in this 12-week fetus measures 0.74 cm (7.4 mm) in thickness. On a follow-up scan at 19 weeks, a major cardiac anomaly—tetralogy of Fallot—was diagnosed. The karyotype was normal.

anomalies were limited. They mainly involved external or body wall abnormalities, such as omphalocele,[39] cystic hygroma,[40,41] and anencephaly.[42] Distinction of omphalocele from physiologic bowel herniation can be suggested based on the size of the herniated mass protruding from the anterior abdominal wall.[11] If the maximum diameter of the mass is more than 7 mm at 10 to 12 weeks, omphalocele should be suspected and confirmatory follow-up scan should be performed in the second trimester. If the measurement is less than or equal to 7 mm, the mass almost certainly represents physiologic bowel herniation and no follow-up is needed.

The introduction of transvaginal sonography markedly improved the ability of ultrasound to visualize fetal anatomy in the late first trimester.[43] By the early 1990s, studies confirmed that the 4-chamber view of the fetal heart can be visualized in most 12- to 14-week fetuses[44] and that cardiac anomalies can be diagnosed.[45] Other fetal structures, including the brain, spine, face, and kidneys, can also be imaged in many fetuses.[46]

Since 2000, studies from numerous centers around the world have confirmed and expanded on these earlier investigations. A fairly extensive fetal anatomic survey can be performed in most 12- to 14-week fetuses using transvaginal sonography.[13,47] In experienced hands, diagnostic views of the 4 cardiac chambers and the great vessel outflow tracts can be obtained in two-thirds of 13-week fetuses.[48] Moreover, in some reports, half or more of major structural anomalies are diagnosable in the first trimester.[49,50] These encompass a broad variety of anomalies, including ones involving the central nervous system, face, heart, ventral wall, kidneys, and skeletal system.

Despite what can be seen and diagnosed in the first trimester, no consensus exists in the United States in 2014 about whether detailed fetal anatomic assessment should be a routine component of late first trimester sonograms. An argument in favor of doing so is that, if a woman is having a scan at that point in her pregnancy for any reason (eg, to measure the nuchal translucency), important information can be gained in little added time by doing a structural survey.[51] An argument against making an anatomic survey a routine part of late first trimester scans, at least for now, is that many ultrasound practitioners do not have the training or experience to do so.[52]

SONOGRAPHIC ASSESSMENT OF GESTATIONAL AGE

A basic rule of sonographic assessment of gestational age is that the earlier in pregnancy a scan is done, the more accurate the age assignment. It follows that gestational age should be assigned at the initial scan in a woman's pregnancy and then not changed at subsequent scans. More specifically, the gestational age at any scan after the first should be assigned as the age from the initial scan plus the intervening time interval. For example, if the best estimate of gestational age is 7.0 weeks at the time of a woman's first scan in her pregnancy, and she then has another scan 28 days later, then the best estimate of gestational age at the time of the latter scan is 11.0 weeks regardless of the findings on that scan.

When the initial sonogram is performed before visualization of an embryo (ie, before 6 weeks' gestation), gestational age can be assigned either via the mean sac diameter or based on the contents of the gestational sac. Age can be predicted via the mean sac diameter using a table that lists the average value of that measurement at each gestational age.[7] An alternative approach is to assign a gestational age of 5.0 weeks if the sonogram shows a gestational sac with no visible yolk sac or embryo, and a gestational age of 5.5 weeks if the gestational sac contains a yolk sac but no embryo.[53]

Once the embryo of the fetus is visible, the CRL is used to assign gestational age. Several tables and formulas have been published to determine gestational age from CRL.[8,9,54] One of the earliest publications appeared in 1975.[8] Despite the major advances in ultrasound technology since that time, assessment of numerous CRL tables using the gold standard of pregnancies with highly accurate dating based on in vitro fertilization[55] shows that the difference between the various tables is generally no more than 3 days.

Overall, the accuracy of sonographic dating in the first trimester is approximately 5 days (95% confidence range).[56]

SUMMARY

Ultrasound plays a major role in the assessment of first trimester pregnancies. In normal pregnancies, first trimester sonography can assist in pregnancy management by accurately dating the pregnancy. Ultrasound is critical to the diagnosis of several abnormalities, including miscarriage and ectopic pregnancy. It also contributes to the identification of aneuploidy and, increasingly, to diagnosis of structural anomalies.

Just as important as correctly diagnosing abnormal pregnancies is avoiding mistakes that can lead to inadvertent harm to normal pregnancies. The most common error in early pregnancy is mistakenly diagnosing, or strongly suggesting, ectopic pregnancy when the pregnancy is in fact intrauterine. This mistake can generally be avoided by recognizing the following 2 points: (1) in a woman with a positive hCG, any round or oval fluid collection is the mid-uterus should be interpreted as a gestational sac, not a pseudogestational sac; and (2) nonvisualization of an intrauterine gestational sac when the hCG is greater than a "discriminatory level" does not rule out a normal intrauterine pregnancy, and therefore treatment should not be initiated based on a single hCG measurement in a hemodynamically stable woman with a pregnancy of uncertain location.

REFERENCES

1. Goldberg BB, Isard HJ, Gershon-Cohen J, et al. Ultrasonic fetal cephalometry. Radiology 1966;87: 328–32.
2. Benson CB, Doubilet PM. The history of imaging in obstetrics. Radiology 2014, in press.
3. Bree RL, Edwards M, Bohm-Velez M, et al. Transvaginal sonography in the evaluation of early pregnancy: correlation with hCG level. Am J Roentgenol 1989;153:75–9.
4. Bradley WG, Fiske CE, Filly RA. The double sac sign of early pregnancy: use in exclusion of ectopic pregnancy. Radiology 1982;143:223–6.
5. Yeh H, Goodman JD, Carr L, et al. Intradecidual sign: a US criterion of early intrauterine pregnancy. Radiology 1986;161:463–7.
6. Doubilet PM, Benson CB. Double sac sign and intradecidual sign in early pregnancy: interobserver reliability and frequency of occurrence. J Ultrasound Med 2013;32:1207–14.
7. Daya S, Woods S, Ward S, et al. Early pregnancy assessment with transvaginal ultrasound scanning. Can Med Assoc J 1991;144:441–6.
8. Robinson HP, Fleming JE. A critical evaluation of sonar "crown–rump length" measurements. Br J Obstet Gynaecol 1975;82:702–10.
9. Hadlock FP, Shah YP, Kanon DJ, et al. Fetal crown–rump length: reevaluation of relation to menstrual age (5–18 weeks) with high-resolution real-time US. Radiology 1992;182:501–5.
10. Cyr DR, Mack LA, Nyberg DA, et al. Fetal rhombencephalon: normal US findings. Radiology 1988; 166:691–2.
11. Bowerman RA. Sonography of fetal midgut herniation: normal size criteria and correlation with crown-rump length. J Ultrasound Med 1993;12:251–4.
12. Nicolaides KH, Azar G, Byrne D, et al. Fetal nuchal translucency: ultrasound screening for chromosomal defects in first trimester of pregnancy. BMJ 1992;304:867–9.
13. Ebrashy A, El Kateb A, Momtaz M, et al. 13-14 week fetal anatomy scan: a 5-year prospective study. Ultrasound Obstet Gynecol 2010;35:292–6.
14. Abdallah Y, Daemen A, Kirk E, et al. Limitations of current definitions of miscarriage using mean gestational sac diameter and crown–rump length measurements: a multicenter observational study. Ultrasound Obstet Gynecol 2011;38:497–502.
15. Doubilet PM, Benson CB, Bourne T, et al. Early first trimester diagnostic criteria for nonviable pregnancy. N Engl J Med 2013;369:1443–51.
16. Kamaya A, Petrovitch I, Chen B, et al. Retained products of conception: spectrum of color Doppler findings. J Ultrasound Med 2009;28:1031–41.
17. Atri M, Rao A, Boylan C, et al. Best predictors of grayscale ultrasound combined with color Doppler in the diagnosis of retained products of conception. J Clin Ultrasound 2011;39:122–7.
18. Casikar I, Lu C, Oates J, et al. The use of power Doppler colour scoring to predict successful expectant management in women with an incomplete miscarriage. Humanit Rep 2011;27:669–75.
19. Centers for Disease Control and Prevention (CDC). Ectopic pregnancy—United States 1990-1992. MMWR Morb Mortal Wkly Rep 1995;44:46–8.
20. Brown DL, Doubilet PM. Transvaginal sonography for diagnosing ectopic pregnancy: positivity criteria and performance characteristics. J Ultrasound Med 1994;13:259–66.
21. Fleischer AC, Pennell RG, McKee MS, et al. Ectopic pregnancy: features at transvaginal sonography. Radiology 1990;174:375–8.
22. Frates MC, Visweswaran A, Laing FC. Comparison of tubal ring and corpus luteum echogenicities: a useful differentiating characteristic. J Ultrasound Med 2001;20:27–31.
23. Barnhart K, van Mello NM, Bourne T, et al. Pregnancy of unknown location: a consensus statement of nomenclature, definitions, and outcome. Fertil Steril 2011;95:857–66.
24. Barnhart KT. Ectopic pregnancy. N Engl J Med 2009;361:379–87.
25. Durfee SM, Frates MC. Sonographic spectrum of the corpus luteum in early pregnancy: gray-scale, color, and pulsed Doppler appearance. J Clin Ultrasound 1999;2:55–9.
26. Blaivas M, Lyon M. Reliability of adnexal mas mobility in distinguishing possible ectopic pregnancy from corpus luteum cysts. J Ultrasound Med 2005;24:599–603.
27. Kadar N, DeVore G, Romero R. Discriminatory hCG zone: its use in the sonographic evaluation for ectopic pregnancy. Obstet Gynecol 1981;58: 156–61.
28. Bateman BG, Nunley WC, Kolp LA, et al. Vaginal sonography findings and hCG dynamics of early intrauterine and tubal pregnancies. Obstet Gynecol 1990;75:421–7.
29. Doubilet PM, Benson CB. Further evidence against the reliability of the human chorionic gonadotropin

discriminatory level. J Ultrasound Med 2011;30: 1637–42.

30. Benson CB, Doubilet PM, Peters HE, et al. Intrauterine fluid with ectopic pregnancy: a reappraisal. J Ultrasound Med 2013;32:389–93.

31. Timor-Tritsch IE, Monteagudo A, Matera C, et al. Sonographic evolution of cornual pregnancies treated without surgery. Obstet Gynecol 1992;79: 1044–9.

32. Timor-Tritsch IE, Monteagudo A, Santos R, et al. The diagnosis, treatment, and follow-up of cesarean scar pregnancy. Am J Obstet Gynecol 2012; 207:44.e1–13.

33. Izquierdo LA, Nicholas C. Three-dimensional transvaginal sonography of interstitial pregnancy. J Clin Ultrasound 2003;31:484–7.

34. Snijders RJ, Noble P, Sebire N, et al. UK multicentre project on assessment of risk of trisomy 21 by maternal age and fetal nuchal-translucency thickness at 10-14 weeks of gestation. Lancet 1998;352: 343–6.

35. Malone FD, Canick JA, Ball RH, et al. First-trimester or second-trimester screening, or both, for Down's syndrome. N Engl J Med 2005;353:2001–11.

36. D'Alton ME, Cleary-Goldman J, Lambert-Messerlian G, et al. Maintaining quality assurance for sonographic nuchal translucency measurement: lessons from the FASTER trial. Ultrasound Obstet Gynecol 2009;33:142–6.

37. Souka AP, Krampl E, Bakalis S, et al. Outcome of pregnancy in chromosomally normal fetuses with increased nuchal translucency in the first trimester. Ultrasound Obstet Gynecol 2001;18:9–17.

38. Atzei A, Gajewska K, Huggon IC, et al. Relationship between nuchal translucency thickness and prevalence of major cardiac defects in fetuses with normal karyotype. Ultrasound Obstet Gynecol 2005;26:154–7.

39. Brown DL, Emerson DS, Shulman LP, et al. Sonographic diagnosis of omphalocele during 10th week of gestation. Am J Roentgenol 1989;153:825–6.

40. Phillips HE, McGahan JP. Intrauterine fetal cystic hygromas: sonographic detection. Am J Roentgenol 1981;136:799–802.

41. Chervanek FA, Isaacson G, Tortora M. A sonographic study of fetal cystic hygromas. J Clin Ultrasound 1985;13:311–5.

42. Johnson A, Losure TA, Weiner S. Early diagnosis of fetal anencephaly. J Clin Ultrasound 1985;13:503–5.

43. Achiron R, Tadmor O. Screening for fetal anomalies during the first trimester of pregnancy: transvaginal versus transabdominal sonography. Ultrasound Obstet Gynecol 1991;1:186–91.

44. Johnson P, Sharland G, Maxwell D, et al. The role of transvaginal sonography in the early detection of congenital heart disease. Ultrasound Obstet Gynecol 1992;2:248–51.

45. Gembruch U, Knopfle G, Bald R, et al. Early diagnosis of fetal congenital heart disease by transvaginal echocardiography. Ultrasound Obstet Gynecol 1993;3:310–7.

46. Whitlow BJ, Economides DL. The optimal gestational age to examine fetal anatomy and measure nuchal translucency in the first trimester. Ultrasound Obstet Gynecol 1998;11:258–61.

47. Timor-Trirsch IE, Bashiri A, Monteagudo A, et al. Qualified and trained sonographers in the US can perform early fetal anatomy scans between 11 and 14 weeks. Am J Obstet Gynecol 2004; 191:1247–52.

48. Vimpelli T, Huhtala H, Acharya G. Fetal echocardiography during routine first trimester screening: a feasibility study in an unselected population. Prenat Diagn 2006;26:475–82.

49. Den Hollander NS, Wessels MW, Niermeijer MF, et al. Early fetal anomaly scanning in a population at increased risk of abnormalities. Ultrasound Obstet Gynecol 2002;19:570–4.

50. Grande M, Arigita M, Borobio V, et al. First-trimester detection of structural abnormalities and the role of aneuploidy markers. Ultrasound Obstet Gynecol 2012;39:157–63.

51. Platt LD. Should the first trimester ultrasound include anatomy survey? Semin Perinatol 2013; 37:310–22.

52. Reddy UM, Abuhamad AZ, Levine D, et al. Fetal imaging: executive summary of a joint Eunice Kennedy Shriver National Institute of Child Health and Human Development, Society for Maternal-Fetal Medicine, American Institute of Ultrasound in Medicine, American College of Obstetricians and Gynecologists, American College of Radiology, Society for Pediatric Radiology, and Society of Radiologists in Ultrasound Fetal Imaging Workshop. Obstet Gynecol 2014;123:1070–82.

53. Benson CB, Doubilet PM. Fetal measurements, normal and abnormal fetal growth. In: Rumack CM, Wilson SR, Charbonneau JW, et al, editors. Diagnostic ultrasound. 4th Edition. Philadelphia: Mosby Elsevier Publishers; 2011. p. 1455–71.

54. Tunon K, Eik-Ness SH, Grottum P, et al. Gestational age in pregnancies conceived after in vitro fertilization: a comparison between age assessed from oocyte retrieval, crown-rump length and biparietal diameter. Ultrasound Obstet Gynecol 2000;15:41–6.

55. Sladkevicius P, Saltvedt S, Almstrom H, et al. Ultrasound dating at 12–14 weeks of gestation: a prospective cross-validation of established dating formulae in in-vitro fertilized pregnancies. Ultrasound Obstet Gynecol 2005;26:504–11.

56. Doubilet PM. Should a first trimester dating scan be routine for all pregnancies? Semin Perinatol 2013; 37:307–9.

Practical Applications of 3D Sonography in Gynecologic Imaging

Rochelle F. Andreotti, MD[a,b,*], Arthur C. Fleischer, MD[a,b]

KEYWORDS

- 3D pelvic sonography • Uterine shape anomalies • IUD malposition

KEY POINTS

- Three-dimensional (3D) sonography of the pelvis provides clinically useful information, especially if any abnormalities associated with the endometrium are suspected.
- 3D sonography is the modality of choice in assessment of uterine congenital anomalies.
- The coronal view of the uterus locates malpositioned intrauterine devices (IUDs) by visualizing the entire IUD and is now considered to be the optimal method of evaluating IUDs.
- The 3D technique can often be used to identify a hydrosalpinx when multiple adjacent cystic structures are demonstrated.

INTRODUCTION

Three-dimensional (3D) sonography has become a popular imaging technique in gynecology answering important questions that could not be previously addressed with traditional 2D imaging due to the constraints of the transvaginal as well as the transabdominal probe. The technique provides rapid acquisition of a volume of data that can be stored, reviewed, and manipulated retrospectively producing images in any desired plane potentially reducing operator dependency. However, reconstructions may be inadequate when accessibility to optimal scan planes for image acquisition is limited.

The most useful clinical 3D applications have evolved from the ability to reconstruct and obtain the coronal plane of the uterus. Applications that have now become a routine part of the standard pelvic imaging protocol in many institutions include the evaluation of uterine shape anomalies and intrauterine device (IUD) location. Problems that arise in the evaluation of masses and adhesions associated with the endometrial cavity may also be solved using this technique. This article concentrates on a variety of indications primarily associated with the uterus and endometrial cavity that have been shown to enhance the diagnostic ability of ultrasound examination of the female pelvis.

EVIDENCE FOR ROUTINE USE OF THE CORONAL PLANE

Reports have suggested that 3D imaging with reconstructions in the coronal plane is better able to characterize some uterine abnormalities and may occasionally detect unsuspected abnormalities. It has also been observed that when 2D imaging is normal, 3D is less likely to be

The authors have nothing to disclose.
[a] Department of Radiology and Radiological Sciences, Vanderbilt University Medical Center, 1161 21st Avenue South, CCC-1118 MCN, Nashville, TN 37232-2675, USA; [b] Department of Obstetrics and Gynecology, Vanderbilt University Medical Center, 1161 21st Avenue South, CCC-1118 MCN, Nashville, TN 37232-2675, USA
* Corresponding author. Department of Radiology and Radiological Sciences, Vanderbilt University Medical Center, 1161 21st Avenue South, CCC-1118 MCN, Nashville, TN 37232-2675.
E-mail address: rochelle.f.andreotti@vanderbilt.edu

Radiol Clin N Am 52 (2014) 1201–1213
http://dx.doi.org/10.1016/j.rcl.2014.07.001

contributory.[1,2] The coronal plane has additionally been found to be more useful when the endometrial thickness is greater than 5 mm because this will provide contrast with the myometrium that is usually more hypoechoic.[2]

Andreotti and colleagues[1] looked at 90 consecutive patients using transvaginal sonography with coronal reconstructions of the uterus. Additional findings using 3D reconstructions in the coronal plane were found in 26 (53%) of 49 patients with abnormalities noted on 2D imaging but only in 2 (5%) of 51 patients with normal 2D imaging. In one of these cases, an IUD location was confirmed, and in the other case, an arcuate uterus was identified. Benacerraf and colleagues[2] demonstrated added value of 3D coronal views compared to traditional 2D imaging in 16 (24%) of 66 consecutive pelvic sonograms. Additional information was identified on the coronal view in 3 (12%) of 25 patients with normal findings on 2D sonography. The 3 patients for whom the coronal view of the uterus was helpful all had arcuate uteri.

The arcuate uterus was a common additional finding in the study by Andreotti and colleagues[1] and the most common additional finding in the report by Benacerraf and colleagues.[2] Because an arcuate uterus is widely considered a variation of normal, whether this adds anything clinically significant remains debatable. However, a report by Woelfer and colleagues[3] has shown that women with an arcuate uterus had a significantly greater risk of second-trimester loss and preterm labor than those with a normal uterine configuration. The diagnosis of a unicornuate uterus, more often associated with pregnancy loss, is also an abnormality that is easily seen with 3D imaging when 2D sonography is interpreted as normal. This information may then be important in the management of the patient with infertility and would support the use of the additional view following even normal 2D imaging in women being evaluated for infertility.

TECHNICAL CONSIDERATIONS

Acquisition of the uterine volume can be obtained via a transabdominal or transvaginal approach. However, the transvaginal approach is the more useful due to the higher frequency of the probe and its closer proximity to the organ being scanned that enhance the resolution of the image. A manual or automated sweep is performed to obtain a volume through the acquisition plane. The images are electronically stored. Three-dimensional images are then processed and displayed on the monitor as a multiplanar format or display showing 3 orthogonal planes with or without a surface rendered image (Fig. 1). The surface rendered image is a thicker slice through volume with depth perception improved by different

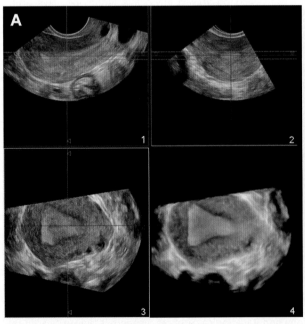
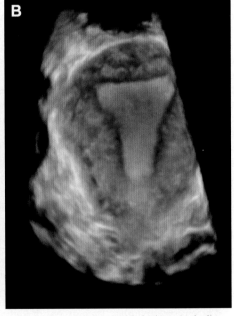

Fig. 1. (A) Multiplanar display following 3D sweep through a normal uterus in the sagittal plane including a surface rendered image. Quadrants demonstrating sagittal plane (1), transverse plane (2), coronal plane (3), and coronal surface rendered image (4). (B) Enlarged surface rendered image of the uterus in the coronal plane that has been rotated so that the fundus is seen as it is routinely viewed, at the top of the image.

computer generated shading and lighting effects. One is then able to slice or rotate using a marker dot or line to select the scan plane from the volume. Abuhamad and colleagues[4] reported a method to obtain the midcoronal view of the uterus that was named the "Z Technique" (Box 1).

Although reconstructed images can give helpful information, the quality of the 3D image can never be as high as the initial 2D image because, at this time, this is usually a mechanical sweep with a single elevation focus so that resolution outside of the focal zone is degraded. As a result, one needs a good 2D image to obtain a diagnostic 3D image.

Like 2D imaging, obesity, prior surgery, and shadowing artifact will degrade the image. Artifacts such as shadowing, enhancement, or volume averaging may also be more confusing or compounded with 3D reconstructions. Shadowing or enhancement can be easily recognized on 2D imaging because the source of the artifact is readily apparent. The source of the enhancement or shadowing may not be seen on the reconstructed plane making the artifact much more difficult to recognize so that it may be mistaken for pathology. With this in mind, it is very important to review the image in the acquisition plane to recognize these artifacts.

Additionally, there are other limitations of 3D sonography that should be considered. There is a substantial learning curve involved although the reconstruction of the coronal plane is one of the easier uses of gynecologic and obstetric 3D imaging. Also, no form of standardization of acquisition, display, and manipulation of the 3D volume presently exists although the "Z Technique" of Abuhamad and colleagues[4] has been well received and is widely used.

CLINICAL APPLICATIONS OF THE CORONAL PLANE OF THE UTERUS
Uterine Shape Anomalies

Uterine anomalies are associated with an increased risk of infertility and obstetric complications. The prevalence of congenital uterine anomalies is as high as 17% in women with recurrent miscarriage compared with 6% in the general population.[5] The correct diagnosis helps to minimize complications and manage infertility. The need for intervention and the type of intervention is determined by the proper classification of the anomaly. Although there are other classification systems, The American Fertility Society's 1988 classification has been widely used as the main classification system for more than 2 decades.[6] This classification is not only based on embryologic factors but also includes clinical factors, prognosis, and treatment. Categories are grouped on the basis of Mullerian development and can only be adequately demonstrated in the coronal plane (Fig. 2).

Traditionally, patients have been initially screened for suspected congenital uterine shape abnormalities by means of hysterosalpingography (HSG), a technique that images only the uterine cavity. If an anomaly was suspected, patients would then proceed to hysteroscopy, which is considered the reference standard for the assessment of the uterine cavity. The assessment of the external contour of the uterus would then require laparoscopy.

The development of MR imaging has recently also played a large role in the evaluation of suspected anomalies. Like hysteroscopy and laparoscopy, MR imaging evaluates both the uterine cavity and the uterine fundus. MR imaging, although costly, is less expensive than surgery

---

Box 1
Reconstruction of the uterine coronal plane

- A manual or automated sweep is performed to obtain a volume through the acquisition plane, the sagittal plane of the uterus.

- A multiplanar format or display will appear on the screen that includes 3 orthogonal planes with or without a surface rendered image.

- Using a marker dot or line, a plane corresponding to the length of the endometrial cavity is selected from the volume in the sagittal plane, with the marker dot placement at the level of the midcavity (see Fig. 1, quadrant 1).

- The marker dot or line is then aligned with the width of the endometrial cavity in the transverse plane, with the marker dot placement at the level of the midcavity (see Fig. 1, quadrant 2).

- The midcoronal plane of the uterus will be displayed in the "Z" plane. Using the marker dot or line, one may slice or rotate through the volume to obtain the desired plane (see Fig. 1, quadrant 3).

- A surface rendered image consisting of a thicker slice, with depth perception improved by different computer generated shading and lighting effects, may be obtained (see Fig. 1, quadrant 4).

Data from Abuhamad AZ. The Z technique: an easy approach to the display of the midcoronal plane of the uterus in volume sonography. J Ultrasound Med 2006;25:607–12.

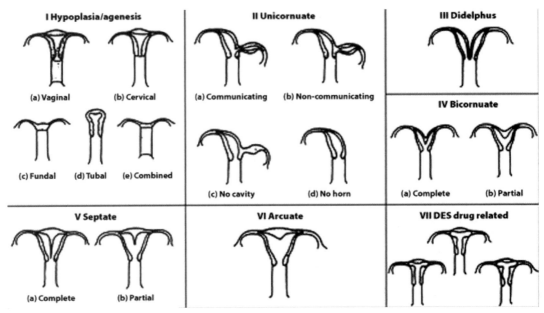

Fig. 2. Classification of uterine malformations according to the American Fertility Society demonstrating how uterine shape anomalies are best viewed in the coronal plane. (*Data from* The American Fertility Society classifications of adnexal adhesions, distal tubal obstruction, tubal occlusion secondary to tubal ligation, tubal pregnancies, mullerian anomalies and intrauterine adhesions. Fertil Steril 1988;49:944–55.)

and is noninvasive. In the diagnosis of congenital uterine anomalies on MR imaging, reported specificities and sensitivities range from 77% to 100% and 33% to 100%, respectively.[7–10]

Although MR imaging is a useful option in the diagnosis of Mullerian anomalies, ultrasound represents a valid alternative[11] due to its lower cost, time saving capability, and better tolerance by patients. In addition, a high degree of concordance between the 2 modalities has been reported. In fact, ultrasound is often now considered to be the initial imaging modality of choice in uterine anomaly assessment.[12]

3D ultrasound has been proved to be beneficial in the workup of infertility often associated with uterine shape anomalies.[13] The technique, like MR imaging, evaluates the fundal contour and cavity in the coronal plane. Most abnormalities will be in the spectrum of arcuate-septate or bicornuate-didelphys, and it is the coronal plane that best differentiate between these different anomalies. In a recent study of 214 patients with infertility and suspected Mullerian anomalies, the sensitivity and specificity of 3D sonography was 86.6% and 96.9%, respectively with an 88.2% accuracy rate.[14] One of the most useful applications in anomaly evaluation is to determine the cause of 2 endometrial cavities seen on 2D imaging (**Fig. 3**). The possible causes would include abnormalities in the spectrum of the septate uterus as well as those

in the spectrum of fusion anomalies. These anomalies can only be completely visualized in the coronal plane favoring the use of 3D reconstructions.

Septate anomalies are the result of the lack of resorption of the uterine septum after complete fusion of the Mullerian ducts. The abnormality may be partial or complete although, with the exception of the arcuate uterus, there is no available literature to support a difference in symptomatology based on the extent of the septum. A smooth fundal contour or minimal undulation of the fundal contour of less than 1 cm is identified (see **Fig. 3**). Management of infertility includes hysteroscopic metroplasty to resect the residual septum when there is history of pregnancy loss.

The mildest form of a septate uterus, the arcuate uterus, is commonly considered a normal variant (see **Fig. 3**). A minimal septum is demonstrated with a central point of indentation at an obtuse angle and a relatively smooth uterine fundus. Although there are no universally accepted criteria for the ultrasound diagnosis of congenital uterine anomalies, criteria such as measuring the vertical distance from a horizontal line drawn across the top of the uterine cavities in the coronal plane to the level where the 2 cavities join (ie, the deepest point of the septum) have been used to differentiate between the 2 shapes (**Fig. 4**). A measured distance of less than 1 cm is considered an arcuate configuration.[3,15]

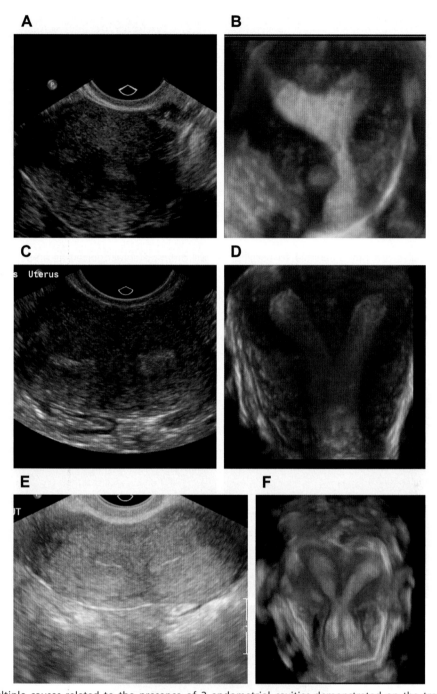

Fig. 3. Multiple causes related to the presence of 2 endometrial cavities demonstrated on the transverse 2D image. Transverse (*A*) and coronal (*B*) images of an arcuate uterus. Transverse (*C*) and coronal (*D*) images of a septate uterus. Transverse (*E*) and coronal (*F*) images of a uterus didelphys.

Fusion anomalies result from the absence of union of the 2 Mullerian ducts forming 2 separate uterine horns (see **Fig. 3**). With a complete duplication anomaly, the uterus didelphys, in addition to the 2 separate horns, 2 entire endometrial cavities and 2 cervices are formed. This may also be accompanied by 2 hemivaginas separated by a longitudinal or transverse septum. The bicornuate uterus is created as a result of incomplete fusion of the Mullerian ducts. This uterus consists of 2 uterine horns with 2 endometrial cavities that join above the internal os of the cervix.

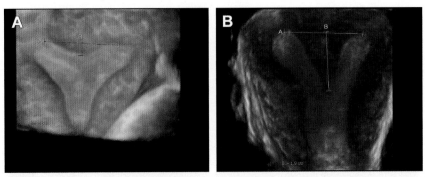

Fig. 4. Differentiation between an arcuate and bicornuate uterus determined by measuring the vertical distance from a horizontal line drawn across the top of the uterine cavities in the coronal plane to the level where the 2 cavities join. The arcuate (*A*) uterus has a vertical distance (line B) of 0.4 cm and the septate (*B*) uterus has a vertical distance of 1.9 cm (line B).

Fusion anomalies are not amenable to surgical management.

Although fusion and septate anomalies are usually at least recognized as uterine shape abnormalities on 2D ultrasound, there is another anomaly associated with increased risk of miscarriage and premature delivery, the unicornuate uterus, which will often go unrecognized as an abnormality unless it is visualized in the coronal plane (**Fig. 5**). This anomaly results from failure of development or incomplete development of 1 of the 2 Mullerian ducts and consists of only 1 uterine horn or a significant difference in size of 1 horn when compared with the other. This second horn is usually referred

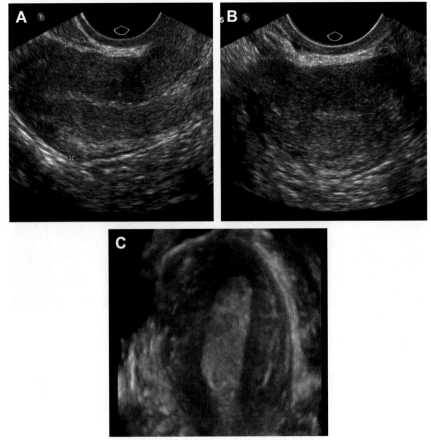

Fig. 5. The unicornuate uterus seen as normal on 2D imaging (*A, B*). The 3D coronal image demonstrates the single uterine horn (*C*).

to as a rudimentary horn on the opposite site. This horn may or may not communicate with the uterine cavity and is linked to the ipsilateral tube. The recognition of such an anomaly could help in the early diagnosis of the rare pregnancy that may implant within such a horn, resulting in a potentially fatal uterine rupture allowing for a timelier surgical resection of the horn.[16]

INTRAUTERINE DEVICES AND TUBAL OCCLUSION PROCEDURES

Two-dimensional transvaginal sonography can confirm the position of an IUD in the uterus and, when abnormally located, may show that part of the IUD is embedded in the myometrium but usually cannot demonstrate the entire IUD. In fact, IUDs that seem to be in satisfactory location in the endometrial cavity on 2D imaging may, in actuality, be embedded in the myometrium. Three-dimensional reconstructions in the coronal plan have been used successfully to improve visualization of the complete IUD including shaft and arms (**Fig. 6**). Imaging the entire IUD can be extremely important because embedded IUDs are a major cause of pelvic pain and abnormal bleeding (**Fig. 7**), although may surprisingly be asymptomatic. In a series of 167 patients presenting with IUDs evaluated in the coronal plane, Benacerraf and colleagues[17] reported that 28 of these patients had side arms embedded in the myometrium, a finding that was detected only in the coronal plane. Seventy five percent of these patients presented with pain or bleeding as opposed to 34.5% of patients with normal placement of the IUD.[17]

Using the coronal plane, it has also been demonstrated that the mean width of the uterine cavity of nulliparous women (27 mm) is narrower than that of a multiparous patient (32 mm) as well

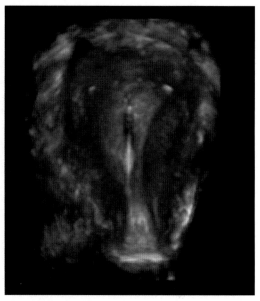

Fig. 6. 3D coronal image of the uterine cavity exhibiting the entire Mirena IUD in satisfactory position.

as narrower than the width of a standard IUD (32 mm) (**Fig. 8**).[18] It has also been reported that the mean uterine cavity width is smaller in patients with embedded IUDs[19]; this would suggest the importance of using the coronal plane to measure the width of the endometrial cavity in patients before placement of a standard device, especially in nulliparous patients.

Tubal occlusion procedures are now often performed in place of traditional tubal ligations in which a soft, flexible coil is placed into each fallopian tube. The device is routed through the vagina and subsequently through the cervix and endometrial cavity using a small scope. Coils are then positioned in the interstitial portion of the fallopian tubes. On occasion, the location of the device

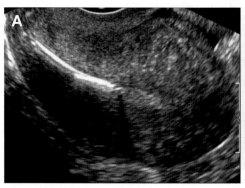
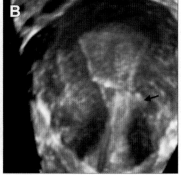

Fig. 7. Malpositioned IUD with the shaft demonstrated within the endometrial cavity on a sagittal 2D image (*A*) but showing the entire IUD lying obliquely with left arm embedded within the myometrium (*arrow*) on the coronal view (*B*).

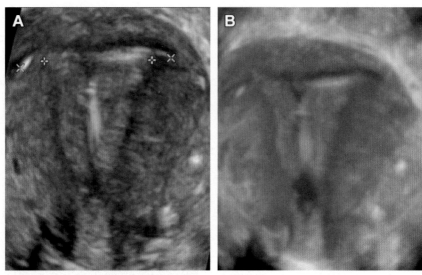

Fig. 8. An endometrial cavity that is too narrow for the width of the arms of the Mirena IUD is identified on 3D thin slice (*A*) and surface rendered (*B*) coronal images. Embedded portions of arms are shown between calipers (*A*).

may be in question. Because the interstitial portions of the fallopian tube are best visualized in the coronal plane, 3D reconstructions may be helpful to confirm the location of the coils (**Fig. 9**).

INTRACAVITARY ABNORMALITIES
Fibroids and Endometrial Polyps

The coronal plane is extremely valuable in the evaluation of the relationship of masses to the

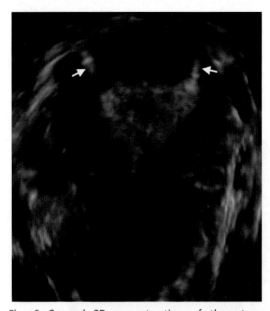

Fig. 9. Coronal 3D reconstruction of the uterus demonstrates coils placed for tubal occlusion in satisfactory location within the interstitial portions of bilateral fallopian tubes (*arrows*).

endometrial cavity. These masses will most commonly be leiomyomas and polyps. Most endometrial polyps are benign masses that cause symptoms of intermenstrual bleeding. They are typically seen as rounded, well circumscribed echogenic structures seen best within the endometrial cavity when there is a contrasting, more hypoechoic, proliferative endometrium. Although the diagnosis can be made by the presence of a vascular pedicle on 2D imaging, frequently, full delineation of the polyp as well as the location and number of polyps can be more accurately determined with a coronal view since nearly the entire endometrial cavity as well as both the cervix and cornua can be seen in the same plane (**Fig. 10**).[20] As with 2D sonography, Doppler can be used to demonstrate blood flow to the polyp on 3D reconstructed views adding benefit to the study.

Leiomyomas are the most common benign tumors of the uterus. Menorrhagia is a common symptom when a leiomyoma is submucosal. The coronal view most accurately demonstrates the exact position of a leiomyoma with respect to the endometrial cavity as well as the serosal surface of the uterus (**Fig. 11**).[21] This information is key in the evaluation of the submucosal extent of the leiomyoma within the cavity and can determine management options. Management options may also depend on the patient's symptoms as well as desire for future pregnancy. Patients wishing to preserve their fertility are best treated by myomectomy. Surgical options would include hysteroscopic myomectomy for those leiomyomas, independent of size, that are submucosal with at

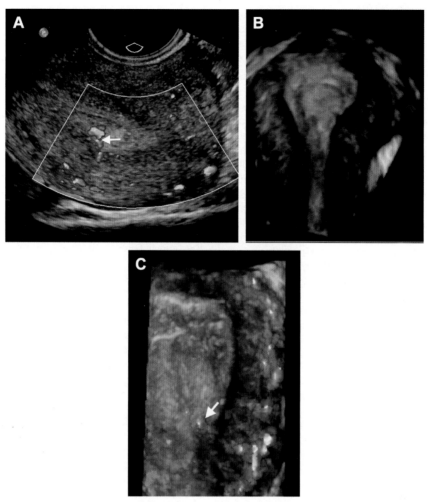

Fig. 10. An endometrial polyp is identified by a vascular pedicle (*arrow*) on a 2D sagittal image of the uterus (*A*) but is much better delineated as an isoechoic mass on the 3D coronal view (*B*). A color Doppler image in the coronal plane (*C*) shows a vascular pedicle (*arrow*).

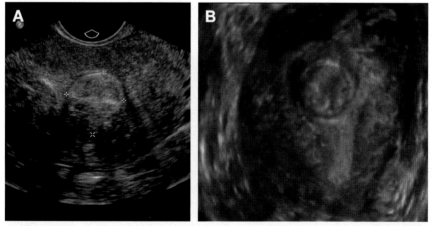

Fig. 11. Leiomyoma (calipers) that is at least partially surrounded by endometrium on a sagittal 2D image of the uterus (*A*). 3D coronal view (*B*) confirms a completely submucosal location because it is entirely surrounded by endometrium.

least 1 cm of intracavitary extension of the leio-myoma with myomectomy by laparotomy or lapa-roscopy reserved for intramural or subserosal leiomyomas or those with a minimal submucosal component.

Uterine Synechiae

The presence of uterine synechiae or adhesions within the endometrial cavity is usually well delin-eated on the coronal plane on 3D imaging and can often be missed on traditional 2D sagittal and transverse images. Adhesions may be sus-pected when focal narrowing or bands within the endometrial echo are seen on 2D imaging, and sonohysterography is often helpful in delineating these bands. However, the true compromise of the width and configuration of the cavity or the bands projecting across the cavity are best delineated on the coronal reconstructed image (**Fig. 12**).

In addition to location and extent of involvement of adhesions, the coronal plane can also illustrate complications of adhesions. A commonly demon-strated symptomatic complication of endometrial adhesions due to an endometrial ablation is the cornual hydrosalpinx (**Fig. 13**). After ablation, there is often an adherent endometrium with little or no functioning tissue within the main cavity but a small amount of residual tissue may still be present in the cornual regions. This tissue bleeds cyclically causing distension and pain if there is occlusion of the more distal fallopian tube, usually due to a prior tubal ligation. The location of this cornual fluid collection can only be well demonstrated on the coronal view.

THREE-DIMENSIONAL RECONSTRUCTIONS WITH SALINE-INSTILLED SONOHYSTEROGRAPHY

Saline-instilled sonohysterography (SIS) consists of instillation of sterile saline within the endometrial cavity through a catheter allowing for evalua-tion of associated endometrial and myometrial processes. The most common indication is abnormal vaginal bleeding although other indica-tions include suspected congenital anomalies, suspected uterine cavity synechiae, further evalu-ation of suspected abnormalities seen on trans-vaginal imaging, and inadequate imaging of the endometrium on transvaginal sonography. Most of these are also indications for 3D reconstructions in the coronal plane.

The question then is what advantages would 3D SIS have over 2D SIS? First, there is fast imaging acquisition of data that decreases the length of time that the patient is undergoing the discomfort of sonohysterography and potentially decreases the time it takes to perform the study. The data can then be manipulated retrospectively and required images reconstructed. Additionally, 3D reconstructions in the coronal plane can more accurately locate and delineate intracavitary ab-normalities with or without saline although saline may give additional information due to enhanced contrast (**Fig. 14**).[22,23]

THE CORONAL VIEW OF THE ADNEXA

Although there are not as many uses for the coro-nal reconstructed view in the adnexa as there are in the uterus, the ability to reconstruct multiple contiguous cystic areas within different planes into a hydrosalpinx in the coronal plane can be extremely valuable. Often, these adjacent adnexal cystic structures are immediately assumed to be ovarian or adnexal cysts and, unless the possibility of a hydrosalpinx is recognized, inappropriate management may be instituted. By placing the horizontal line representing the "Z" (coronal) plane through the cystic areas, a plane that elongates into a tubular structure may be found. Because there may not be a single plane within the volume

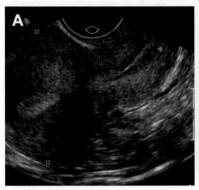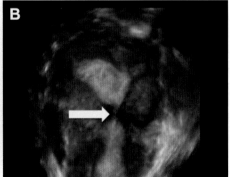

Fig. 12. Adhesions causing narrowing of the endometrial cavity are not appreciated on the 2D sagittal image (*A*) but narrowing of the cavity (*arrow*) is well seen on the 3D coronal view (*B*).

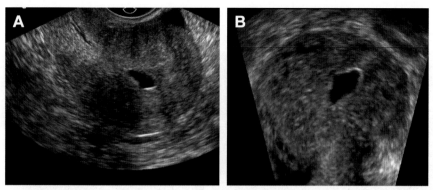

Fig. 13. A cornual hydrosalpinx is seen as fluid within the endometrial cavity on the 2D sagittal image (*A*) but more clearly and accurately located within the left uterine cornua on the 3D coronal image (*B*).

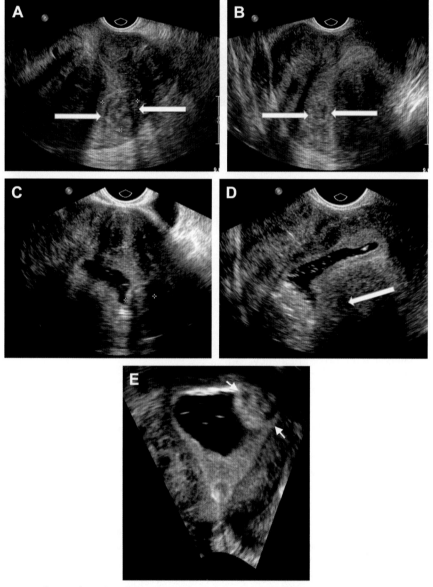

Fig. 14. Leiomyoma (*arrows*) causing distortion of the right cornual endometrium on transverse (*A*) and sagittal (*B*) 2D images. Following 2D SIS, transverse (*C*) and sagittal (*D*) images show a portion of the leiomyoma (calipers in *C* and *arrow* in *D*) surrounded by fluid, although the 3D coronal image (*E*) more accurately depicts the leiomyoma's location within the cornua of the endometrial cavity confirming a completely submucosal location (*arrows*).

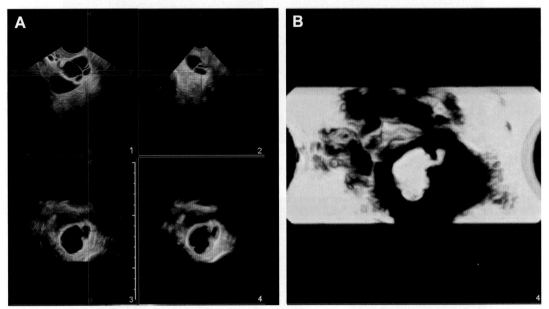

Fig. 15. Multiformat display (A) of the 3D coronal reconstruction of a hydrosalpinx with the acquisition plane (quadrant 1) demonstrating cystic structures and coronal thin slice and surface rendered images (quadrants 3 and 4) exhibiting the reconstructed hydrosalpinx. The inversion mode (B) establishes a cast of the tube confirming its shape.

that demonstrates the tubular configuration well, the surface rendered image with an inverse mode can be used to produce an echogenic cast of the cystic area displaying enough of the tube to be diagnostic (Fig. 15). Alternatively, all manipulations may continue to show relatively round structures more consistent with cysts.

The location of structures within the interstitial portion of the fallopian tube is also better visualized in the coronal plane of the uterus. This would be extremely important when differentiating between an interstitial ectopic pregnancy, an eccentric intrauterine pregnancy, and a pregnancy within a uterine horn of a didelphys or bicornuate uterus.

SUMMARY

Volume imaging in the pelvis has been well demonstrated as an extremely useful technique, largely based on its ability to reconstruct the coronal plane of the uterus that usually cannot be visualized using traditional 2D imaging due to the constraints of manipulation of the vaginal probe. Three-dimensional imaging of the uterus is now the modality of choice for congenital uterine anomaly assessment, surpassing MR imaging since it is faster, cheaper, and similar in accuracy. Three-dimensional imaging improves visualization of the entire IUD as well as other methods of tubal contraception and can be used with or

without SIS to better delineate and locate abnormalities associated with the endometrium. In the adnexa, another useful application includes differentiating a hydrosalpinx from ovarian or adnexal cysts.

REFERENCES

1. Andreotti RF, Fleischer AC, Mason LE Jr. Three-dimensional sonography of the endometrium and adjacent myometrium: preliminary observations. J Ultrasound Med 2006;25(10):1313–9.
2. Benacerraf BR, Shipp TD, Bromley B. Which patients benefit from a 3D reconstructed coronal view of the uterus added to standard routine 2D pelvic sonography? AJR Am J Roentgenol 2008;190(3): 626–9. http://dx.doi.org/10.2214/AJR.07.2632.
3. Woelfer B, Salim R, Banerjee S, et al. Reproductive outcomes in women with congenital uterine anomalies detected by three-dimensional ultrasound screening. Obstet Gynecol 2001;98(6):1099–103.
4. Abuhamad AZ, Singleton S, Zhao Y, et al. The Z technique: an easy approach to the display of the midcoronal plane of the uterus in volume sonography. J Ultrasound Med 2006;25:607–12.
5. Saravelos SH, Cocksedge KA, Li TC. Prevalence and diagnosis of congenital uterine anomalies in women with reproductive failure: a critical appraisal. Hum Reprod Update 2008;14(5):415–29.
6. The American Fertility Society classifications of adnexal adhesions, distal tubal obstruction, tubal

occlusion secondary to tubal ligation, tubal pregnancies, mullerian anomalies and intrauterine adhesions. Fertil Steril 1988;49:944–55.

7. Fedele L, Dorta M, Brioschi D, et al. Magnetic resonance evaluation of double uteri. Obstet Gynecol 1989;74:844–7.

8. Carrington BM, Hricak H, Nuruddin RN, et al. Mullerian duct anomalies: MR imaging evaluation. Radiology 1990;176:715–20.

9. Pellerito JS, McCarthy SM, Doyle MB, et al. Diagnosis of uterine anomalies: relative accuracy of MR imaging, endovaginal sonography and hysterosalpingography. Radiology 1992;183:795–800.

10. Fischetti SG, Politi G, Lomeo E, et al. Magnetic resonance in the evaluation of mullerian duct anomalies. Radiol Med 1995;89:105–11.

11. Bermejo C, Martínez Ten P, Cantarero R, et al. Three-dimensional ultrasound in the diagnosis of Müllerian duct anomalies and concordance with magnetic resonance imaging. Ultrasound Obstet Gynecol 2010;35:593–601.

12. Bocca SM, Abuhamad AZ. Use of 3-dimensional sonography to assess uterine anomalies. J Ultrasound Med 2013;32(1):1–6.

13. Bocca SM, Oehninger S, Stadtmauer L, et al. A study of the cost, accuracy, and benefits of 3-dimensional sonography compared with hysterosalpingography in women with uterine abnormalities. J Ultrasound Med 2012;31(1):81–5.

14. Moini A, Mohammadi S, Hosseini R, et al. Accuracy of 3-dimensional sonography for diagnosis and classification of congenital uterine anomalies. J Ultrasound Med 2013;32(6):923–7.

15. Letterie GS. Structural abnormalities and reproductive failure: effective techniques of diagnosis and management. New York: Blackwell Science; 1998.

16. Dhar H. Rupture of non-communicating rudimentary uterine horn pregnancy. J Coll Physicians Surg Pak 2008;18(1):53–4.

17. Benacerraf BR, Shipp TD, Bromley B. Three-dimensional ultrasound detection of abnormally located intrauterine contraceptive devices which are a source of pelvic pain and abnormal bleeding. Ultrasound Obstet Gynecol 2009;34(1):110–5.

18. Benacerraf BR, Shipp TD, Lyons JG, et al. Width of the normal uterine cavity in premenopausal women and effect of parity. Obstet Gynecol 2010;116:305–10.

19. Shipp TD, Bromley B, Benacerraf BR. The width of the uterine cavity is narrower in patients with an embedded intrauterine device (IUD) compared to a normally positioned IUD. J Ultrasound Med 2010; 29(10):1453–6.

20. LaTorre R. Transvaginal sonographic evaluation of endometrial polyps: a comparison with two-dimensional and three dimensional contrast sonography. Clin Exp Obstet Gynecol 1999;26:171–3.

21. Benacerraf BR, Benson CB, Abuhamad AZ, et al. Three- and 4-dimensional ultrasound in obstetrics and gynecology: proceedings of the American Institute of Ultrasound in Medicine Consensus Conference. J Ultrasound Med 2005;24(12):1587–97.

22. Lev-Toaff AS, Pinheiro LW, Bega G, et al. Three-dimensional multiplanar sonohysterography: comparison with conventional two-dimensional sonohysterography and X-ray hysterosalpingography. J Ultrasound Med 2001;20(4):295–306.

23. Kowalczyk D, Guzikowski W, Więcek J, et al. Clinical value of real time 3D sonohysterography and 2D sonohysterography in comparison to hysteroscopy with subsequent histopathological examination in perimenopausal women with abnormal uterine bleeding. Neuro Endocrinol Lett 2012;33(2):212–6.

Ultrasound Evaluation of Pelvic Pain

Smbat Amirbekian, MD*, Regina J. Hooley, MD

KEYWORDS

- Ultrasound • Pelvic • Pain • Acute • Chronic • Pregnant

KEY POINTS

- Pelvic pain is a very common complaint in women of all ages.
- Obtaining a thorough clinical history is important to help narrow the wide differential diagnosis for acute and chronic pelvic pain.
- Determination of pregnancy status using a serum hCG level test is also of utmost importance in women of reproductive age; nevertheless, clinical and laboratory results are often inconclusive.
- Pelvic ultrasound (US) is the initial imaging modality of choice and can often diagnose specific abnormalities without the need for additional imaging.
- Familiarity with the differential diagnosis of pelvic pain and knowledge of the associated US features is essential for both US technologists and radiologists to make an accurate diagnosis and facilitate appropriate clinical management.

INTRODUCTION

Pelvic pain is a common symptom in women of all ages and is often associated with morbidity and even mortality. Pelvic pain may be either acute or chronic and may be due to a wide spectrum of causes. No matter what the underlying cause is, a thorough history and physical examination are critical. However, the absence of physical findings does not negate the significance of a patient's pain, because a normal clinical examination does not preclude the possibility of underlying pelvic pathologic abnormality.[1] Ultrasound (US) is the imaging modality of choice in women presenting with pelvic pain. Transabdominal (TA) and transvaginal (TV) US are ideal for diagnosis in both the emergency room and the outpatient setting given the relatively high sensitivity, lack of ionizing radiation, relatively low cost, and widespread availability.

US SCANNING TECHNIQUE

A routine female pelvic US examination should include both TA and TV sonography (TVS). The TA technique is typically performed first, allowing visualization of the uterus and ovaries usually using the fluid-filled bladder as an acoustic window. The initial TA scan provides a wider field-of-view for improved visualization of large masses or fluid collections. Because free fluid will collect dependently, the right hepatorenal space (ie, Morrison pouch) should also be evaluated at this time. After completion of the TA scan, the patient should void, and TVS is performed, unless contraindicated or not desired by the patient. Because of the improved resolution of the higher-frequency TV probe, TVS provides a more detailed evaluation of structures not well seen by the TA study, including the ovaries and endometrial canal. Moreover, the TV probe can be used in a manner similar to a bimanual gynecologic examination, with the examiner holding the probe in one hand and performing palpation of the pelvis transabdominally with the other hand. This technique may separate adjacent structures from a lesion to help identify its origin as well as determine organ mobility, determine site of maximal pelvic tenderness, and compress the bowel, thereby eliminating artifact

Department of Diagnostic Radiology, Yale University School of Medicine, New Haven, CT 06520-8042, USA
* Corresponding author. Department of Diagnostic Radiology, Yale New Haven Hospital, 333 Cedar Street, New Haven, CT 06515.
E-mail address: smbat.amirbekian@yale.edu

Radiol Clin N Am 52 (2014) 1215–1235
http://dx.doi.org/10.1016/j.rcl.2014.07.008
0033-8389/14/$ – see front matter © 2014 Elsevier Inc. All rights reserved.

from overlying bowel gas.[2] Therefore, the TA and TV examinations are complementary: both are required to perform a complete pelvic US examination.

ACUTE PELVIC PAIN

Acute pelvic pain (APP) is defined as noncyclic lower abdominal or pelvic pain lasting less than 3 months and is often associated with nausea, vomiting, and/or leukocytosis.[3] Women with APP pose a challenging clinical scenario because history and physical examination findings are often nonspecific, and the differential diagnosis includes a broad range of gynecologic and nongynecologic causes (Box 1). The gynecologic causes of APP differ significantly based on pregnancy status, and therefore, a serum β-human chorionic gonadotropin (hCG) level should be obtained in all women of reproductive age presenting with APP.

Box 1
Differential diagnoses for acute gynecologic and nongynecologic pelvic pain

Acute pelvic pain: US findings

1. Gynecologic pelvic pain
   a. Nonobstetric
      Large ovarian cysts[a]
      Ruptured/hemorrhagic ovarian cysts
      Ovarian torsion[a]
      Pelvic inflammatory disease[a]
      Malpositioned IUD
      Degenerating fibroids
   b. Obstetric[b]
      Ectopic pregnancy
      Ovarian hyperstimulation syndrome
      Threatened/spontaneous abortion
      Retained products of conception
      Ovarian vein thrombophlebitis
      Uterine rupture
      Degenerating fibroids
2. Nongynecologic pelvic pain
      Ureteral calculi
      Appendicitis
      Diverticulitis

   [a] May be seen in postmenopausal women.
   [b] Most causes of nonobstetric and nongynecologic pelvic pain can also be seen during pregnancy.

Acute Gynecologic Pelvic Pain

Gynecologic causes of APP can be subcategorized into nonobstetric and obstetric causes. Nonobstetric causes include large simple ovarian cysts, hemorrhagic and ruptured ovarian cysts, ovarian/adnexal torsion, pelvic inflammatory disease (PID), a malpositioned intrauterine device (IUD), and degenerating fibroids. Obstetric causes of pelvic pain include ectopic pregnancy (EP), pregnancy of unknown location (PUL), spontaneous abortion (SAB), subchorionic hemorrhage, pain associated with ovarian hyperstimulation syndrome (OHSS), and degenerating fibroids. Postpartum patients may also develop pelvic pain secondary to retained products of conception (RPOC), endometritis, and ovarian vein thrombophlebitis.

Simple ovarian cysts

Most ovarian follicles measure less than 1 cm in diameter. At ovulation, the dominant follicle usually measures 2.0 to 2.5 cm, but can measure up to 3.0 cm.[4–6] Follicles that fail to release an oocyte or do not regress can enlarge into follicular cysts, which are greater than 3 cm in maximum diameter, accounting for most simple ovarian cystic lesions. Although small ovarian cysts are often asymptomatic, large ovarian cysts are a common source of APP. Furthermore, cysts greater than 5 cm in diameter increase the risk of ovarian torsion.[3] Simple or follicular cysts appear on US as anechoic intraovarian or exophytic ovarian masses with an imperceptible wall and associated posterior acoustic enhancement. However, if harmonic imaging or spatial compounding is used, posterior enhancement will be less apparent. When large, a cyst can compress adjacent ovarian parenchyma, which may be nearly imperceptible (Fig. 1). In such cases, color and spectral Doppler can identify typical low-velocity, low-resistance peripheral ovarian blood flow. Most simple ovarian cysts will spontaneously resolve over time and US follow-up is not necessary for asymptomatic simple cysts less than 5 cm in maximal diameter in premenopausal women, although yearly US follow-up is advised for simple cysts measuring 5 to 7 cm in diameter. In premenopausal women, MRI is also recommended for asymptomatic simple cysts greater than 7 cm in diameter due to the risk of missing malignant mural nodularity because of potential US sampling error in large lesions.[7]

Hemorrhagic and ruptured ovarian cysts

A ruptured or hemorrhagic ovarian cyst is the most common cause of APP in an afebrile, premenopausal woman presenting to the emergency room.[3] Although hemorrhagic cysts are

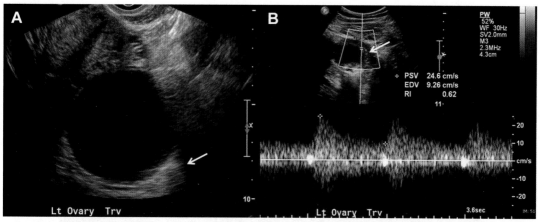

Fig. 1. Simple/follicular ovarian cyst. A 31-year-old woman presenting with APP. (*A*) TVS demonstrates an anechoic 6.0-cm cyst with a thin wall and posterior acoustic enhancement (*arrow*). (*B*) Pulsed Doppler interrogation demonstrates no internal vascularity. Normal low-velocity, low-resistance waveforms are seen in the compressed and thin rim of ovarian tissue (*arrow*). Due to its size, a 1-year follow-up US examination was advised.

more common in nonpregnant women, they may also occur during pregnancy. The associated pain may be due to mass effect, stretching of the capsule of the ovary or cyst, torquing of the ovarian pedicle, or leakage of fluid/blood. If the cyst is leaking fluid, rebound tenderness may be present. If there is significant hemoperitoneum, patients may become hypotensive and present with syncope. The cyst may have a crenated or angular appearance with adjacent free fluid. Hemoperitoneum is most often diagnosed by the presence of free intraperitoneal fluid containing low-level echoes within the cul-de-sac, Morrison pouch, or the left upper quadrant. Echogenic subacute clot may be distinguished from adjacent loops of bowel by lack of vascularity and absence of peristalsis as well as the presence of air within bowel or the elongated tubular appearance of bowel. A critical differential diagnosis for such a constellation of findings is a ruptured EP. However, US features of hemoperitoneum are nonspecific, because echoes within free fluid may also be due to infection or debris.

Hemorrhagic cysts typically develop because of hemorrhage within a corpus luteum. The US appearance of a hemorrhagic cyst varies depending on time course, although hemorrhagic cysts should always exhibit a thin wall (which may be vascular), posterior acoustic enhancement, and absence of internal vascularity. In the acute state, hemorrhagic cysts often exhibit diffuse low-level internal echoes.[8] A fluid/fluid level due to layering of the dependent red blood cells (RBCs) and/or debris may be observed. As the

RBCs lyse, thin echogenic fibrin strands in a reticular or lacelike pattern will form. Clot will form, which is initially echogenic. Subsequently, the echogenic thrombus will retract and pull away from the cyst wall, developing a straight, scalloped, or concave contour (**Fig. 2**).[5] Retractile clot with a concave margin has a 100% specificity for a benign hemorrhagic cyst.[9]

Like simple ovarian cysts, most hemorrhagic cysts resolve spontaneously. In women of reproductive age, US follow-up of classic hemorrhagic cysts (ie, those with the reticular fibrin strand pattern or retractile clot) is not necessary unless they are greater than 5 cm in size. If greater than 5 cm in size, hemorrhagic cysts should be followed in 6 to 12 weeks with repeat US to assure resolution.[7] Hemorrhagic cysts in perimenopausal women are less common and should be followed with repeat sonography in 6 to 12 weeks no matter what their size or pattern of internal echoes. Because hemorrhagic cysts should not occur during late menopause, surgical evaluation should be considered for any apparent hemorrhagic cyst in this age group. A cystic structure that does not conform to the above described classic pattern should be further evaluated with short-interval follow-up US or MRI depending on exact US appearance, clinical presentation, and risk factors for malignancy.

Ovarian torsion

Ovarian torsion is the fifth most common gynecologic emergency, accounting for approximately 3% of all causes of acute pelvic pain.[10,11] Affected women often present with nonspecific

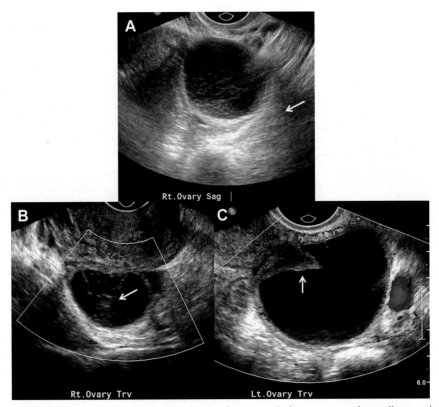

Fig. 2. Hemorrhagic ovarian cysts. Hemorrhagic cysts can have a varied appearance depending on their stage of hemorrhage. (*A*) TVS demonstrates a hypoechoic cyst with a thin wall and a "lacelike" pattern of internal low-level echoes representing fibrin formation from lysis of RBCs and posterior acoustic enhancement (*arrow*). (*B, C*) TVS demonstrating a later stage of hemorrhagic cysts, which contain retractile clot seen as heterogeneous iso-echoic to hypo-echoic irregular-shaped mural-based foci with straight and angular margins (*arrows*) without any evidence of flow on color Doppler interrogation.

clinical symptoms, including APP, nausea, vomiting, and adnexal tenderness. The degree of pelvic pain may be severe, mild, or intermittent and can occur over the course of a few hours, days, or even weeks. Ovarian torsion is a surgical emergency requiring timely diagnosis and intervention to preserve vascularity and prevent ovarian necrosis. The chance of tissue salvage is markedly diminished if symptoms persist longer than 48 hours.

Ovarian torsion is due to partial or complete twisting of the ovary or fallopian tube around its vascular pedicle and occurs more commonly on the right side.[12] The twisting of the vascular pedicle initially causes lymphatic and venous obstruction and, if not relieved, progresses to compromised arterial flow and necrosis. The most common risk factor is an ipsilateral adnexal mass greater than 5 cm in size, reported to be present in 22% to 73% of cases occurring in pre-menopausal women.[3] Ovarian dermoids are the most commonly associated mass, present in

approximately 20%.[12] Masses greater than 10 cm are less likely to undergo torsion, likely because of decreased mobility with fixation by compression from adjacent pelvic structures.[3] Other associated risk factors include OHSS, polycystic ovarian syndrome, prior tubal ligation (likely due to adhesions), and hypermobility of adnexal structures, which is more common in children.[10,12,13] Ovarian torsion occurs in approximately 1 in 1800 pregnancies and approximately 25% of adnexal torsions occur in pregnant patients.[14]

The sonographic features of ovarian torsion are variable, depending on the degree and tension of the torquing, the duration of torsion, whether the fallopian tube is involved, and whether the torsion is intermittent.[3,15] The classic gray-scale US features of ovarian torsion include the presence of an enlarged midline ovary with peripherally displaced small follicles and heterogeneous central stroma due to hemorrhage and edema (**Fig. 3**).[15] A long-standing infarcted ovary

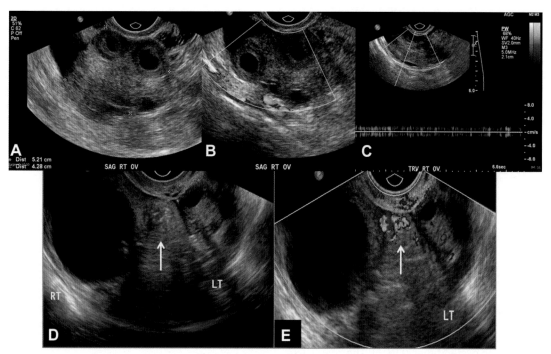

Fig. 3. Ovarian torsion. (*A*) Gray-scale TVS image of a 30-year-old female patient with APP demonstrating an enlarged right ovary measuring up to 5.2 cm, with peripheral follicles and heterogeneous central stroma (for comparison, the patient's left ovary measured up to 2.9 cm). (*B*) Color and (*C*) power with spectral Doppler images from the same patient in (*A*) demonstrating lack of discernible arterial flow. (*D*) Gray-scale TVS image from a different patient with ovarian torsion demonstrating the "target" sign of the twisted vascular pedicle (*arrow*). (*E*) Color Doppler image from same patient in (*D*), demonstrating the "whirlpool" sign (*arrow*), representing the color Doppler appearance of the twisted vascular pedicle. (*From* Scoutt LM, Baltarowich OH, Lev-Toaff AS. Imaging of adnexal torsion. US Clin 2007;2:315; with permission.)

may have a more complex appearance with cystic degeneration. Despite a variable US appearance, in all cases the ovary should be very tender. A thickened, twisted, edematous, tubular vascular pedicle may also be seen between the ovary and uterus. In cross-section, this may have the appearance of alternating echogenic and hypoechoic rings, termed the target sign.[16]

The twisted vessels within the vascular ovarian pedicle may be identified with color Doppler, described as the "whirlpool" sign (see **Fig. 3**).[16] Spectral Doppler findings are variable, but the absence of arterial flow is highly specific with a positive predictive value of 94% in premenopausal women.[17] Unfortunately, this is a late finding, often indicating nonviability of the ovary. However, it may be difficult to detect ovarian flow in a perimenopausal or postmenopausal woman or in a deep ovary. Hence, one should be cautious about making the diagnosis of ovarian torsion because of the inability to detect blood flow on Doppler US unless the ovary is enlarged or painful. Decreased or absent diastolic flow and absent

venous flow can be seen in early ovarian torsion. Importantly, because the ovary has a dual blood supply, a normal Doppler examination does not exclude ovarian torsion. Moreover, the presence of arterial flow in a torsed ovary may also be due to an intermittent, partial, or loosely twisted torsion. Therefore, if the gray-scale appearance is suggestive of ovarian torsion, or if the ovary is markedly tender during the TV scan, the diagnosis should be suspected despite a normal Doppler examination.

PID

PID is a spectrum of ascending sexually transmitted infection that begins with cervicitis and progresses to endometritis, salpingitis, and tubo-ovarian abscess (TOA). The most commonly isolated pathogens are *Neisseria gonorrhoeae* and *Chlamydia trachomatis*, but polymicrobial infection is the most common.[3,18,19] PID is commonly encountered in premenopausal women, presenting with APP, cervical motion tenderness, vaginal discharge, fever, and leukocytosis. Pain may be variable in intensity, ranging from no symptoms to severe bilateral lower quadrant pain, dyspareunia, cramping, dysuria, and abnormal and/or postcoital bleeding.[19] Less commonly, patients may present with right upper quadrant pain due to perihepatitis, known as Fitz-Hugh–Curtis syndrome.[19]

Patients presenting with mild signs and symptoms of PID may be managed clinically without imaging. However, in uncertain cases or to evaluate disease extent, US can be useful. In isolated early cervicitis, the pelvic US examination is usually normal, although the patient may experience marked pain during endovaginal scanning. In cases of endometritis, fluid and gas may be seen distending the endometrial canal (Fig. 4). Heterogeneous thickening, increased vascularity, and indistinctness of the endometrial stripe may be noted. Pulsed Doppler waveforms may reveal low-resistance vascularity within the endometrium.[3] If PID involves the fallopian tube, wall thickening, distension with fluid, incomplete septa, and increased vascularity may be seen. In cases of pyosalpinx, US will demonstrate low-level echoes or multiple fluid-fluid levels with echogenic debris in the dilated tubes (Fig. 5). The "cogwheel sign" may also be seen, which describes the echogenic edematous walls and associated echogenic mucosal folds, representing the dilated and acutely inflamed fallopian tube, as seen in cross-section.[20]

In a minority of cases, a hypoechoic rim surrounding the serosal surface of the uterus will be noted because of uterine serositis. A tuboovarian complex (TOC) or a TOA will result if the ascending infection progresses. TOC is the term used if the ovary and tube are discernible as separate structures within the inflammatory mass. The term TOA is used if the ovary and tube are confluent and cannot be identified as separate structures within the thick-walled, multilocular, complex vascular adnexal collections.[21] TOAs are most commonly bilateral. There may be increased echogenicity of the surrounding pelvic fat, representing inflammatory changes, and purulent echogenic debris containing fluid within the cul-de-sac (Fig. 6).[3,22] In all cases, the patient will experience marked pain and tenderness during TVS.

An untreated TOA may progress to form a pelvic abscess, which may also result from prior surgery, trauma, instrumentation, or gastrointestinal abnormalities. On US, pelvic abscesses are complex, multilocular fluid collections containing low-level echoes. Occasionally, if the clinical findings are nonspecific, it may be difficult to differentiate pelvic abscesses from hematomas, and needle aspiration may be required for definitive diagnosis.[3]

IUDs

IUDs are commonly used for contraception or treatment of menorrhagia. These devices are most often "T" shaped with the long stem oriented along the long axis of the endometrial canal and the 2 limbs located transversely within the uterine fundus. A malpositioned IUD can cause pelvic pain and bleeding: in a single study cohort, 75% of patients with an abnormally located IUD presented with bleeding or pain

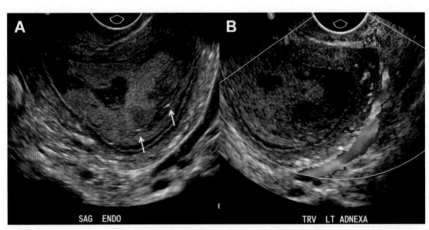

Fig. 4. Endometritis and pyometria. This 78-year-old patient presented with cervical motion tenderness and thick yellow vaginal discharge. (*A*) TVS demonstrates significant distention of the endometrial cavity, which is filled with heterogeneous echogenic debris and pockets of fluid. Echogenic foci (*arrows*) are consistent with air. (*B*) Color Doppler image demonstrates the lack of vascularity within the debris in the endometrial canal, helping exclude an underlying soft tissue lesion. These findings resolved on follow-up US obtained 4 weeks after completion of antibiotic therapy.

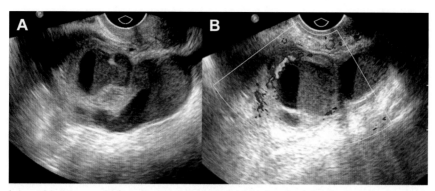

Fig. 5. Pyosalpinx. This 36-year-old female patient presented with lower abdominal tenderness, fever, and leuko-cytosis. Gray-scale (A) and color (B) images demonstrate a dilated, serpiginous tubular structure in the adnexa, which demonstrates avascular, echogenic debris with fluid-fluid levels within. Given the patient's history, these findings are diagnostic for pyosalpinx.

compared with 35% of those with a normally placed IUD.[23]

On TVS, the echogenic, shadowing long stem of a well-positioned IUD should be visualized entirely within the endometrial canal on the sagittal view and the echogenic limbs visualized within the fundus on the transverse or coronal view. Three-dimensional (3D) US can visualize an entire IUD, including the string within the endocervical canal, on a single coronal image, and is now becoming standard practice for routine US evaluation.[24] Complications of IUD placement include expulsion, displacement, myometrial penetration, and myometrial perforation (Fig. 7). In all cases, symptoms may range from no symptoms to severe pain and bleeding.

Displacement and myometrial penetration are often encountered in the presence of uterine structural abnormalities or large fibroids. Myometrial penetration is also more common in women with

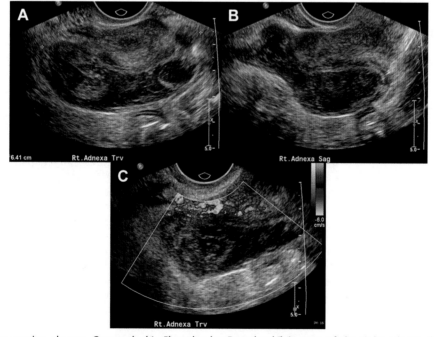

Fig. 6. Tubo-ovarian abscess. Gray-scale (A, B) and color Doppler (C) images of the right adnexa demonstrate a tubular, heterogeneous fluid collection with echogenic debris and lack of internal vascularity and peripheral hyperemia. The right ovary is not visualized and not clearly discerned within this collection.

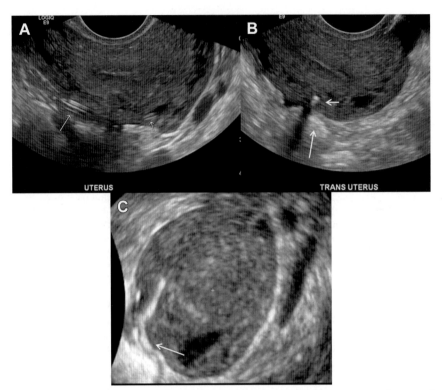

Fig. 7. Malpositioned IUD. Sagittal and transverse gray-scale images (*A, B*) of a retroverted uterus demonstrates parts of the echogenic stems of the IUD within the myometriun (*short arrows*) and external to the myometrium, along the anterior serosal surface of the uterine body and fundus (*long arrows*). (*C*) 3D US image more clearly demonstrates the echogenic linear stem of the IUD extending through the myometrium and the serosal surface (*arrow*). These findings are consistent with myometrial penetration and perforation because this IUD was partially located within the peritoneal cavity.

small endometrial cavities.[25] Complete perforation of the IUD can lead to serious complications including adhesions and intestinal obstruction. If the IUD is not visualized after a TV and TA scan, an abdominal radiograph may be obtained to differentiate IUD expulsion from myometrial perforation.

EP

EP results when a fertilized ovum implants outside the endometrial cavity and occurs in 0.65% to 2% of all pregnancies.[26] A tubal location accounts for greater than 90% of EPs, with 70% of these located in the ampulla.[27] Less common locations include the fimbrial, isthmic, and interstitial portions of the fallopian tube, as well as the ovary, cervix, C-section scars, or peritoneal cavity.[3,27] Early diagnosis made by the combination of TVS, clinical history, and serial hCG levels can significantly reduce morbidity and mortality. A ruptured EP can compromise a woman's future fertility and accounts for 6% of all maternal deaths in the first trimester.[3,28,29]

Risk factors for EP include a prior history of EP, PID, infertility treatment, pelvic surgery, endometriosis, prior cesarean section, and IUD placement (**Fig. 8**). However, 50% of women do not have known risk factors.[28] Therefore, EP should be considered in all pregnant women with APP and/or vaginal bleeding in the first trimester, although in more than 70% of these symptomatic women, a normal early intrauterine pregnancy (IUP) will be identified on TVS,[3] effectively excluding EP. Rarely, a coexisting IUP and EP may occur; this is called a heterotopic pregnancy and has an estimated frequency of approximately 1/7000 to 1/30,000 of all pregnancies.[30,31] However, patients undergoing assisted reproduction have a higher incidence of heterotopic pregnancy, estimated at approximately 1 in 100 to 500 pregnancies.[30] The serum hCG levels in women with ectopic pregnancies are highly variable, but are typically lower than expected for gestational age, often less than 1000 mIU/mL.[32]

The most specific US finding of an EP is an extra-uterine gestational sac containing a yolk

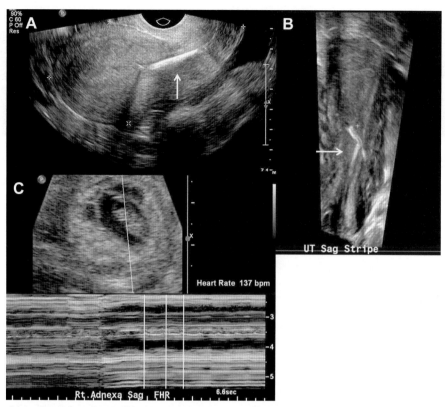

Fig. 8. EP with malpositioned IUD. (*A*) TV sagittal US image demonstrating an IUD (*arrow*) malpositioned within the lower uterine segment. (*B*) 3D US sagittal image demonstrating the IUD (*arrow*) asymmetrically positioned within the lower uterine segment. (*C*) M-mode image of the right adnexa demonstrating a live EP. Having an IUD is a known risk factor for EP.

sac or embryo. An EP may also present as a solid or partially cystic extra-ovarian adnexal mass, usually located between the ovary and uterus or within the cul-de-sac. Enlargement of the fallopian tube may be noted because of hemorrhage within the wall.[33] The most common US appearance of an EP is an echogenic tubal ring, which may exhibit a high-velocity, low-resistance spectral Doppler waveform (**Fig. 9**) However, this is a nonspecific finding that may be mimicked by a normal corpus luteum.[33] In such cases, bimanual scanning can help distinguish between an intra-ovarian or exophytic corpus luteum and an extra-ovarian EP. Intra-ovarian lesions will move synchronously with the ovary, whereas extra-ovarian lesions will move separately from the ovary. Identification of a thin rim of ovarian tissue surrounding the lesion, known as the claw sign, is also typical of a corpus luteum.

If no IUP or EP is identified after TVS, the symptomatic pregnant woman is said to have a PUL. Most of these cases will eventually progress to a normal viable early pregnancy, although the differential diagnosis also includes an EP and nonviable

IUP. Approximately 2% to 10% of women with PUL will eventually be diagnosed with EP.[34,35] Management of PUL includes close clinical follow-up, serial hCG levels, and serial TVS.[34] In cases of a normal early IUP, the hCG level should approximately double every 48 hours, whereas in cases of an EP, the hCG level will plateau, increase, or decrease slightly in 48 hours. Typically, hCG levels will drop more quickly in the setting of a failed IUP.

Spontaneous and threatened abortion

SAB (also known as miscarriage) is defined as a spontaneous loss of an IUP, the majority occurring before 16 weeks of gestation.[36,37] It is a very common complication of pregnancy, often associated with fetal chromosomal abnormalities, inherited blood disorders, and uterine structural abnormalities. Patients typically present with vaginal bleeding associated with pelvic pain and cramping. US plays an important role in establishing fetal viability. In women with a complete SAB, the uterus often appears normal or may contain a small amount of blood or debris within the endometrial canal

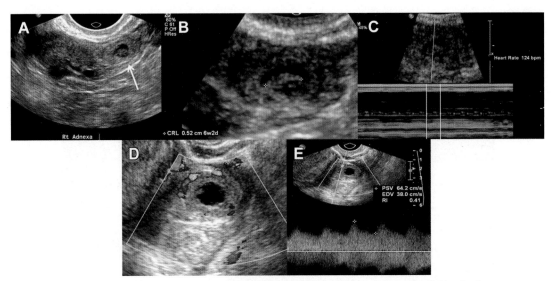

Fig. 9. EP. (*A*) TVS of the right adnexa in a patient with a positive pregnancy test and pelvic pain demonstrates a round structure with an echogenic rim (*arrow*) separate from the right ovary. (*B*) Magnified gray-scale image of lesion in (*A*) reveals a gestational sac with a fetus with cardiac activity on M-mode imaging (*C*) confirming a live EP. (*D*) TVS in another patient with a positive pregnancy test and pelvic pain demonstrates a tubal ring separate from the ovary (not shown) in the left adnexa with high-velocity, low-resistance trophoblastic flow on spectral Doppler interrogation (*E*) consistent with an EP.

without evidence of trophoblastic flow or RPOC. However, in many cases, an incomplete SAB may be discovered, with evidence of a nonviable fetus or an abnormal, irregular, or empty gestational sac (**Fig. 10**). In addition to these findings, the presence of trophoblastic flow on Doppler imaging, characterized by increased systolic and diastolic flow, suggests an incomplete abortion.[38]

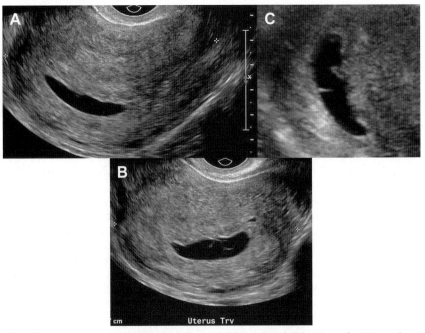

Fig. 10. SAB. This 30-year-old female patient presented with a reported history of a 10-week pregnancy and vaginal bleeding and pain. (*A, B*) Sagittal and transverse gray-scale US images demonstrate an irregular-shaped intrauterine gestational sac with echogenic foci within, which are not readily identifiable. (*C*) Magnified view of the abnormal gestational sac demonstrates irregular shape and margins without any identifiable normal fetus or yolk sac. These findings are compatible with fetal demise and an incomplete abortion.

In cases of threatened abortion, a subchorionic hemorrhage surrounding the intrauterine gestational sac may be identified on TVS. Although a small subchorionic hemorrhage may be asymptomatic, women with larger collections may present with vaginal bleeding, pelvic pain, and/or cramping. These collections have a variable appearance on US, depending on the age and size of the hemorrhage. Acute hemorrhage appears echogenic and may be difficult to differentiate from the adjacent chorion, but is usually hypoechoic when subacute or chronic.[39] The size of the hemorrhage can be measured according to the percentage of chorionic sac circumference elevated by the hemorrhage and is considered large if greater than two-thirds of the chorionic sac circumference.[40] The potential for fetal viability in the presence of a subchorionic hemorrhage is multifactorial, likely related to size, maternal and gestational age, as well as maternal pelvic pain and vaginal bleeding.

RPOC

RPOC is defined as the presence of persistent placental or trophoblastic tissue within the endometrial cavity following delivery, SAB, or pregnancy termination. Patients typically present in the postpartum or posttermination period with excessive vaginal bleeding, pelvic pain, and/or fever.

A positive serum hCG and an elevated white blood cell (WBC) count (especially in cases complicated by endometritis) may be seen in patients with suspected RPOC, but these are nonspecific markers because they can also be seen in a normal postpartum state.[41] However, US with color Doppler also plays an important diagnostic role. The endometrial stripe is typically thickened and heterogeneous, with a masslike appearance. An endometrial stripe greater than 10 mm in thickness has a reported sensitivity of greater than 80%,[41] although the specificity is low because this finding is also characteristic of both endometritis and normal postpartum debris or hemorrhage. Color Doppler can help accurately distinguish RPOC, because the presence of vascularity extending from the myometrium into the endometrium is reported to have a positive predictive value of 96%.[42] Vascularity may exhibit high-velocity, low-resistance trophoblastic spectral Doppler waveforms, although any degree of vascularity is suspicious (**Fig. 11**).[41] The absence of endometrial vascularity does not exclude the diagnosis of RPOC and there is wide overlap of

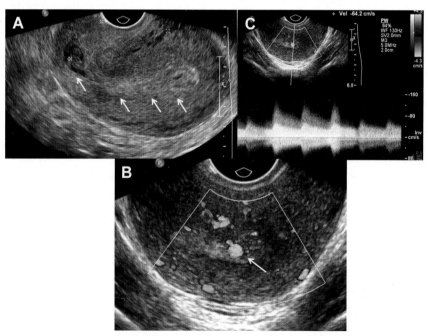

Fig. 11. RPOC. This 20-year-old female patient presented with pelvic pain and vaginal bleeding 3 days after a miscarriage. (*A*) TV sagittal gray-scale image of the uterus demonstrates a thickened heterogeneous endometrial stripe (*arrows*). (*B*) Color gray-scale image of the endometrial stripe demonstrates significant vascularity within it (*arrow*), differentiating this from bland blood products/clot. (*C*) Spectral Doppler interrogation of the thickened endometrial stripe demonstrates trophoblastic flow typically seen within RPOC, classified by high diastolic flow with low-resistance waveforms.

the Doppler findings with normal postpartum and posttermination findings, making the confident diagnosis or RPOC problematic.

Ovarian vein thrombophlebitis

Ovarian vein thrombosis or thrombophlebitis is a rare cause of APP in the postpartum period, occurring in less than 0.05% of vaginal deliveries and 0.1% to 0.2% of cesarean sections.[43] Patients most often present with nonspecific symptoms, including fever, pelvic or back pain, and right lower quadrant pain.[44] It is more common on the right and best imaged with TA scanning. Sonographic findings include a tubular or serpiginous avascular, hypoechoic, or anechoic structure in the adnexa adjacent to the ovarian artery and leading to the inferior vena cava.

Other causes of post-partum and pregnancy related APP

Large fibroids, uterine rupture, OHSS, and hematomas may also cause APP. Uterine rupture is life threatening and often associated with a prior cesarean delivery. US may identify an intraperitoneal or extraperitoneal hematoma, fluid in the uterus extending through the myometrium, or even extra-uterine fetal parts.[45] Finally, although most fibroids do not change during pregnancy, approximately 30% will grow and may cause APP secondary to degeneration, torsion, or infarction following delivery.[46] Because fibroids are a common cause of chronic pelvic pain (CPP), they are discussed in detail in a later section.

OHSS is a rare and usually self-limiting disorder due to an exaggerated response to ovulation induction therapy. The characteristic feature of OHSS is an increase in capillary permeability leading to third spacing of fluid. Symptoms are variable, ranging from mild pelvic discomfort, nausea, and vomiting to tense ascites, pleural effusions, oliguria, and hemodynamic instability.[47] APP can result from rapid enlargement of multiple ovarian follicles with stretching of the ovarian capsule or hemorrhage/rupture of a follicle. The ovaries may exceed 10 cm in size. There is also an increased risk of ovarian torsion.[3] On pelvic US, the ovaries typically are enlarged, containing multiple cysts of varying sizes, some of which may contain low-level echoes and fluid/fluid levels due to hemorrhage.

Rectus sheath and bladder flap hematomas are uncommon complications of cesarean deliveries. In these cases, patients will present with dropping hematocrit, fever, and/or pelvic pain. Bladder flap hematomas are typically located in the lower uterine segment within the cesarean section incision and are best seen with TA scans.[42] Rectus sheath hematomas occur in the lower pelvis adjacent to the rectus muscle. Because of their superficial location, they are best visualized transabdominally using a high-resolution linear transducer. On US, rectus sheath hematomas typically are hypoechoic and complex masses with cystic and/or echogenic components (Fig. 12).

Nongynecologic Causes of APP

Common nongynecologic causes of APP include ureteral obstruction, appendicitis, and diverticulitis. These causes of APP can be seen in women, independent of age and pregnancy status, and can coexist with gynecologic disease.

Ureteral calculi

An obstructing distal ureteral stone is a frequently overlooked cause of APP in women. TVS can identify the stone and is particularly useful in obese or pregnant patients. The dilated distal ureter, containing an echogenic, shadowing calculus, should be identified anterior and slightly lateral to the upper vagina at the ureterovesical junction and is best visualized with a partially distended bladder (Fig. 13).[48] In cases of complete obstruction, the normal ureteral jet will be absent, confirmed by placing color or power Doppler over the bladder trigone. If a distal ureteral calculus is found or suspected, the ipsilateral kidney should be assessed for pelvicaliectasis, although this finding may be absent in approximately 25% of patients.[48]

Appendicitis

Appendicitis is a frequent cause of emergent abdominal surgery. Patients usually present with anorexia, fever, elevated WBCs, and periumbilical pain that migrates to the right lower quadrant. Compression US of the right lower quadrant, using a TA approach with a high-resolution linear array transducer, can identify the abnormal painful appendix, which will appear as a noncompressible, blind-ending, nonperistalsing, thick-walled tubular structure greater than 6 to 7 mm in diameter.[49] The wall may be vascular. The abnormal appendix may be associated with adjacent free fluid, inflamed echogenic periappendiceal fat, or an echogenic appendicolith with posterior acoustic shadowing. The appendix can be located in unusual positions, including retrocecal, retroilieal, or within the pelvis. A patient with pelvic appendicitis may present with suprapubic pain and may be referred for pelvic US to evaluate for uterine or adnexal pathologic

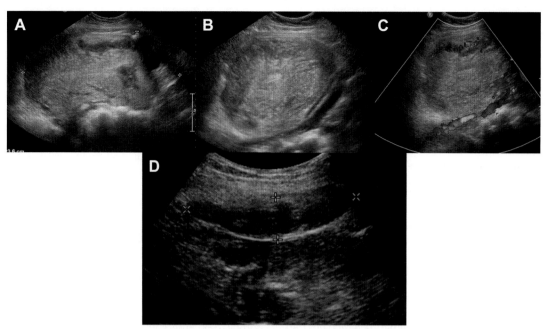

Fig. 12. Rectus sheath hematoma. (*A, B*) TA US images of the mid and right lower anterior abdominal wall in a patient with right pelvic pain demonstrating a large, heterogeneous, predominantly hyperechoic lesion without any significant evidence of internal vascularity on color Doppler imaging. (*C*) Clinically, a hematoma was suspected and this showed complete resolution on 2-month follow-up US examination, confirming the clinical diagnosis. (*D*) Gray-scale TA image of the anterior abdominal wall in a different patient demonstrates an ovoid, predominantly hypoechoic fluid collection (*calipers*). This lesion was shown to be another rectus sheath hematoma on a follow-up abdominal CT scan, likely of longer duration than that seen in (*A–C*).

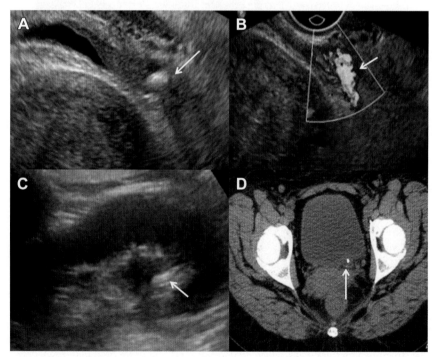

Fig. 13. Ureteral calculus. (*A*) TV gray-scale image demonstrating a dilated distal left ureter with an echogenic focus at the end of the dilated segment (*arrow*) with associated mild posterior shadowing. Adjacent proximal debris and ureteral wall thickening are noted. (*B*) Color Doppler image correlated to image in (*A*) demonstrating twinkle artifact (*arrow*) posterior to the echogenic focus, suggesting that this finding is most consistent with a calculus. (*C*) Sagittal image of the left kidney demonstrating mild hydronephrosis involving the lower pole (*arrow*). (*D*) Axial CT image through the ureterovesical junction confirming an obstructing calculus at this level (*arrow*).

abnormality. The unsuspected pelvic appendix can be identified on either TA or TVS within the right adnexa (separate from the ovary) or cul-de-sac (**Fig. 14**). TVS diagnostic criteria for the diagnosis of acute appendicitis are the same as for the TA approach, although compression cannot be evaluated with TVS.

Diverticulitis

Although diverticulitis and other sources of bowel inflammation are usually clinically evident and confirmed with CT, an atypical clinical presentation, particularly in premenopausal women, may be discovered on pelvic US. The sensitivity of US in the diagnosis of diverticulitis has been shown to be 84%.[50,51] In cases of diverticulitis, an inflamed, nonperistalsing segment of sigmoid colon is usually found deep within the left lower quadrant, surrounded by prominent echogenic pericolonic fat or free fluid (**Fig. 15**). Right-sided diverticulitis is rare. An inflamed diverticulum can be seen as a bright echogenic focus of shadowing gas, stool, or fecalith projecting beyond the colonic margin.[52]

CCP

CPP is defined as noncyclic pelvic pain lasting longer than 6 months and is of sufficient severity to cause functional disability and lead to medical care.[1] In a survey of 18- to 50-year-old American women, 15% reported CPP within the last 3 months, and 61% of these women reported that the cause of their pelvic pain was unknown.[53] However, US is useful in the diagnostic workup, because a wide variety of underlying causes can be readily identified (**Box 2**).

Endometriosis

Endometriosis is defined as the presence of ectopic endometrial tissue outside of the uterus, most commonly implanted on the ovary, uterus, fallopian tubes, and peritoneal surfaces. Endometriosis is found in approximately 10% of reproductive age women who most often present with chronic pain and/or infertility.[54] However, patients may be asymptomatic. Hormonal stimulation of these ectopic foci is associated with repetitive cycles of hemorrhage, resorption, and fibrosis,

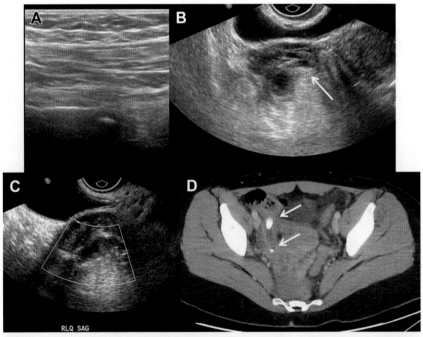

Fig. 14. Appendicitis. (*A*) TA image of the right lower quadrant in this patient with right lower quadrant pain failed to demonstrate any obvious findings. (*B*) TV gray-scale image of the right lower quadrant/adnexa demonstrates a tubular structure with thick walls, which demonstrates echogenic foci within (*arrow*). Corresponding color Doppler image (*C*) demonstrates slight peripheral vascularity surrounding this tubular structure. Also, note the increased echogenicity of the surrounding soft tissues in (*B, C*) consistent with inflamed peri-appendiceal fat. Appendicitis was highly suspected on this US examination and a follow-up CT study (*D*) confirmed the finding of a pelvic appendix with appendicoliths (*arrows*), extending from the right lower quadrant into the right adnexa.

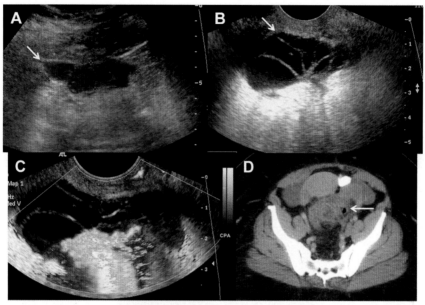

Fig. 15. Diverticulitis. This 35-year-old female patient presented with diffuse lower abdominal and rectal pain. TA (A) and TV (B) images of the left adnexa demonstrate a complex fluid collection (arrows) with echogenic material and septations, better seen on the TV images. Also, note the increased echogenicity of the adjacent bowel loops and pelvic fat, consistent with inflammatory changes in the region. (C) Power Doppler image of same lesion in (B) demonstrates hyperemia of the adjacent bowel loops and soft tissues. Concurrent CT (D) shows an inflamed segment of the sigmoid colon with a small focus of extracolonic air (arrow), pericolonic fat-stranding, and small focal pockets of free fluid. These findings confirm the diagnosis of sigmoid diverticular abscess.

resulting in scarring, adhesions, and cystic ovarian lesions called endometriomas.[3]

The gold standard for diagnosis and staging of endometriosis is laparoscopy. Small implants and adhesions are difficult to visualize on US (or MRI) and the reported sensitivity of US for detection of small implants is as low as 11%.[55] However, TVS can be helpful in the diagnosis of endometriomas, which classically appear as complex cystic avascular masses with homogenous low-level echoes, the so-called ground-glass appearance. Shading may be observed as the

RBCs and products of hemorrhage settle dependently, although true layering is uncommon. They are typically unilocular, although are often multiple, exhibiting angular margins and small echogenic mural foci. These echogenic mural foci are highly specific and have a high positive likelihood ratio for endometriomas (Fig. 16).[56]

Endometriomas may mimic the US appearance of hemorrhagic cysts. However, endometriomas rarely present with acute clinical symptoms and do not resolve over time. Interestingly, even though there is repeated hemorrhage within endometriomas, findings related to acute hemorrhage, such as fibrinous strands and retractile clot, are only seen in 8% of cases.[56] A newly discovered endometrioma should be rescanned in 6 to 12 weeks to document stability and, if not surgically excised, yearly US follow-up is recommended because there is a small risk of malignant transformation.[7]

Adenomyosis

Adenomyosis is histologically defined as the presence of ectopic endometrial glands located in the myometrium, usually within the subendometrial tissue, and is associated with adjacent smooth muscle hyperplasia.[3,57] The clinical

---

Box 2
Differential diagnoses of CPP
CCP: US findings
Endometriosis[a]
Adenomyosis[a]
Fibroids
Pelvic congestion syndrome
Peritoneal inclusion cysts
Periurethral cysts/diverticula
[a] Premenopausal-/perimenopausal women only.

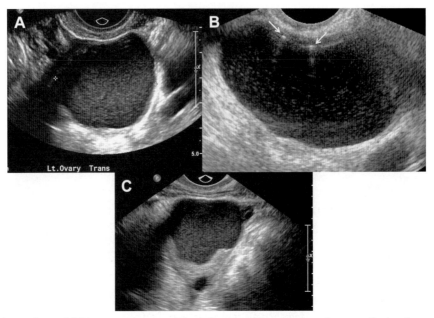

Fig. 16. Endometrioma. (A) Transverse image of the left ovary demonstrates a large cystic structure with diffuse homogeneous low-level echoes throughout typical of an endometrioma. (B) Magnified image of lesion in (A) again demonstrating this cystic structure with diffuse low-level echoes and a few echogenic foci within the wall (arrows). Given this additional finding, this lesion has a very high likelihood of being an endometrioma. On follow-up examination 6 months later (C), this lesion showed no significant change.

presentation includes dysfunctional uterine bleeding, dysmenorrhea, infertility, and/or pelvic pain. TVS has been reported to have sensitivities ranging from 80% to 85% and specificities ranging from 50% to 96% for the detection of adenomyosis.[58–60]

Adenomyosis may be focal or diffuse, although focal adenomyosis is less common. Diffuse adenomyosis is associated with US findings of an enlarged uterus, heterogeneity of the myometrium with poorly marginated heterogeneous hypoechoic or echogenic areas, as well as asymmetric thickening of the subendometrial halo.[3] In addition, there may be small subendometrial myometrial cysts, echogenic nodules, or linear striations extending from the endometrium into the myometrium, with poor definition of the endometrial-myometrial interface (**Fig. 17**).[3] The subendometrial cysts and nodules, thought to represent ectopic endometrial glands, have been shown to be the most specific US findings.[61]

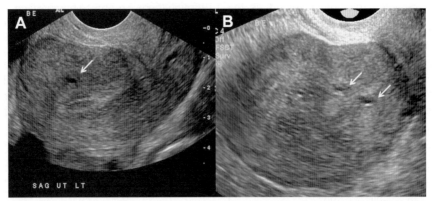

Fig. 17. Adenomyosis. (A) TV sagittal gray-scale image of the uterus demonstrates a small subendometrial myometrial cyst (arrow). Similar additional cysts (arrows in B) were seen in this patient in a parasagittal plane, again in the region of the junctional zone.

Fibroids

Uterine fibroids (leiomyomas) are the most common female genital tract tumor and are composed of smooth muscle cells, fibrous connective tissue, and collagen.[62] Hormonally responsive, fibroids may enlarge secondary to increased estrogen levels (particularly during pregnancy) and often regress during menopause or following delivery.[2] They may be submucosal, myometrial, or subserosal in location. Small fibroids are usually well characterized on TVS, although large fibroids are usually better evaluated using the TA approach.

Symptoms related to fibroids depend on size and location. Large subserosal fibroids can be painful due to torsion, necrosis, or mass effect/compression on adjacent structures. Degenerating fibroids may also be painful and are most commonly seen during pregnancy or following delivery. Although fibroid-associated pain is usually chronic, mild and due to mass effect on adjacent structures, rapid enlargement, often seen during pregnancy, may also result in acute pain due to hemorrhagic infarction.[62]

Leiomyomas are often multiple, and echogenicity is variable. The most frequent US finding is a homogeneously or heterogeneous solid, hypoechoic or isoechoic mass, although rarely leiomyomas will be echogenic.[62] The uterine serosal surface may appear lobulated. Large fibroids, greater than 3 to 5 cm, often have focal areas of degeneration or calcification. Edge refraction, marked posterior acoustic shadowing, as well as "comblike" striated posterior acoustic shadowing are common findings. Subserosal pedunculated leiomyomas can be found in the adnexa, and these cases may be differentiated from other adnexal masses by using color Doppler interrogation to demonstrate a vascular pedicle originating from the uterus.

Pelvic Congestion Syndrome

Pelvic congestion syndrome (PCS) is an often underdiagnosed cause of CCP due to dilated, tortuous, and congested pelvic veins or varices produced by retrograde flow through incompetent valves in the ovarian veins.[57] The pain may be unilateral or bilateral but is often asymmetric and usually seen in premenopausal, usually multiparous women.[63]

TV US is useful in demonstrating pelvic varices. Ovarian vein diameters measuring greater than 5 to 6 mm have a positive predictive value of 71% to 83% for the diagnosis.[64] Direct connection to the arcuate veins in the myometrium, low-velocity flow, and increase in venous diameter after the Valsalva maneuver are all US findings associated with symptoms of PCS (**Fig. 18**). Treatment options include hormonal suppression and sclerotherapy.

Peritoneal inclusion cysts

Peritoneal inclusion cysts are a cause of CCP and may be associated with a mass palpated on bimanual pelvic examination, although 10% are discovered incidentally on unrelated imaging or surgery.[65] Peritoneal inclusion cysts are found in premenopausal women and occur secondary to pelvic adhesions, which trap serous fluid produced by the ovaries likely at ovulation. Risk factors include a history of pelvic surgery, PID, endometriosis, appendicitis, or trauma. Typical US features include a large irregular cystic mass with thin septations and no discrete outer wall or margin that conforms to surrounding structures. A normal-appearing ovary should be seen within or at the periphery of the mass (**Fig. 19**). These cysts are hormonally sensitive and may resolve spontaneously during menopause. Symptomatic peritoneal inclusion cysts

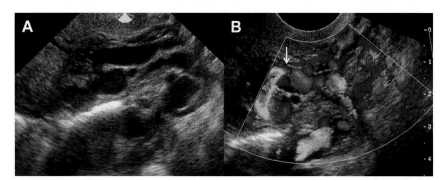

Fig. 18. PCS. This 56-year-old woman presented with pelvic pain of several months. (*A*) TVS gray-scale images of the left adnexa demonstrate pelvic veins that measure up to 7 mm and are even more prominent during Valsalva maneuver (*B*). The connection to the uterine arcuate veins, which are easily seen here (*arrow*), is the most specific findings for PCS.

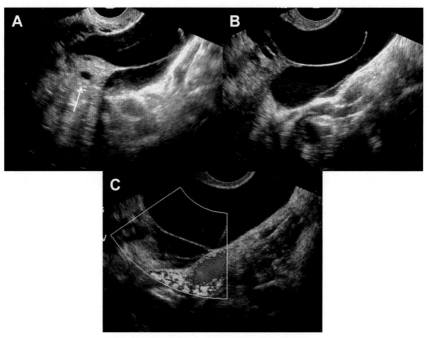

Fig. 19. Peritoneal inclusion cyst in a 31-year-old woman with a history of C-section. (*A, B*) TVS demonstrates the left ovary (*arrow*) at the periphery of an anechoic septated fluid collection. The margins of the cystic collection conform to the surrounding structures. Color Doppler image of the septations (*C*) shows no internal vascularity.

may be treated with oral contraceptives, US or CT-guided aspiration, and sclerotherapy. Surgical resection is associated with 30% to 50% risk of recurrence.[66]

Perineal cysts, periurethral cysts, and urethral diverticula

Gartner cysts, Bartholin gland cysts, and urethral diverticula are rare causes of CPP. Large cysts are associated with obstruction, urinary urgency, urinary frequency, and recurrent urinary tract infection. Gartner cysts are remnants of the mesonephric ducts and are located in the antero-lateral wall of the proximal vagina.[57,67] Bartholin gland cysts are located in the vulva and can become painful if infected. Symptomatic periurethral cysts and urethral diverticula may arise from inflamed periurethral glands that drain into the urethra.[57] Occasionally, an echogenic calculus can be seen in a chronically inflamed urethral diverticulum. Although all of these cysts are best evaluated on MR, they can also be identified using TVS or translabial US using a high-resolution linear array transducer (**Fig. 20**).

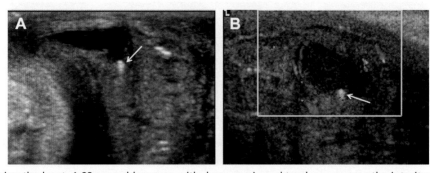

Fig. 20. Periurethral cyst. A 23-year-old woman with dyspareunia and tender mass near the introitus on physical examination. Translabial sagittal (*A*) and transverse (*B*) US demonstrates a cystic mass with internal echoes and ring down artifact (*arrows*) and peripheral vascularity. This mass was located anterior and inferior to the urethra and is likely a urethral diverticulum with a stone or inflamed Bartholin gland.

SUMMARY

Pelvic pain is a common complaint in women of all ages. Obtaining a thorough clinical history is important to help narrow the wide differential diagnosis for acute and chronic pelvic pain. Determination of pregnancy status using serum hCG levels testing is also of utmost importance in women of reproductive age. Nevertheless, clinical and laboratory results are often inconclusive. Pelvic US is the initial imaging modality of choice and can often diagnose specific abnormalities without the need for additional imaging. Familiarity with the differential diagnosis of pelvic pain and knowledge of the associated US features is essential for both US technologists and radiologists to make an accurate diagnosis and facilitate appropriate clinical management.

REFERENCES

1. ACOG Committee on Practice Bulletins–Gynecology. ACOG Practice Bulletin No. 51. Chronic pelvic pain. Obstet Gynecol 2004;103:589–605.

2. Laing FC, Brown DL, DiSalvo DN. Gynecologic ultrasound. Radiol Clin North Am 2001;39: 523–40.

3. Cicchiello LA, Hamper UM, Scoutt LM. Ultrasound evaluation of gynecologic causes of pelvic pain. Obstet Gynecol Clin North Am 2011;38: 85–114, viii.

4. Ritchie WG. Sonographic evaluation of normal and induced ovulation. Radiology 1986;161:1–10.

5. Laing FC, Allison SJ. US of the ovary and adnexa: to worry or not to worry? Radiographics 2012;32: 1621–39 [discussion: 1640–2].

6. Bakos O, Lundkvist O, Wide L, et al. Ultrasonographical and hormonal description of the normal ovulatory menstrual cycle. Acta Obstet Gynecol Scand 1994;73:790–6.

7. Levine D, Brown DL, Andreotti RF, et al. Management of asymptomatic ovarian and other adnexal cysts imaged at US: Society of Radiologists in Ultrasound Consensus Conference Statement. Radiology 2010;256:943–54.

8. Jain KA. Sonographic spectrum of hemorrhagic ovarian cysts. J Ultrasound Med 2002;21: 879–86.

9. Patel MD, Feldstein VA, Filly RA. The likelihood ratio of sonographic findings for the diagnosis of hemorrhagic ovarian cysts. J Ultrasound Med 2005;24: 607–14 [quiz: 615].

10. Houry D, Abbott JT. Ovarian torsion: a fifteen-year review. Ann Emerg Med 2001;38:156–9.

11. Hibbard LT. Adnexal torsion. Am J Obstet Gynecol 1985;152:456–61.

12. Albayram F, Hamper UM. Ovarian and adnexal torsion: spectrum of sonographic findings with pathologic correlation. J Ultrasound Med 2001; 20:1083–9.

13. White M, Stella J. Ovarian torsion: 10-year perspective. Emerg Med Australas 2005;17: 231–7.

14. Cappell MS, Friedel D. Abdominal pain during pregnancy. Gastroenterol Clin North Am 2003;32: 1–58.

15. Graif M, Shalev J, Strauss S, et al. Torsion of the ovary: sonographic features. AJR Am J Roentgenol 1984;143:1331–4.

16. Vijayaraghavan SB. Sonographic whirlpool sign in ovarian torsion. J Ultrasound Med 2004;23: 1643–9 [quiz: 1650–1].

17. Ben-Ami M, Perlitz Y, Haddad S. The effectiveness of spectral and color Doppler in predicting ovarian torsion. A prospective study. Eur J Obstet Gynecol Reprod Biol 2002;104:64–6.

18. Barrett S, Taylor C. A review on pelvic inflammatory disease. Int J STD AIDS 2005;16:715–20 [quiz: 721].

19. Gradison M. Pelvic inflammatory disease. Am Fam Physician 2012;85:791–6.

20. Romosan G, Valentin L. The sensitivity and specificity of transvaginal ultrasound with regard to acute pelvic inflammatory disease: a review of the literature. Arch Gynecol Obstet 2014;289(4): 705–14.

21. Timor-Tritsch IE, Lerner JP, Monteagudo A, et al. Transvaginal sonographic markers of tubal inflammatory disease. Ultrasound Obstet Gynecol 1998; 12:56–66.

22. Horrow MM. Ultrasound of pelvic inflammatory disease. Ultrasound Q 2004;20:171–9.

23. Benacerraf BR, Shipp TD, Bromley B. Three-dimensional ultrasound detection of abnormally located intrauterine contraceptive devices which are a source of pelvic pain and abnormal bleeding. Ultrasound Obstet Gynecol 2009;34: 110–5.

24. Boortz HE, Margolis DJ, Ragavendra N, et al. Migration of intrauterine devices: radiologic findings and implications for patient care. Radiographics 2012;32:335–52.

25. Shipp TD, Bromley B, Benacerraf BR. The width of the uterine cavity is narrower in patients with an embedded intrauterine device (IUD) compared to a normally positioned IUD. J Ultrasound Med 2010;29:1453–6.

26. Hoover KW, Tao G, Kent CK. Trends in the diagnosis and treatment of ectopic pregnancy in the United States. Obstet Gynecol 2010;115: 495–502.

27. Bouyer J, Coste J, Fernandez H, et al. Sites of ectopic pregnancy: a 10 year population-based study of 1800 cases. Hum Reprod 2002;17:3224–30.

28. Barnhart KT. Clinical practice. Ectopic pregnancy. N Engl J Med 2009;361:379–87.

29. Chang J, Elam-Evans LD, Berg CJ, et al. Pregnancy-related mortality surveillance–United States, 1991–1999. MMWR Surveill Summ 2003; 52:1–8.

30. Anastasakis E, Jetti A, Macara L, et al. A case of heterotopic pregnancy in the absence of risk factors. A brief literature review. Fetal Diagn Ther 2007;22:285–8.

31. Hann LE, Bachman DM, McArdle CR. Coexistent intrauterine and ectopic pregnancy: a reevaluation. Radiology 1984;152:151–4.

32. Doubilet PM, Benson CB, Bourne T, et al. Diagnostic criteria for nonviable pregnancy early in the first trimester. N Engl J Med 2013;369: 1443–51.

33. Levine D. Ectopic pregnancy. Radiology 2007;245: 385–97.

34. Barnhart K, van Mello NM, Bourne T, et al. Pregnancy of unknown location: a consensus statement of nomenclature, definitions, and outcome. Fertil Steril 2011;95:857–66.

35. Kirk E, Condous G, Bourne T. Pregnancies of unknown location. Best Pract Res Clin Obstet Gynaecol 2009;23:493–9.

36. Jurkovic D, Overton C, Bender-Atik R. Diagnosis and management of first trimester miscarriage. BMJ 2013;346:f3676.

37. Paspulati RM, Turgut AT, Bhatt S, et al. Ultrasound assessment of premenopausal bleeding. Obstet Gynecol Clin North Am 2011;38:115–47, viii.

38. Nyberg DA, Laing FC, Filly RA. Threatened abortion: sonographic distinction of normal and abnormal gestation sacs. Radiology 1986;158:397–400.

39. Dogra V, Paspulati RM, Bhatt S. First trimester bleeding evaluation. Ultrasound Q 2005;21:69–85 [quiz: 149–50, 153–4].

40. Bennett GL, Bromley B, Lieberman E, et al. Subchorionic hemorrhage in first-trimester pregnancies: prediction of pregnancy outcome with sonography. Radiology 1996;200:803–6.

41. Sellmyer MA, Desser TS, Maturen KE, et al. Physiologic, histologic, and imaging features of retained products of conception. Radiographics 2013;33: 781–96.

42. Steinkeler J, Coldwell BJ, Warner MA. Ultrasound of the postpartum uterus. Ultrasound Q 2012;28: 97–103.

43. Brown CE, Stettler RW, Twickler D, et al. Puerperal septic pelvic thrombophlebitis: incidence and response to heparin therapy. Am J Obstet Gynecol 1999;181:143–8.

44. Kamaya A, Shin L, Chen B, et al. Emergency gynecologic imaging. Semin Ultrasound CT MR 2008; 29:353–68.

45. Shanbhogue AK, Menias CO, Lalwani N, et al. Obstetric (nonfetal) complications. Radiol Clin North Am 2013;51:983–1004.

46. Lee HJ, Norwitz ER, Shaw J. Contemporary management of fibroids in pregnancy. Rev Obstet Gynecol 2010;3:20–7.

47. Practice Committee of American Society for Reproductive Medicine. Ovarian hyperstimulation syndrome. Fertil Steril 2008;90:S188–93.

48. Laing FC, Benson CB, DiSalvo DN, et al. Distal ureteral calculi: detection with vaginal US. Radiology 1994;192:545–8.

49. Jeffrey RB, Jain KA, Nghiem HV. Sonographic diagnosis of acute appendicitis: interpretive pitfalls. AJR Am J Roentgenol 1994;162:55–9.

50. Pradel JA, Adell JF, Taourel P, et al. Acute colonic diverticulitis: prospective comparative evaluation with US and CT. Radiology 1997;205:503–12.

51. Zielke A, Hasse C, Nies C, et al. Prospective evaluation of ultrasonography in acute colonic diverticulitis. Br J Surg 1997;84:385–8.

52. Baltarowich OH, Scoutt LM, Hamper UM. Nongynecologic findings on pelvic ultrasound: focus on gastrointestinal diseases. Ultrasound Q 2012;28: 65–85.

53. Mathias SD, Kuppermann M, Liberman RF, et al. Chronic pelvic pain: prevalence, health-related quality of life, and economic correlates. Obstet Gynecol 1996;87:321–7.

54. Chamie LP, Blasbalg R, Pereira RM, et al. Findings of pelvic endometriosis at transvaginal US, MR imaging, and laparoscopy. Radiographics 2011; 31:E77–100.

55. Friedman H, Vogelzang RL, Mendelson EB, et al. Endometriosis detection by US with laparoscopic correlation. Radiology 1985;157:217–20.

56. Patel MD, Feldstein VA, Chen DC, et al. Endometriomas: diagnostic performance of US. Radiology 1999;210:739–45.

57. Kuligowska E, Deeds L 3rd, Lu K 3rd. Pelvic pain: overlooked and underdiagnosed gynecologic conditions. Radiographics 2005;25:3–20.

58. Bromley B, Shipp TD, Benacerraf B. Adenomyosis: sonographic findings and diagnostic accuracy. J Ultrasound Med 2000;19:529–34 [quiz: 535–6].

59. Dueholm M. Transvaginal ultrasound for diagnosis of adenomyosis: a review. Best Pract Res Clin Obstet Gynaecol 2006;20:569–82.

60. Reinhold C, Tafazoli F, Mehio A, et al. Uterine adenomyosis: endovaginal US and MR imaging features with histopathologic correlation. Radiographics 1999;19(Spec No):S147–60.

61. Atri M, Reinhold C, Mehio AR, et al. Adenomyosis: US features with histologic correlation in an in-vitro study. Radiology 2000;215:783–90.

62. Webb EM, Green GE, Scoutt LM. Adnexal mass with pelvic pain. Radiol Clin North Am 2004;42: 329–48.

63. Durham JD, Machan L. Pelvic congestion syndrome. Semin Intervent Radiol 2013;30:372–80.

64. Park SJ, Lim JW, Ko YT, et al. Diagnosis of pelvic congestion syndrome using transabdominal and transvaginal sonography. AJR Am J Roentgenol 2004;182:683–8.

65. Vallerie AM, Lerner JP, Wright JD, et al. Peritoneal inclusion cysts: a review. Obstet Gynecol Surv 2009;64:321–34.

66. Ross MJ, Welch WR, Scully RE. Multilocular peritoneal inclusion cysts (so-called cystic mesotheliomas). Cancer 1989;64:1336–46.

67. Hosseinzadeh K, Heller MT, Houshmand G. Imaging of the female perineum in adults. Radiographics 2012;32:E129–68.

Ultrasonography Evaluation of Pelvic Masses

Linda C. Chu, MD[a],*, Stephanie F. Coquia, MD[a],
Ulrike M. Hamper, MD, MBA[b]

KEYWORDS

- Pelvic sonography • Uterine fibroid • Adenomyosis • Endometrial hyperplasia
- Endometrial carcinoma • Cervical cancer • Ovarian cysts • Ovarian neoplasms

KEY POINTS

- Ultrasonography is the primary imaging modality for evaluation of pelvic masses.
- Both real-time imaging and three-dimensional ultrasonography are important in identifying the organ of origin, which helps narrow the differential diagnosis.
- Many pelvic masses have characteristic sonographic appearances that allow confident diagnosis.
- Clinical factors such as age, menstrual status, and symptoms are important in the management of pelvic masses.

INTRODUCTION

Ultrasonography (US) is the primary imaging modality for evaluation of pelvic masses, both for symptomatic pelvic masses and asymptomatic pelvic masses that are incidentally detected on physical examination or other imaging modalities. US has the advantage of being inexpensive, widely available, and offering superior tissue characterization compared with computed tomography (CT). The real-time imaging ability of US and three-dimensional US (3DUS) also has the advantage of being better able to identify the organ of origin of the pelvic mass compared with CT and magnetic resonance (MR). Many pelvic masses have characteristic sonographic appearances that allow confident diagnosis and management (**Box 1**). This article reviews the sonographic appearances and management of common pelvic masses encountered in a nonpregnant women, and is organized based on anatomic location: uterus, cervix, ovaries, and fallopian tubes.

NORMAL ANATOMY AND IMAGING TECHNIQUE

Pelvic US is optimally performed using both the transabdominal (TA) and transvaginal (TV) techniques. The TA examination is performed using transducers with frequencies of up to 5 MHz through the anterior abdominal wall using the distended urinary bladder as an acoustic window. The TV examination is performed with the patient's bladder empty using an endovaginal transducer with frequencies of 7.5 MHz or higher.[1] The TA examination serves as a general overview of the pelvic anatomy. The TV examination provides better anatomic detail, tissue characterization, and evaluation of vascular flow at the cost of a more limited field of view.

Disclosures: The authors have nothing to disclose.
[a] The Russell H. Morgan Department of Radiology and Radiological Science, Johns Hopkins University School of Medicine, Johns Hopkins Medical Institutions, JHOC 3142, 601 North Caroline Street, Baltimore, MD 21287, USA; [b] The Russell H. Morgan Department of Radiology and Radiological Science, Johns Hopkins University School of Medicine, 1800 Orleans Street, Suite 4030A, Baltimore, MD 21287, USA
* Corresponding author.
E-mail address: lindachu@jhmi.edu

Radiol Clin N Am 52 (2014) 1237–1252
http://dx.doi.org/10.1016/j.rcl.2014.07.003

The normal uterus can have different orientations within the pelvis but is most commonly anteverted with the entire uterus tilted forward toward the anterior abdominal wall. The uterus is composed of the endometrium, junctional zone, and myometrium. The sonographic appearance of the endometrium varies during the monthly menstrual cycle. During the proliferative phase, the hyperechoic endometrial complex increases from 2 to 3 mm to 8 mm in thickness. A trilaminated appearance with alternating hyperechoic (3) and hypoechoic (2) layers is typically seen at midcycle. During the proliferative phase, the endometrium further thickens to 15 mm or more and becomes more homogeneous.[1] The junctional zone, which represents the innermost layer of the myometrium, is the anatomic boundary between the endometrium and the myometrium and is not always detected by US.

The ovaries vary in size during each menstrual cycle because of the varying number and sizes of follicles. The reported maximum volumes of the ovaries are 9.0 mL for nulliparous and 15.0 mL for parous women. During the estrogen phase (before ovulation), the dominant follicle progressively grows in size and attains a diameter of 20 to 25 mm by midcycle. This mature follicle ruptures and releases its egg at midcycle and becomes the corpus luteum of menses during the progesterone phase.[2] The normal fallopian tubes are not usually identified on US unless surrounded by ascites.

IMAGING FINDINGS AND DISORDERS
Uterine Masses

Uterine fibroids or leiomyomas are the most common benign uterine tumors, observed on US in up to 24% of premenopausal women.[3] Predictors of increased incidence of fibroids include African American race, nulliparity, obesity, and positive family history of fibroids.[4] The most common sonographic appearance of a fibroid is a solid hypoechoic mass with posterior acoustic shadowing and/or edge refraction (**Fig. 1**, **Table 1**).[5] Fibroids, especially if greater than 3 to 5 cm in diameter, can occasionally undergo necrosis and calcification, which may result in a more heterogeneous echotexture. Areas of calcifications can be identified as well-defined hyperechoic areas with posterior acoustic shadowing.[1] Although most fibroids are intramural and are surrounded by myometrium, fibroids can also be submucosal or subserosal in location, and may mimic an endometrial (**Fig. 2**) or adnexal mass, respectively.[5] Real-time examination is important in showing the attachment of a subserosal fibroid to the myometrium or a tissue plane separating a submucosal fibroid from the endometrial complex. In rare cases, a saline infusion sonohysterogram (SIS) or 3DUS (see **Fig. 2**) is helpful in differentiating a submucosal fibroid from an endometrial mass. The claw sign and visualization of bridging vessels crossing between the uterus and an adnexal mass are important clues to the diagnosis of an exophytic subserosal fibroid rather than a solid ovarian mass.[5]

Adenomyosis is the presence of ectopic endometrial glands and stroma within the myometrium.[6] Both diffuse and focal forms of adenomyosis can be confused with uterine fibroids.[7] Sonographic findings of adenomyosis include globular uterine enlargement, cystic anechoic spaces in the myometrium (**Fig. 3**), linear hyperechoic bands or nodules extending deep into the myometrium, diffuse

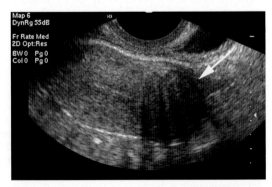

Fig. 1. Uterine fibroid. Gray-scale transverse US image shows classic hypoechoic mass with posterior acoustic shadowing (*arrow*).

Table 1 Differential diagnosis and classic sonographic features of uterine masses	
Fibroid	Solid hypoechoic mass with posterior acoustic shadowing Necrosis and calcifications can result in heterogeneous echotexture
Adenomyosis	Diffuse heterogeneous echotexture of myometrium without discrete mass Cystic anechoic spaces in myometrium
Lipoleiomyoma	Hyperechoic uterine mass indicates fat content
Sarcoma	Unusually large heterogeneous mass Increase in size in postmenopausal woman

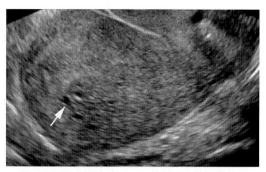

Fig. 3. Adenomyosis. Gray-scale sagittal US image shows diffuse heterogeneous echotexture of the uterus with cystic anechoic spaces within the myometrium (*arrow*).

heterogeneous echotexture of the myometrium without a discrete mass, comblike shadowing from the myometrium, and thickening of the junctional zone (see **Table 1**).[6,7] In uncertain cases, pelvic MR can be helpful in differentiating adenomyosis from fibroids.

A lipoleiomyoma is a rare benign tumor composed of smooth muscle, fat, and fibrous tissue, with a reported incidence of 0.03%.[5] The characteristic echogenic appearance with posterior attenuation indicates fat content within the uterine mass and is diagnostic of a lipoleiomyoma (**Fig. 4**, see **Table 1**).

Uterine sarcomas may develop de novo or be caused by malignant degeneration of a uterine fibroid. There is no specific sonographic finding that can reliably differentiate a uterine sarcoma

from a benign uterine fibroid. Visualization of a large heterogeneous vascular myometrial mass, rapid increase in size of a fibroid in a postmenopausal woman, and associated ascites may suggest the diagnosis of uterine sarcoma (see **Table 1**).[1,5]

Endometrial Masses

The normal thickness of the endometrial complex varies greatly during the menstrual cycle. The endometrial complex should measure 5 mm or less in a postmenopausal woman. The risk of endometrial carcinoma is related to the thickness of the endometrial complex, premenopausal or postmenopausal status, and any associated vaginal bleeding. Risk factors for endometrial cancer include obesity, diabetes, polycystic ovarian syndrome, nulliparity, hypertension, unopposed estrogen replacement therapy, and tamoxifen therapy.[8] In women with postmenopausal bleeding, an endometrial thickness of 5 mm has been reported to have a 96% sensitivity in the

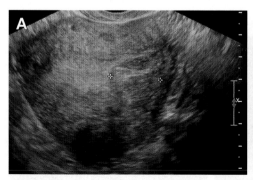

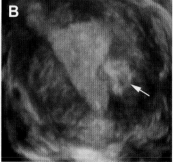

Fig. 2. Submucosal fibroid. (*A*) Gray-scale coronal US image shows a mass arising from the junction of the myometrium and endometrium (*calipers*), which may represent a submucosal fibroid or an endometrial mass. (*B*) 3DUS rendering more clearly shows that the submucosal fibroid (*arrow*) is separate from the endometrial complex.

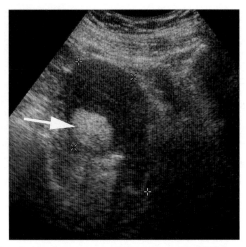

Fig. 4. Lipoleiomyoma. Gray-scale sagittal US image shows a well-circumscribed hyperechoic mass (*arrow*) arising from the uterus, with hyperechoic component indicating fat content of the mass.

Table 2 Differential diagnosis and classic sonographic features of endometrial masses	
Endometrial hyperplasia	Focal or diffuse thickening of endometrial complex Preservation of endometrial-myometrial interface
Endometrial polyp	Hyperechoic mass with vascular stalk
Endometrial carcinoma	Thickened heterogeneous endometrium with increased internal vascularity Disruption of endometrial-myometrial interface
Tamoxifen effect	Thickened endometrium with multiple cystic spaces

detection of endometrial cancer and a 92% sensitivity in the detection of endometrial disease, including cancer, polyp, and atypical hyperplasia.[9] However, the findings are nonspecific and other causes of a thickened endometrium in a postmenopausal woman include endometrial hyperplasia, endometrial polyp, and endometrial carcinoma.

Endometrial hyperplasia is a histologic diagnosis characterized by overgrowth of glands with or without stromal proliferation. Endometrial hyperplasia appears as focal or diffuse thickening of the endometrial complex with preservation of the endometrial-myometrial interface (**Table 2**).[10] However, because endometrial hyperplasia cannot reliably be differentiated from endometrial cancer, a thickened endometrium greater than 5 mm in a woman with postmenopausal bleeding warrants endometrial biopsy.[10] The risk of endometrial cancer in postmenopausal women without vaginal bleeding is low compared with symptomatic women with postmenopausal bleeding. An endometrium thickness of greater than 11 mm has been proposed as a threshold for pursuing endometrial biopsy in postmenopausal women without vaginal bleeding.[11]

An endometrial polyp (**Fig. 5**) is a circumscribed overgrowth of endometrial mucosa. Polyps may be single or multiple, and may be sessile or pedunculated.[10,12] The prevalence of endometrial polyps increases with age and ranges from 7.8% to 34.9%. Risk factors for endometrial polyps include hypertension, obesity, and tamoxifen use.[12] The classic appearance of an endometrial polyp is a hyperechoic mass surrounded by more hypoechoic endometrium with a vascular stalk (see **Fig. 5**, **Table 2**). However, polyps may appear sonographically as diffusely thickened endometrium without identification of a discrete mass mimicking the sonographic appearance of endometrial hyperplasia.

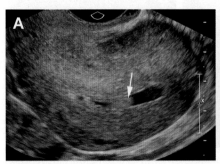
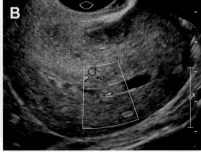

Fig. 5. Endometrial polyp. (*A*) Gray-scale sagittal US image shows a polypoid mass within the endometrial cavity (*arrow*), outlined by spontaneously occurring fluid within the endometrial cavity. (*B*) Color Doppler sagittal US image shows presence of internal vascularity within the endometrial polyp.

A   **B**

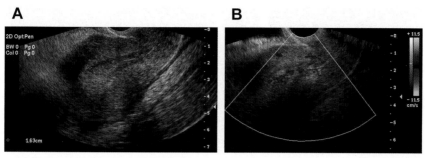

Fig. 6. Endometrial cancer. Gray-scale sagittal US image shows abnormal thickening of the endometrial complex measuring 16 mm (*calipers*) without a discrete focal mass in a postmenopausal woman (*A*), with markedly increased internal vascularity on color Doppler image (*B*).

SIS and/or 3DUS may be helpful in differentiating an endometrial polyp from endometrial hyperplasia in such cases.[10,13,14] A small amount of spontaneous endometrial fluid, if present, may be helpful, simulating a naturally occurring sonohysterogram (see **Fig. 5**).[14] Most endometrial polyps are benign, with malignant transformation reported in up to 12.9% of polyps.[12]

Endometrial carcinoma is the fourth most common cancer and the most common invasive gynecologic cancer in the United States.[15] Sonographic features of endometrial carcinoma (**Fig. 6**) include a focal endometrial mass, an enlarged or globular uterus,[10] thickened endometrium and increased endometrium volume,[16] heterogeneous echotexture of the endometrium,[17,18] increased internal vascularity, fluid collection in the endometrial cavity, and disruption of the endometrial-myometrial interface (see **Table 2**).[19] Disruption of the endometrial-myometrial interface is the most specific sonographic finding. Transvaginal US may be helpful in evaluating myometrial invasion to differentiate between stage IA disease (<50% myometrial invasion) and stage IB disease (>50% myometrial invasion). Studies have compared the accuracy of preoperative transvaginal US in assessment of myometrial invasion with surgical specimens, with reported accuracies ranging from 73% to 84%.[20,21] Contrast-enhanced MR imaging has the highest reported overall staging accuracy, ranging from 85% to 93%, and remains the preferred imaging modality for preoperative planning.[15]

Patients with estrogen receptor–positive breast cancer are frequently treated with long-term tamoxifen or other serum estrogen receptor modulator therapies. Tamoxifen is a mixed estrogen agonist/antagonist that has antagonist effects on estrogen receptors in breast tissue and agonist effects on the endometrium. Tamoxifen can cause endometrial hyperplasia, polyps, and endometrial carcinoma. The most common sonographic

appearance of tamoxifen's effect is thickening of the endometrium with multiple anechoic small cystic spaces (**Fig. 7**, see **Table 2**).[22] In two-thirds of patients the endometrial thickness measures greater than 8 mm on transvaginal US, but half of these women have endometrial atrophy on hysteroscopy and/or curettage. This discordance between apparent increased endometrial thickness on US and hysteroscopy may be caused by subendometrial changes rather than true endometrial growth.[23] Therefore, US screening of endometrial cancer is considered problematic in current clinical practice in such patients despite the increased risk of endometrial cancer, and most clinicians recommend that postmenopausal women on tamoxifen therapy with vaginal bleeding should be screened with hysteroscopy.[13]

Cervical Masses

Cervical polyps are the most common mass lesions of the cervix, with a reported prevalence of 1.5% to 10%. Cervical polyps are considered to be focal hyperplastic protrusions of endocervical

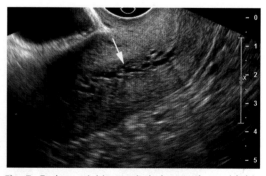

Fig. 7. Endometrial hyperplasia in a patient with history of tamoxifen treatment of breast cancer with characteristic cystic appearance of thickened endometrial complex measuring up to 10 mm (*arrow*) on gray-scale sagittal US image.

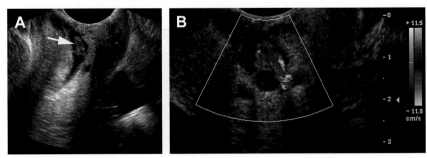

Fig. 8. Cervical polyp. (*A*) Gray-scale sagittal US image shows a polypoid mass (*arrow*) in the cervical canal. Differential diagnosis includes cervical polyp, cervical cancer, prolapsing endometrial polyp, and prolapsing fibroid. (*B*) Color Doppler transverse US image shows vascular stalk attaching to cervix, confirming diagnosis of cervical polyp.

folds rather than true neoplasms.[24] Most patients present during the perimenopausal period in the fifth decade of life. Patients may present with menorrhagia, postmenopausal bleeding, and vaginal discharge.[25] On US, cervical polyps appear as sessile or pedunculated well-circumscribed, hypoechoic or echogenic masses within the endocervical canal (**Fig. 8**).[26] Differential diagnosis of a polypoid mass within the cervical canal includes cervical polyp, cervical cancer, prolapsing endometrial polyp, and prolapsing fibroid. Identification of the vascular stalk attaching the polyp to the cervical wall helps to confirm the diagnosis of cervical polyp (see **Fig. 8**). Approximately 0.1% of cervical polyps are associated with malignancy, and approximately 10% of patients with cervical polyps also have coexisting endometrial disorders (eg, hyperplasia, polyp, and carcinoma).[24]

Cervical cancer is the third most common cancer in women worldwide and is most common in developing countries. Risk factors for cervical cancer include infections with high-risk human papillomavirus (types 16 and 18), oral contraceptive pills, low socioeconomic status, smoking, multiple sexual partners, human immunodeficiency virus

infection, and other sexually transmitted diseases.[8] Cervical cancer arises almost exclusively along the squamocolumnar junction between the columnar cells of the endocervical glands and the squamous epithelium of the cervix. In young women, the squamocolumnar junction is located outside the external os and cervical cancers tend to grow outward. In elderly patients, the squamocolumnar junction is located within the cervical canal and tumors tend to grow inward along the cervical canal.[25] On US, cervical cancer appears as a heterogeneous mass in the cervix (**Fig. 9**) that may show increased internal vascularity.[27] With locally advanced disease, tumor infiltrates the fibrous cervical stroma and invades the parametrium. Although cervical cancer is staged clinically, MR and US may be helpful in identifying resectable disease (stage IIA and below) versus locally advanced disease (stage IIB and above) by identification of tumor size (<4 cm vs >4 cm), parametrial invasion, and tumor invasion into lower one-third of vagina and adjacent pelvic organs. The presence of hydronephrosis implies stage IIIB disease with tumor extending to the pelvic side wall.

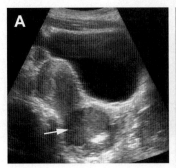
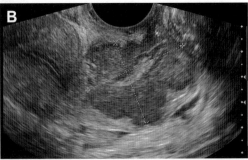

Fig. 9. Cervical cancer. (*A*) Transabdominal sagittal US image shows a mass (*arrow*) with heterogeneous echotexture arising from the cervix. (*B*) Transvaginal sagittal US image betters shows the heterogeneous echotexture and contour irregularity of the cervical cancer (*calipers*).

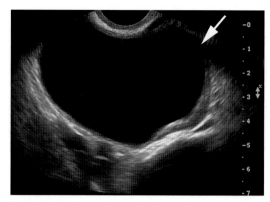

Fig. 10. Simple ovarian cyst. Gray-scale transverse US image shows a 7.9 cm × 4.8 cm well-circumscribed thin-walled anechoic structure (*arrow*).

> Box 2
> **Differential diagnosis of ovarian masses**
>
> Simple cyst
>
> Hemorrhagic cyst
>
> Endometrioma
>
> Tubo-ovarian abscess
>
> Ovarian torsion
>
> Ovarian neoplasms

Ovarian Masses

Optimal management of ovarian masses depends on sonographic features of the masses, menopausal status of the patient, and patients' clinical symptoms. In 2010, the Society of Radiologists in Ultrasound published guidelines regarding management of ovarian and adnexal cysts in asymptomatic women (**Box 2**).[28]

A simple cyst on US appears as a round or oval anechoic structure with smooth, thin walls; posterior acoustic enhancement; no solid component or septations; and no internal vascularity on color Doppler (**Box 3, Fig. 10**).[28] Simple cysts of up to 10 cm in a patient of any age are highly likely to be benign.[29,30] In premenopausal women, simple cysts less than or equal to 3 cm in diameter are considered physiologic and do not require follow-up.[31] Simple cysts greater than 3 cm and less than or equal to 5 cm are almost certainly benign and do not need follow-up, although they should be mentioned in the report. Annual follow-up is recommended for simple cysts greater than 5 cm and less than or equal to 7 cm in diameter. In postmenopausal women, simple cysts greater than 1 cm and less than or equal to 7 cm are almost certainly benign, and yearly follow-up is recommended, at least initially. For simple cysts greater than 7 cm, MR or surgical evaluation is recommended for further evaluation because small mural nodules can be missed in these large lesions (**Table 3**).[28]

Hemorrhagic ovarian cysts are caused by hemorrhage within a corpus luteum or other functional cysts. Imaging appearances can be variable depending on the age of the blood products. Hemorrhagic cysts are classically described on US as complex cystic masses with reticular or lacelike internal echoes or more homogeneous solid-appearing areas with straight or concave margins. In either case, no internal blood flow should be demonstrable on Doppler interrogation (**Box 4, Fig. 11**).[32,33] Hemorrhagic cysts usually resolve within 8 weeks.[34] According to current guidelines, in premenopausal women, hemorrhagic cysts less than or equal to 5 cm in diameter with a classic US appearance (lacelike reticular pattern of internal echoes or retractile clot) do not need follow-up, and hemorrhagic cysts greater than 5 cm should be followed up with US in 6 to 12 weeks to ensure resolution or expected change in appearance. Early in menopause, women may occasionally ovulate and develop hemorrhagic cysts, but they are less common. Therefore, in this age group it is recommended that even classic-appearing hemorrhagic cysts less than or equal to 5 cm should get US follow-up in 6 to 12 weeks to ensure

> Box 3
> **Classic sonographic features of simple ovary cyst**
>
> Anechoic structure with smooth, thin walls
>
> Posterior acoustic enhancement
>
> No solid component or septations
>
> No internal flow

Table 3 Management of simple ovarian cysts	
Premenopausal Women	**Postmenopausal Women**
≤5 cm: no follow-up necessary >5 and ≤7 cm: yearly follow-up	>1 and ≤7 cm: yearly follow-up
>7 cm: MR or surgical evaluation	>7 cm: MR or surgical evaluation

Box 4
Classic sonographic features of hemorrhagic ovarian cysts

Complex cystic mass with reticular internal echoes

Homogeneous-appearing areas with concave margins

No internal flow

Table 4
Management of hemorrhagic ovarian cysts

Premenopausal Women	Early Menopause	Late Menopause
≤5 cm: no follow-up necessary >5 cm: follow-up in 6–12 wk	Any size: follow-up in 6–12 wk	Any size: surgical evaluation

resolution. In late menopause, women do not ovulate and should not develop hemorrhagic cysts. Hence, any ovarian masses in women in late menopause that resemble hemorrhagic cysts should be considered neoplastic and surgical evaluation or MR imaging is recommended (**Table 4**).[28]

Endometriomas are focal cystic fluid collections arising from functional endometrial glands outside the uterus. Endometriomas usually present as unilocular single or multiple complex cystic structures with homogeneous low-level internal echoes (the so-called ground-glass appearance), without solid components or internal flow (**Box 5, Fig. 12**).[28] The presence of multiple lesions and/or tiny echogenic mural foci can help differentiate endometriomas from acute hemorrhagic cysts.[33,35,36] In premenopausal women, follow-up in 6 to 12 weeks can be useful to help differentiate acute hemorrhagic cysts from endometriomas. If an endometrioma is not removed surgically, it should be followed up with US at least yearly to ensure stability in size and sonographic appearance.[28] About 1% of endometriomas are thought to undergo

Box 5
Classic sonographic features of endometriomas

Cystic mass with low-level internal echoes, with or without tiny echogenic wall foci

No solid component

No internal flow

malignant transformation, typically developing endometrioid or clear cell carcinomas.[37] Malignancy is uncommon in endometriomas smaller than 6 cm, with most malignancies occurring in endometriomas larger than 9 cm.[37,38]

Pelvic inflammatory disease is an ascending infection from the vagina involving the cervix, uterus, fallopian tubes, and/or ovaries, usually caused by polymicrobial infection (*Chlamydia trachomatis* or *Neisseria gonorrhoeae*). Patients typically present with fever, acute pelvic pain, cervical motion tenderness, vaginal discharge, and leukocytosis.[39,40] Infection involving the fallopian tube and ovary can lead to formation of a tubo-ovarian

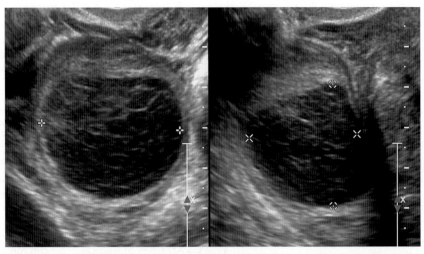

Fig. 11. Hemorrhagic cyst. Gray-scale coronal and sagittal US images show a well-circumscribed 3.6 cm × 2.8 cm × 3.0 cm cystic structure with characteristic fishnet or lacelike appearance of a hemorrhagic cyst (*calipers*).

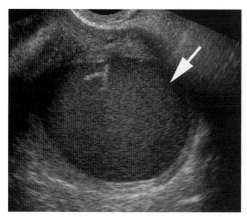

Fig. 12. Endometrioma. Gray-scale coronal US image shows a well-circumscribed cystic structure with homogeneous low-level internal echoes; the so-called ground-glass appearance (arrow).

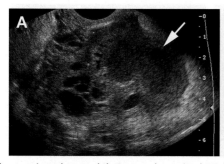 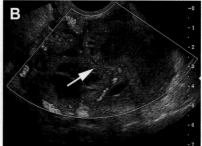

Fig. 13. Tubo-ovarian abscess. (A) Gray-scale sagittal US image shows a heterogeneous thick-walled mass with low-level internal echoes (arrow) intimately associated with the ovary. (B) Color Doppler sagittal US image shows increased vascularity along the periphery of the tubo-ovarian abscess (arrow).

Box 6
Classic sonographic features of tubo-ovarian abscess

Complex thick-walled fluid collection

Internal septations and fluid debris levels

Increased peripheral vascularity

abscess. The typical sonographic appearance of a tubo-ovarian abscess is of a multiseptated, complex, thick-walled fluid collection in the adnexa (Fig. 13), which may contain internal septations, fluid debris levels, gas, and increased peripheral vascularity on color Doppler images (Box 6).[39,41]

Ovarian torsion is defined as partial or complete twisting of the ovary or fallopian tube around its vascular pedicle and accounts for 3% of all gynecologic emergencies.[42] Patients present with sudden-onset abdominal pain, nausea, vomiting, palpable pelvic mass, and sometimes mild leukocytosis or low-grade fever.[40] The presence of an ipsilateral adnexal mass larger than 5 cm is the most common risk factor for ovarian torsion in adults and has been reported in 22% to 73% of cases.[39] The sonographic appearance of ovarian torsion is variable and depends on the degree and chronicity of the vascular compromise. The typical sonographic appearance of acute ovarian torsion is an enlarged ovary with multiple peripheral follicles from vascular congestion (Fig. 14).

Absence of arterial flow is a highly specific finding for ovarian torsion (see Fig. 14); however, the presence of arterial and venous flow does not exclude torsion, because torsion can be intermittent. Additional sonographic findings include an abnormal, often midline location of the torsed ovary with the twisted ovarian vessels seen adjacent to the ovary creating a target sign on gray-scale US or the whirlpool sign on color Doppler US. Chronic torsion can result in a more heterogeneous appearance caused by necrosis and hemorrhage that may mimic a cystic ovarian mass (Box 7). Absence of vascular flow and clinical presentation are important clues to the correct diagnosis.

Ovarian neoplasms can be categorized based on cell type of origin into epithelial tumors (75%), germ cell tumors (15%–20%), sex cord–stromal tumors (5%–10%), and metastatic tumors (1%–5%). Epithelial ovarian tumors can be subclassified as benign, borderline, or malignant, according to their histologic features and clinical behavior.[31] Serous tumors are the most common epithelial tumors and serous epithelial cystadenocarcinomas account for 60% to 80% of all epithelial malignancies of the ovary. Serous cystadenomas generally present as unilocular cystic adnexal lesions. Serous epithelial cystadenocarcinomas (Fig. 15) are typically more heterogeneous in appearance, with solid components, papillary projections, and internal vascularity (Table 5).[31] Mucinous tumors are typically large and multilocular with numerous smooth, thin septations containing mucoid

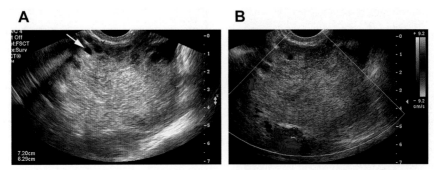

Fig. 14. Ovarian torsion. (*A*) Gray-scale sagittal US image shows a 7.2 cm × 6.3 cm enlarged right ovary with heterogeneous echotexture and multiple peripheral follicles (*arrow*). (*B*) Color Doppler sagittal US image shows lack of vascular flow within the ovary, which is highly concerning for ovarian torsion.

Box 7
Classic sonographic features of ovarian torsion

Unilaterally enlarged ovary with multiple peripheral follicles

Absence of arterial and/or venous flow

Twisted vascular pedicle with target or whirlpool sign

Heterogeneous appearance from necrosis and hemorrhage in chronic torsion

Table 5
Differential diagnosis and sonographic features of ovarian neoplasms

Serous cystadenoma/ cystadenocarcinomas	Cystic solid mass with papillary projections Internal vascularity
Mucinous cystadenoma/ cystadenocarcinoma	Large multilocular cystic mass Thin-walled cysts with low-level internal echoes Thin, multiple septations
Mature cystic teratoma	Focal or diffuse hyperechoic components Hyperechoic lines and dots Acoustic shadowing No internal flow
Sex cord–stromal tumors	Homogeneous solid mass

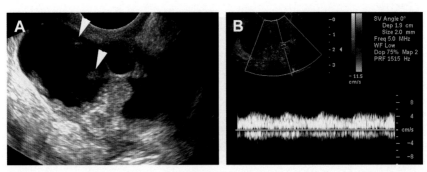

Fig. 15. Ovarian serous cystadenocarcinoma. Gray-scale coronal US image (*A*) shows a complex cystic mass with thick papillary projections along the periphery of the mass (*arrowheads*). Color Doppler coronal image (*B*) shows flow within the solid nodular components of the mass.

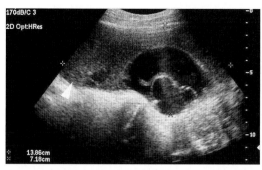

Fig. 16. Ovarian mucinous cystadenoma. Gray-scale sagittal US image shows a 13.9 cm × 7.2 cm complex cystic mass with mixed anechoic and hypoechoic components (*arrowhead*) and multiple thick internal septations. There is no reliable sonographic feature that can differentiate this benign ovarian neoplasm from malignant ovarian neoplasm.

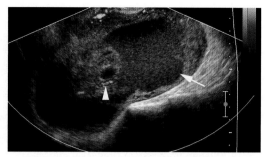

Fig. 17. Ovarian mucinous cystadenocarcinoma. Power Doppler sagittal US image shows a 15.1 cm × 10.1 cm × 11.1 cm complex cystic and solid mass with low-level internal echoes within the cystic component (*arrow*) and internal vascularity within the solid component (*arrowhead*).

material with low-level internal echoes (**Figs. 16** and **17**, see **Table 5**). Different locules may have different levels of echogenicity.

The most common germ cell tumors are mature cystic teratomas, which account for 15% to 20% of ovarian neoplasms and are bilateral in 10% to 15% of patients. Classic sonographic features of a mature cystic teratoma, or dermoid, include focal or diffuse hyperechoic components with posterior attenuation, fat-fluid levels, hyperechoic lines and dots (dot-dash or dermoid mesh appearance), hyperechoic areas with posterior acoustic shadowing, (caused by bone or teeth), mobile spherical masses (caused by hair balls), mural hyperechoic Rokitansky nodules, and absence of internal flow on color Doppler imaging (**Fig. 18**, see **Table 5**).[43–45] Complications include torsion, rupture causing chemical peritonitis, and malignant transformation. Malignant transformation has been reported in 0.17% to 2% of dermoids, and is almost exclusively caused by squamous cell carcinoma. Malignant transformation tends to occur in

women older than 50 years and in tumors larger than 10 cm. Sonographic features suggesting malignant transformation include presence of solid components with Doppler-detectable internal blood flow and invasion of adjacent organs. Ovarian masses with features classic for a dermoid should be followed at an initial interval of between 6 months and 1 year, and then yearly, if they are not surgically removed.[28]

Sex cord–stromal tumors include granulosa cell tumors, thecomas, fibromas, and Sertoli-Leydig cell tumors. These tumors are usually unilateral and appear homogeneous and mostly solid (**Fig. 19**, see **Table 5**). These tumors may appear as partly solid, partly cystic masses.[31] Granulosa cell tumors are divided into adult and juvenile types. The adult type accounts for 95% of all granulosa cell tumors and occurs predominantly in perimenopausal and postmenopausal women, with peak prevalence at 50 to 55 years of age. Juvenile granulosa cell tumors occur in patients younger than 30 years of age.[46] Granulosa cell tumors produce estrogen and the hyperestrogenemia may result in endometrial hyperplasia and

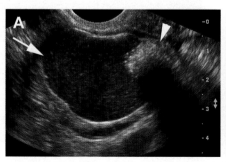
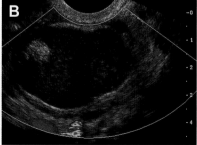

Fig. 18. Mature ovarian teratoma. (*A*) Gray-scale sagittal US image shows a well-circumscribed mass with heterogeneous echotexture with cystic component with low-level internal echoes (*arrow*) and hyperechoic component with posterior shadowing from fat (*arrowhead*). (*B*) Color Doppler coronal US image shows absence of internal vascularity.

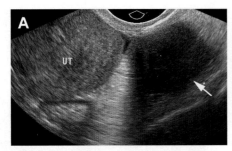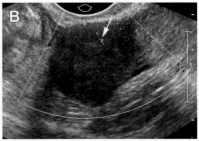

Fig. 19. Ovarian fibroma. (A) Gray-scale sagittal US image shows a well-circumscribed hypoechoic ovarian mass with posterior acoustic shadowing that mimics a fibroid (*arrow*). This mass is separate from the uterus (UT). (B) Color Doppler transverse US image shows internal vascularity within this mass (*arrow*).

polyps, and is associated with endometrial carcinoma in 3% to 25% of patients. Adult patients may present clinically with irregular menstrual bleeding or postmenopausal bleeding. Premenarchal girls with granulosa cell tumors may present with precocious puberty.[46] The sonographic appearance of granulosa cell tumors varies widely, ranging from solid masses, to tumors with varying degrees of hemorrhage or fibrotic changes, to multilocular cystic masses, to completely cystic tumors. Compared with epithelial neoplasms, granulosa cell tumors are unlikely to have intracystic papillary projections, have a lesser propensity for peritoneal seeding, and are usually confined to the ovary at the time of diagnosis.[47]

Fibroma, fibrothecoma, and thecoma form a spectrum of benign ovarian tumors. Fibromas have no thecal cells and have no estrogen activity, whereas lipid-rich thecomas have estrogen activity and few fibroblasts.[46,48] Thecomas or fibrothecomas tend to occur in older women than granulosa cell tumors, with mean age of 59 years. Approximately two-thirds of patients are postmenopausal. Similar to adult granulosa cell tumors, patients with these tumors commonly present with vaginal bleeding and are associated with endometrial hyperplasia and endometrial carcinoma.[46] Imaging appearance of thecomas without prominent fibrosis is similar to that of other solid ovarian tumors and is nonspecific.[46] The presence of collagen and fibrous contents in fibromas leads to the specific sonographic findings of a homogeneous hypoechoic solid mass with posterior shadowing (see Fig. 19).[46] Identification of a feeding vessel may be helpful in distinguishing between an ovarian fibroma and a subserosal fibroid.[47]

Sertoli-Leydig cell tumors are rare, virilizing ovarian tumors and account for less than 0.5% of ovarian tumors. Approximately 75% of Sertoli-Leydig cell tumors occur in patients younger than 30 years of age and 30% of patients present with clinical signs of increased androgen activity, including amenorrhea and virilized secondary sexual characteristics. These tumors have variable imaging appearances, including solid, solid and cystic, and cystic ovarian masses.[48]

Aside from mature cystic teratomas and fibromas, there usually are no distinct sonographic features that can distinguish benign from malignant ovarian neoplasms. In general, ovarian masses with thick, vascular, and numerous internal septations, solid component, and internal vascularity are more worrisome for malignancy and surgical consultation is recommended.[28]

Nonovarian Adnexal Masses

Fallopian tube masses

Hydrosalpinx can develop secondary to obstruction from pelvic adhesions or postinflammatory scarring. It appears as a tubular anechoic adnexal structure that folds on itself showing an incomplete septation sign (Fig. 20) and can mimic a multiseptated adnexal mass. Real-time US or 3DUS imaging is helpful in appreciating the serpiginous tubular structure as a fluid-distended fallopian tube.

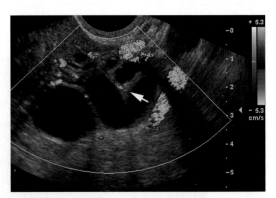

Fig. 20. Hydrosalpinx. Color Doppler coronal image shows a serpiginous anechoic tubular structure in the adnexa. Real-time imaging helps differentiate this tubular structure from complex adnexal cystic mass. Note the incomplete septation sign (*arrow*).

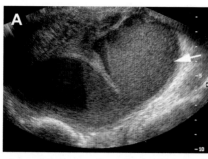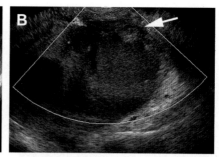

Fig. 21. Pyosalpinx. (*A*) Gray-scale sagittal US image shows serpiginous tubular structure (*arrow*) in the adnexa with low-level internal echoes in a patient with symptoms of pelvic inflammatory disease that indicate pyosalpinx. (*B*) Color Doppler sagittal US image shows peripheral vascularity along the inflamed fallopian tube (*arrow*).

In the setting of pelvic inflammatory disease, presence of low-level echoes or fluid debris levels in a dilated fluid-filled fallopian tube suggest the diagnosis of pyosalpinx (**Fig. 21**). A beads-on-a-string or cogwheel appearance on transverse images with multiple small mural protrusions resulting from inflamed tubal mucosa has also been described.[39]

Primary fallopian tube carcinoma is one of the rarest gynecologic malignancies and accounts for 0.15% to 1.8% of gynecologic malignancies.[49] It can be difficult to differentiate between primary fallopian tube carcinoma and serous epithelial ovarian carcinoma that secondarily involves the fallopian tubes. The proposed diagnostic criteria for primary fallopian tube carcinoma requires at least 1 of the following: (1) main tumor is in the tube and arises from the endosalpinx; (2) on histology the pattern is similar to the epithelium of the tubal mucosa and often shows a papillary pattern; (3) if tubal wall is involved, the transition between benign and malignant epithelium should be demonstrable; and (4) the ovaries and endometrium are either normal or contain less tumor than the tube.[50] Patients usually present in the sixth or seventh decades with pelvic pain, vaginal bleeding, or discharge and pelvic mass. Primary fallopian tube carcinoma usually presents as hydrosalpinx with papillary projections or solid mural nodules.[51,52] The hydrosalpinx may be anechoic or show low-level echoes. Presence of vascularity in the solid mural nodules on color Doppler helps to differentiate tumor from blood clot or debris.[52] Less frequently, primary fallopian tube carcinoma presents as a sausage-shaped solid mass with heterogeneous echogenicity.[51,52] Another characteristic finding of primary fallopian tube carcinoma is the change in shape on serial imaging studies caused by change in the degree of tubal distention.[53]

Paraovarian masses

Paraovarian cysts are benign intraperitoneal mesothelial cysts that arise from the broad ligament of the uterus (hydatid of Morgagni) and account for 10% to 20% of all adnexal masses. The typical sonographic appearance of a paraovarian cyst is a simple, anechoic, unilocular, round or oval cyst that is separate from the ipsilateral ovary (**Fig. 22**).[31] Real-time images are helpful in distinguishing a paraovarian cyst from the adjacent ovary. The recommended follow-up thresholds for simple paraovarian cysts are the same as for simple ovarian cysts.[28] Paraovarian cysts are mostly asymptomatic, but can be complicated by rupture, torsion, and hemorrhage in rare cases.[54–56] The presence of a soft tissue nodule in the cyst may indicate development of a benign or malignant neoplasm, which is a rare complication.[54]

Peritoneal inclusion cysts are intraperitoneal mesothelial cysts that arise secondary to peritoneal insult such as surgery, trauma, endometriosis, and infection. Peritoneal inclusion cysts occur almost exclusively in premenopausal women with active ovaries, pelvic adhesions, and impaired absorption of peritoneal fluid, which leads to formation of fluid-filled cysts that conform to the shape of the peritoneal cavity.[55] Peritoneal inclusion

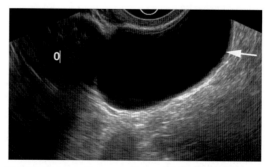

Fig. 22. Paraovarian cyst. Gray-scale sagittal US image shows a 4.5 cm × 2.8 cm well-circumscribed anechoic cystic structure (*arrow*) that is separate from the adjacent normal-appearing ovary (O).

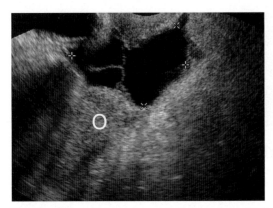

Fig. 23. Peritoneal inclusion cyst. Gray-scale sagittal US image shows a well-circumscribed anechoic cystic structure that is separate from the adjacent normal-appearing ovary (O) in a patient with a history of hysterectomy.

cysts appear as multiloculated, lobular cystic lesions with thin septations with the ovary either at the edge or suspended within the cystic area, which conforms to the appearance of the surrounding pelvic structures (**Fig. 23**).[31]

SUMMARY

Management of pelvic masses often depends on clinical information such as age, menstrual status, and symptoms. US should be the first-line imaging modality for pelvic masses and can narrow the differential diagnosis based on organ of origin and characteristic sonographic appearance of these pelvic masses. Familiarity with a variety of typical sonographic appearances and management of these pelvic masses enables the radiologist to help referring clinicians manage this commonly encountered clinical problem.

REFERENCES

1. Middleton WD, Kurtz AB, Hertzberg BS. Pelvis and uterus. Ultrasound: the requisites. 2nd edition. St Louis (MO): Mosby; 2004. p. 530–57.
2. Middleton WD, Kurtz AB, Hertzberg BS. Adnexa. Ultrasound: the requisites. 2nd edition. St Louis (MO): Mosby; 2004. p. 558–86.
3. Lurie S, Piper I, Woliovitch I, et al. Age-related prevalence of sonographically confirmed uterine myomas. J Obstet Gynaecol 2005;25(1):42–4.
4. Shwayder J, Sakhel K. Imaging for uterine myomas and adenomyosis. J Minim Invasive Gynecol 2014; 21(3):362–76.
5. Maizlin ZV, Vos PM, Cooperberg PL. Is it a fibroid? Are you sure? Sonography with MRI assistance. Ultrasound Q 2007;23(1):55–62.
6. Sakhel K, Abuhamad A. Sonography of adenomyosis. J Ultrasound Med 2012;31(5):805–8.
7. Valentini AL, Speca S, Gui B, et al. Adenomyosis: from the sign to the diagnosis. Imaging, diagnostic pitfalls and differential diagnosis: a pictorial review. Radiol Med 2011;116(8):1267–87.
8. Tirumani SH, Shanbhogue AK, Prasad SR. Current concepts in the diagnosis and management of endometrial and cervical carcinomas. Radiol Clin North Am 2013;51(6):1087–110.
9. Smith-Bindman R, Kerlikowske K, Feldstein VA, et al. Endovaginal ultrasound to exclude endometrial cancer and other endometrial abnormalities. JAMA 1998;280(17):1510–7.
10. Davidson KG, Dubinsky TJ. Ultrasonographic evaluation of the endometrium in postmenopausal vaginal bleeding. Radiol Clin North Am 2003;41(4):769–80.
11. Smith-Bindman R, Weiss E, Feldstein V. How thick is too thick? When endometrial thickness should prompt biopsy in postmenopausal women without vaginal bleeding. Ultrasound Obstet Gynecol 2004;24(5):558–65.
12. Salim S, Won H, Nesbitt-Hawes E, et al. Diagnosis and management of endometrial polyps: a critical review of the literature. J Minim Invasive Gynecol 2011;18(5):569–81.
13. Dreisler E, Poulsen LG, Antonsen SL, et al. EMAS clinical guide: assessment of the endometrium in peri and postmenopausal women. Maturitas 2013; 75(2):181–90.
14. Goldstein SR. Sonography in postmenopausal bleeding. J Ultrasound Med 2012;31(2):333–6.
15. Lee JH, Dubinsky T, Andreotti RF, et al. ACR Appropriateness Criteria® pretreatment evaluation and follow-up of endometrial cancer of the uterus. Ultrasound Q 2011;27(2):139–45.
16. Gruboeck K, Jurkovic D, Lawton F, et al. The diagnostic value of endometrial thickness and volume measurements by three-dimensional ultrasound in patients with postmenopausal bleeding. Ultrasound Obstet Gynecol 1996;8(4):272–6.
17. Hulka CA, Hall DA, McCarthy K, et al. Endometrial polyps, hyperplasia, and carcinoma in postmenopausal women: differentiation with endovaginal sonography. Radiology 1994;191(3):755–8.
18. Sheikh M, Sawhney S, Khurana A, et al. Alteration of sonographic texture of the endometrium in postmenopausal bleeding. A guide to further management. Acta Obstet Gynecol Scand 2000;79(11): 1006–10.
19. Dubinsky TJ. Value of sonography in the diagnosis of abnormal vaginal bleeding. J Clin Ultrasound 2004;32(7):348–53.
20. Arko D, Takac I. High frequency transvaginal ultrasonography in preoperative assessment of myometrial invasion in endometrial cancer. J Ultrasound Med 2000;19(9):639–43.

21. Savelli L, Ceccarini M, Ludovisi M, et al. Preoperative local staging of endometrial cancer: transvaginal sonography vs. magnetic resonance imaging. Ultrasound Obstet Gynecol 2008;31(5):560–6.

22. Hulka CA, Hall DA. Endometrial abnormalities associated with tamoxifen therapy for breast cancer: sonographic and pathologic correlation. AJR Am J Roentgenol 1993;160(4):809–12.

23. Liedman R, Lindahl B, Andolf E, et al. Disaccordance between estimation of endometrial thickness as measured by transvaginal ultrasound compared with hysteroscopy and directed biopsy in breast cancer patients treated with tamoxifen. Anticancer Res 2000;20(6C):4889–91.

24. Esim Buyukbayrak E, Karageyim Karsidag AY, Kars B, et al. Cervical polyps: evaluation of routine removal and need for accompanying D&C. Arch Gynecol Obstet 2011;283(3):581–4.

25. Okamoto Y, Tanaka YO, Nishida M, et al. MR imaging of the uterine cervix: imaging-pathologic correlation. Radiographics 2003;23(2):425–45 [quiz: 534–5].

26. Sahdev A. Cervical tumors. Semin Ultrasound CT MR 2010;31(5):399–413.

27. Byun JM, Kim YN, Jeong DH, et al. Three-dimensional transvaginal ultrasonography for locally advanced cervical cancer. Int J Gynecol Cancer 2013;23(8):1459–64.

28. Levine D, Brown DL, Andreotti RF, et al. Management of asymptomatic ovarian and other adnexal cysts imaged at US: Society of Radiologists in Ultrasound Consensus Conference Statement. Radiology 2010;256(3):943–54.

29. Ekerhovd E, Wienerroith H, Staudach A, et al. Preoperative assessment of unilocular adnexal cysts by transvaginal ultrasonography: a comparison between ultrasonographic morphologic imaging and histopathologic diagnosis. Am J Obstet Gynecol 2001;184(2):48–54.

30. Modesitt SC, Pavlik EJ, Ueland FR, et al. Risk of malignancy in unilocular ovarian cystic tumors less than 10 centimeters in diameter. Obstet Gynecol 2003;102(3):594–9.

31. Ackerman S, Irshad A, Lewis M, et al. Ovarian cystic lesions: a current approach to diagnosis and management. Radiol Clin North Am 2013; 51(6):1067–85.

32. Patel MD, Feldstein VA, Filly RA. The likelihood ratio of sonographic findings for the diagnosis of hemorrhagic ovarian cysts. J Ultrasound Med 2005;24(5): 607–14 [quiz: 615].

33. Valentin L. Use of morphology to characterize and manage common adnexal masses. Best Pract Res Clin Obstet Gynaecol 2004;18(1):71–89.

34. Okai T, Kobayashi K, Ryo E, et al. Transvaginal sonographic appearance of hemorrhagic functional ovarian cysts and their spontaneous regression. Int J Gynaecol Obstet 1994;44(1):47–52.

35. Patel MD, Feldstein VA, Chen DC, et al. Endometriomas: diagnostic performance of US. Radiology 1999;210(3):739–45.

36. Sokalska A, Timmerman D, Testa AC, et al. Diagnostic accuracy of transvaginal ultrasound examination for assigning a specific diagnosis to adnexal masses. Ultrasound Obstet Gynecol 2009;34(4):462–70.

37. Kawaguchi R, Tsuji Y, Haruta S, et al. Clinicopathologic features of ovarian cancer in patients with ovarian endometrioma. J Obstet Gynaecol Res 2008;34(5):872–7.

38. Kobayashi H, Sumimoto K, Kitanaka T, et al. Ovarian endometrioma–risks factors of ovarian cancer development. Eur J Obstet Gynecol Reprod Biol 2008;138(2):187–93.

39. Cicchiello LA, Hamper UM, Scoutt LM. Ultrasound evaluation of gynecologic causes of pelvic pain. Obstet Gynecol Clin North Am 2011;38(1): 85–114, viii.

40. Kamaya A, Shin L, Chen B, et al. Emergency gynecologic imaging. Semin Ultrasound CT MR 2008; 29(5):353–68.

41. Griffin Y, Sudigali V, Jacques A. Radiology of benign disorders of menstruation. Semin Ultrasound CT MR 2010;31(5):414–32.

42. Hibbard LT. Adnexal torsion. Am J Obstet Gynecol 1985;152(4):456–61.

43. Caspi B, Appelman Z, Rabinerson D, et al. Pathognomonic echo patterns of benign cystic teratomas of the ovary: classification, incidence and accuracy rate of sonographic diagnosis. Ultrasound Obstet Gynecol 1996;7(4):275–9.

44. Mais V, Guerriero S, Ajossa S, et al. Transvaginal ultrasonography in the diagnosis of cystic teratoma. Obstet Gynecol 1995;85(1):48–52.

45. Patel MD, Feldstein VA, Lipson SD, et al. Cystic teratomas of the ovary: diagnostic value of sonography. AJR Am J Roentgenol 1998;171(4): 1061–5.

46. Outwater EK, Wagner BJ, Mannion C, et al. Sex cord-stromal and steroid cell tumors of the ovary. Radiographics 1998;18(6):1523–46.

47. Jung SE, Lee JM, Rha SE, et al. CT and MR imaging of ovarian tumors with emphasis on differential diagnosis. Radiographics 2002;22(6):1305–25.

48. Jung SE, Rha SE, Lee JM, et al. CT and MRI findings of sex cord-stromal tumor of the ovary. AJR Am J Roentgenol 2005;185(1):207–15.

49. Rosen A, Klein M, Lahousen M, et al. Primary carcinoma of the fallopian tube–a retrospective analysis of 115 patients. Austrian Cooperative Study Group for Fallopian Tube Carcinoma. Br J Cancer 1993;68(3):605–9.

50. Hu CY, Taymor ML, Hertig AT. Primary carcinoma of the fallopian tube. Am J Obstet Gynecol 1950; 59(1):58–67. illust.

51. Patlas M, Rosen B, Chapman W, et al. Sono-graphic diagnosis of primary malignant tumors of the fallopian tube. Ultrasound Q 2004;20(2): 59–64.

52. Shaaban AM, Rezvani M. Imaging of primary fallopian tube carcinoma. Abdom Imaging 2013;38(3): 608–18.

53. Hosokawa C, Tsubakimoto M, Inoue Y, et al. Bilateral primary fallopian tube carcinoma: findings on sequential MRI. AJR Am J Roentgenol 2006; 186(4):1046–50.

54. Kim JS, Woo SK, Suh SJ, et al. Sonographic diagnosis of paraovarian cysts: value of detecting a separate ipsilateral ovary. AJR Am J Roentgenol 1995;164(6):1441–4.

55. Moyle PL, Kataoka MY, Nakai A, et al. Nonovarian cystic lesions of the pelvis. Radiographics 2010; 30(4):921–38.

56. Kiseli M, Caglar GS, Cengiz SD, et al. Clinical diagnosis and complications of paratubal cysts: review of the literature and report of uncommon presentations. Arch Gynecol Obstet 2012;285(6):1563–9.

Fetal CNS
A Systematic Approach

Julie A. Ritner, MD*, Mary C. Frates, MD

KEYWORDS

• CNS • Ultrasound • Ventriculomegaly • Intracranial hemorrhage • Central nervous system

KEY POINTS

- As many abnormalities of central nervous system (CNS) can carry a poor neurologic prognosis for the fetus, accurate prenatal diagnosis is important for parental counseling and pregnancy management.
- A systematic approach to the fetal CNS starting with the size and appearance of the lateral ventricles will allow optimal diagnostic characterization of various abnormalities.

LEARNING OBJECTIVES

1. Review normal fetal central nervous system (CNS) anatomy and sonographic views.
2. Review technique for accurate measurement of lateral ventricles.
3. Describe a systematic approach for evaluating intracranial findings in the setting of ventriculomegaly to diagnose specific underlying abnormalities.
4. Review selected CNS abnormalities using the described approach.

INTRODUCTION

Routine sonographic evaluation of the fetal head should include biometric measurement as well as evaluation of intracranial anatomy.[1] The nuchal fold is often routinely measured, because an enlarged nuchal thickness may be associated with aneuploidy.[2] Typical evaluation of the fetal head can be achieved with a minimum of 3 images: an axial image at the level of the cerebral ventricles, an axial image at the level of the thalami and cavum septum pellucidum (CSP) for head biometry, and an axial image through the posterior fossa, oriented slightly more caudally from the biometric view.

NORMAL SONOGRAPHIC ANATOMY/ MEASUREMENT TECHNIQUE

Fetal head biometry measurements should be obtained in an axial plane at the level of the paired thalami and CSP and should not include the cerebellar hemispheres. Measurement of either the biparietal diameter (outer proximal skull to inner distal skull) or head circumference (around the outer perimeter of the calvarium) can be used to determine gestational age. The head circumference may be a more reliable measurement in the setting of variant head shape.[1] Normal anatomic structures that can be assessed on this view include the CSP, falx, thalami, third ventricle, cortex, temporal horns of the lateral ventricles, and calvarium.

Imaging at the level of the cerebral ventricles provides assessment of the choroids, lateral ventricles, midline falx, cerebral cortex, and calvarium. The normal fetal lateral ventricle measures 10 mm or less throughout gestation.[3] Accurate measurement of the lateral ventricle is the foundation for diagnosing ventriculomegaly and therefore strict adherence to measurement criteria should be practiced. The standard measurement should be obtained in a true axial plane at the atria of the

Disclosures: The authors have nothing to disclose.
Department of Ultrasound, Brigham and Women's Hospital, Harvard Medical School, 75 Francis Street, Boston, MA 02115, USA
* Corresponding author. 36 Woodley Avenue, West Roxbury, MA 02132.
E-mail address: jritner@partners.org

Radiol Clin N Am 52 (2014) 1253–1264
http://dx.doi.org/10.1016/j.rcl.2014.07.012

lateral ventricle and glomus of the choroid plexus. Measurement calipers are placed from the inner margin of the medial ventricular wall to the inner margin of the lateral ventricular wall and should be oriented perpendicular to the long axis of the ventricle (**Fig. 1**).[4] Measurement error is a source of false-positive diagnoses, and numerous pitfalls have been described including off-axis image, angled placement of the calipers, and misidentification of the medial or lateral ventricular borders (**Fig. 2**).[5,6] False-negative results are not reported, as undermeasurement of the ventricle is not a source of error.

Posterior fossa abnormalities are an important cause of obstructive ventriculomegaly, and accurate evaluation of posterior fossa anatomy is essential. Evaluation of the posterior fossa should include assessment of the cerebellar hemispheres, cerebellar vermis, cisterna magna, occipital calvarium, and nuchal skin thickness. The normal cerebellum is dumbbell shaped with a slightly echogenic vermis in the center (**Fig. 3**). The cisterna magna may be subjectively assessed or directly measured and should be less than 10 mm throughout gestation. Scanning in a semicoronal plane may simulate an enlarged cisterna magna or absent cerebellar vermis leading to misdiagnosis.[7] Additionally, because the cerebellar vermis is not fully formed until after 18 weeks, a false diagnosis of vermian hypoplasia or agenesis is a pitfall in scans before this gestational age.[8]

SYSTEMATIC APPROACH TO VENTRICULOMEGALY

Ventriculomegaly is often considered the "tip of the iceberg", because it is a finding frequently associated with numerous CNS anomalies. It has been reported to have an 88% sensitivity for detection of an underlying anomaly of the fetal brain and spinal cord.[9] Ventriculomegaly can be characterized as mild (10–12 mm), moderate (12.1–15 mm), or severe (>15 mm) (**Fig. 4**).[10] In the setting of mild ventriculomegaly without associated CNS structural anomaly, abnormal karyotype, or other identifiable cause, the clinical outcome is favorable. As the degree of ventriculomegaly increases, there is increased association with other abnormalities.

The causes of ventriculomegaly are varied, but may be divided into 3 general categories: obstructive, dysgenesis, or destructive causes (**Table 1**).

Obstructive causes lead to enlargement of a normally formed supratentorial ventricular system. The ventricles, cortex, and midline structures are normally developed but altered in appearance due to excess fluid within the ventricular system. Dysgenesis causes frequently show enlargement of the ventricular system as a result of cerebral maldevelopment. Clues to this diagnosis are abnormalities in ventricular shape or orientation and a spectrum of absent midline structures ranging from the CSP alone to complete absence of all midline divisional structures creating a fused appearance of many structures. Destructive changes result from an in utero insult to a normally formed ventricular system and brain; therefore midline structures are always present. With destructive causes, ventricular enlargement is often a result of ex-vacuo dilatation, although specific imaging findings vary depending on the acuity and magnitude of the insult. Clues to this diagnosis are symmetric or asymmetric enlarged portions of the ventricles, nodularity of the ventricular wall indicating prior hemorrhage, altered cortical echogenicity, and variable amounts of absent cortex.

When ventriculomegaly is detected, a detailed search for an underlying explanation is warranted. A systematic approach evaluating the ventricles, surrounding cortex, midline structures, and posterior fossa may be helpful to determine the general cause category and subsequently arrive at a correct diagnosis, as outlined in **Table 2**.

Obstructive causes lead to ventriculomegaly as a result of hydrocephalus: dilatation of normally formed ventricles. Sonographic findings demonstrate smooth-walled ventricles and a normal ventricular orientation angled slightly toward the midline anteriorly. With mild hydrocephalus, the CSP is normal, although in severe hydrocephalus the CSP may be absent, possibly due to pressure necrosis with subsequent fenestration and disintegration of the septum pellucidi.[12] The falx is seen in all types of hydrocephalus, confirming presence of midline structures. Evaluation of the cerebral

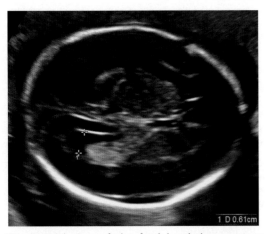

Fig. 1. Axial view of the fetal head demonstrates appropriate technique for accurate measurement of the lateral ventricle.

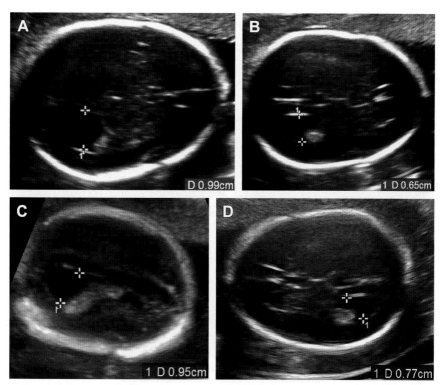

Fig. 2. Technique for lateral ventricular measurement. (*A*) Axial image in an 18-week-old fetus misidentifies the medial ventricular border overestimating lateral ventricle size. (*B*) Adjustment of technical parameters allows visualization of the medial ventricular border demonstrating normal ventricular size. (*C*) Off-axis image plane overestimates ventricular size. (*D*) Angled placement of the calipers overestimates normal ventricle size.

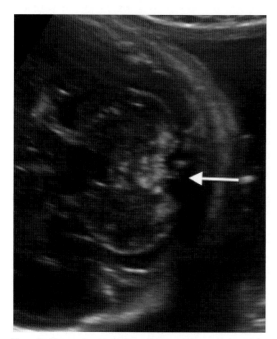

Fig. 3. Normal posterior fossa demonstrates the dumbbell-shaped cerebellum with central echogenic vermis (*arrow*) and anechoic cisterna magna posteriorly.

cortex shows a uniform hypoechoic cortical mantle that may be compressed with severe hydrocephalus. Examination of the posterior fossa often reveals the obstructive abnormality. In the setting of a normal posterior fossa, aqueductal stenosis is the presumed diagnosis. It should be noted, however, that the hydrocephalus associated with aqueductal stenosis is often massive and may make identification of most structures challenging.

Ventriculomegaly related to cerebral dysgenesis often shows abnormal configuration, such as the parallel orientation and colpocephaly seen with agenesis of the corpus callosum (ACC) or the monoventricle of alobar holoprosencephaly. The ventricle walls are typically smooth and the cerebral cortex demonstrates a uniform appearance. The key finding that is consistently noted with cerebral dysgenesis causes is absence of the CSP. As the ventricles are followed anteriorly, the frontal horns demonstrate a fused appearance, which is a paramount finding to indicate cerebral dysgenesis. In some diagnoses, such as septo-optic dysplasia and lobar holoprosencephaly, this abnormality may be the only obvious sonographic finding. Although the septum pellucidi should be visualized

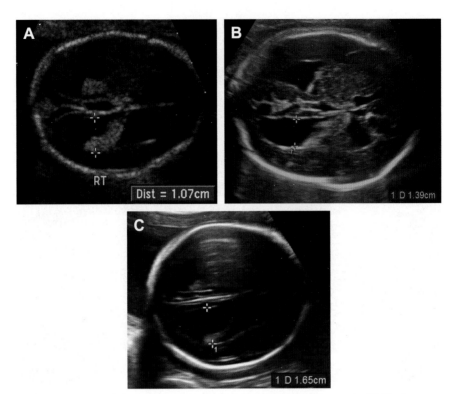

Fig. 4. Cerebral ventriculomegaly in 3 different patients. (*A*) Mild ventriculomegaly. (*B*) Moderate ventriculomegaly. (*C*) Severe ventriculomegaly.

by 18 weeks,[13] it has also been shown that patients with callosal agenesis can have normal scans before 22 weeks.[14] Possible pitfalls in this diagnosis include misinterpretation of the columns of the fornix as the CSP and linear artifact from the walls of nondilated lateral ventricles mimicking the septum pellucidi (**Fig. 5**).[15,16] The posterior fossa is usually normal in patients with cerebral dysgenesis unless a concurrent abnormality is also present.

Destructive causes occur in the setting of a structurally normal ventricular system and include hemorrhagic, ischemic, and infectious causes. Imaging findings vary depending on the magnitude and timing of the initial insult. Ventricular enlargement may be symmetric or asymmetric, focal or diffuse, and typically is due to ex-vacuo dilatation

from loss of cortical tissue. A clue to prior hemorrhage is a nodular appearance to the ventricle walls. By contrast, periventricular leukomalacia (PVL) is a result of ischemia of the white matter tracts and does not affect the appearance of the ventricular wall. Acute changes are typically echogenic and as the process evolves, the findings become more heterogeneous and finally hypoechoic and cystic. Although both hemorrhage and PVL frequently result in regions of porencephaly, communication with the ventricle is more commonly seen following hemorrhage. Destructive processes typically occur in the setting of a normally formed CNS and therefore midline and posterior fossa structures should be present and normal, although in the setting of severe

Table 1
Ventriculomegaly: cause

Obstructive	Dysgenesis	Destructive
Chiari II malformation	Agenesis of the corpus callosum	Intracranial hemorrhage
Dandy-Walker malformation	Septo-optic dysplasia	Periventricular leukomalacia
Aqueductal stenosis	Holoprosencephaly	Hydranencephaly
Mass lesions	Schizencephaly	Infection

Table 2
Ventriculomegaly: approach

	Obstruction	Dysgenesis	Destruction
Ventricle orientation	Normal	Abnormal	Normal
Ventricle walls	Smooth	Smooth	Abnormal
Cortex	Intact	Intact[a]	Abnormal
Falx	Present	+/− Absent	Present
CSP	+/− Present	Absent	Present
Posterior fossa	+/− Abnormal	Normal	Normal

Findings may overlap between categories due to coexistent diagnoses.

[a] Exception: The cortex in open-lip schizencephaly can have a variable appearance ranging from normal to absence of large areas that can be difficult to differentiate from destructive causes.[11]

hydrocephalus, the CSP is often partially or completely destroyed due to pressure necrosis.[12]

Depending on the stage or severity of the abnormality, the presentation may be that of a large amount of cerebrospinal fluid (CSF) in the head, making diagnosis of a particular cause challenging.

In this situation, assessment of the ventricular system and visualization of the CSP may not be possible. Identification of several key structures, specifically the falx and cortex, can help the imager differentiate between the most common causes (**Table 3**). Use of a high-frequency transducer

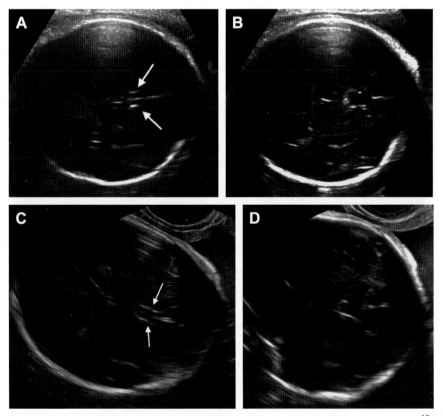

Fig. 5. (*A*) Columns of the fornix (*arrows*) with central linear reflection (3 white lines) mimics CSP.[13] (*B*) Axial image [same patient as (*A*)] oriented slightly more cranially demonstrates normal fluid-filled CSP (2 lines). (*C*) Axial transvaginal image in a different patient demonstrates columns of the fornix (*arrows*) mimicking the CSP. (*D*) Axial transvaginal image more cranial [same patient as (*C*)] shows the fused frontal horn appearance consistent with absent CSP.

Table 3
Large amount of CSF in head

	Falx	Cortex
Hydrocephalus	+	+
Holoprosencephaly	−	+
Hydranencephaly	+	−[a]

[a] Depending on the timing of the insult, destruction of the cortex may be incomplete and variable amounts of cortex may be present in an irregular distribution.

and/or transvaginal scanning may allow better identification of the potentially thin cortical mantle and thus help distinguish severe hydrocephalus from hydranencephaly.

CASE REVIEW
Arnold-Chiari (Type II) Malformation (Obstructive)

The intracranial appearance of this malformation is consistently recognizable (**Fig. 6**). The malformation develops as a cascade of findings that are the result of an open lumbosacral myelomeningocele. The spinal defect causes downward displacement of the cerebellum through the foramen magnum leading to a small posterior fossa with an inferiorly displaced cerebellum and obliterated cisterna magna (banana sign). This malformation

obstructs flow of CSF through the fourth ventricle and posterior fossa leading to classic severe hydrocephalus. Anterior angulation of the frontal bones is also frequently seen (lemon sign), although this is not a specific finding and may be seen in normal fetuses.

Dandy-Walker Malformation (Obstructive)

Dandy-Walker malformation (DWM) is classically defined as cystic dilatation of the fourth ventricle, agenesis of the cerebellar vermis, and an enlarged posterior fossa with upward displacement of the torcula and tentorium (**Fig. 7**). Dandy Walker (DW) variant typically demonstrates hypoplasia of the cerebellar vermis and mildly enlarged or normal-sized posterior fossa. Although DWM or DW variant may be suspected during the second trimester, a conclusive diagnosis cannot be made until at least 18 weeks, as the cerebellar vermis is not fully formed before this.[8] Numerous structural and genetic abnormalities are frequently associated with these complexes. The most important prognostic factor is the presence or absence of associated abnormalities and gestational age at diagnosis.[17,18] Although ventricle size may be normal, ventriculomegaly is the most common associated finding. The cerebral cortex is intact and the falx is present.

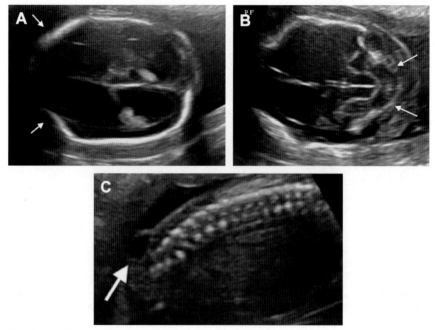

Fig. 6. Arnold-Chiari malformation (*A*). Angulation of the frontal bones (*arrows*, lemon sign), severe hydrocephalus with intact cortex, dangling choroid, and presence of the falx. (*B*) Posterior fossa is small with abnormally shaped cerebellum (*arrows*, banana sign) and effaced cisterna magna. (*C*) Sagittal spine image demonstrates lumbosacral myelomeningocele (*arrow*).

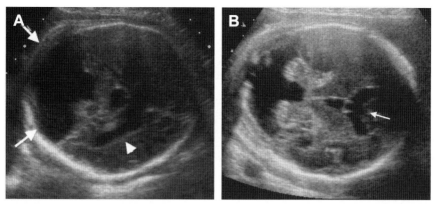

Fig. 7. Dandy-Walker malformation (*A*). Axial image demonstrates ventriculomegaly (*arrowhead*), intact cortical mantle, and midline falx. Posterior fossa (*arrows*) is partially imaged showing a large cyst. (*B*) Oblique axial image through the posterior fossa demonstrates small dysplastic cerebellar hemispheres and absent vermis. Fused frontal horns are also noted (*arrow*) consistent with absent CSP and partial dysgenesis of the corpus callosum.

Aqueductal Stenosis (Obstructive)

Congenital aqueductal stenosis is due to the blockage of normal CSF flow through the aqueduct of Sylvius, often resulting in severe obstructive hydrocephalus (**Fig. 8**, see **Table 3**). Although the exact cause is not known, the obstruction may result from a web or stricture in the aqueduct of Sylvius or less commonly may

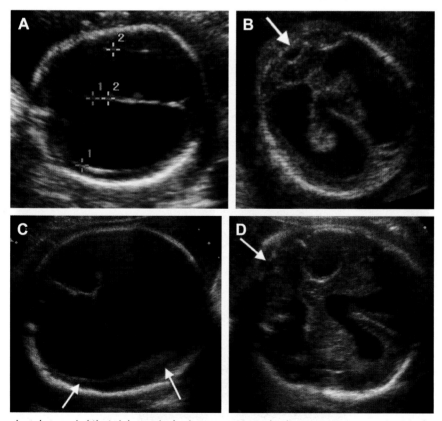

Fig. 8. Aqueductal stenosis (*A*). Axial ventricular image at 18 weeks demonstrates severe ventriculomegaly with intact cortex and falx. (*B*) Posterior fossa (*arrow*) at 18 weeks is normal; therefore aqueductal stenosis is suspected. (*C*) Axial ventricular image at 32 weeks in the same patient demonstrates a massive amount of fluid with intact cortical mantle (*arrows*) and partially visualized falx consistent with obstructive cause. (*D*) The normal posterior fossa (*arrow*) confirms aqueductal stenosis.

be X linked or related to other genetic abnormalities. When ventriculomegaly is seen at imaging, hydrocephalus can be diagnosed when the ventricles are normal in orientation, have smooth walls, cortex is present and compressed appearing, and midline structures are present (CSP may not be present with severe hydrocephalus). When subsequent examination of the posterior fossa is normal, blockage at the aqueduct is assumed.

Agenesis of the Corpus Callosum (Dysgenesis)

ACC may be partial or complete and the constellation of imaging findings may be seen in varying degrees (**Fig. 9**). Even with complete callosal agenesis, findings may not be apparent until after 22 weeks,[14] making diagnosis challenging. Ventriculomegaly presents as disproportionate dilatation of the posterior portion of the lateral ventricles (colpocephaly) with more normal width of the anterior portion leading to a teardrop configuration. Additionally, the ventricles assume a parallel orientation, creating a steer horn appearance of the frontal horns in the coronal plane. The ventricular walls are smooth and cortex is intact. A midline falx is present, although an absent

CSP is the rule with complete ACC. The third ventricle is often high riding and an interhemispheric cyst, which may enlarge throughout gestation, may also be seen. Although the posterior fossa should be normal in isolated ACC, it should be noted that ACC is frequently associated with other malformations, most notably DWM, which will affect the posterior fossa. Once ACC is suspected, direct evaluation of the corpus callosum should be attempted in coronal and sagittal planes, often aided by the use of transvaginal scanning in vertex fetuses to better visualize the intracranial structures.

Schizencephaly (Dysgenesis)

Schizencephaly is a rare CNS abnormality that is thought to arise from an abnormality in neuronal migration, although other causes have also been proposed (**Fig. 10**). Closed-lip and open-lip types are described, although the findings of closed-lip schizencephaly are subtle and preclude prenatal sonographic diagnosis. At imaging, open-lip schizencephaly is seen as a CSF cleft that extends through the cortex from the ventricle to the pial surface. Findings may be unilateral or bilateral

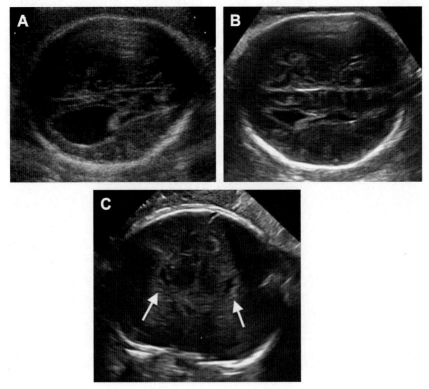

Fig. 9. Agenesis of the corpus callosum in 3 different patients. (*A*) Teardrop configuration of lateral ventricle due to colpocephaly (dilated posterior horn). (*B*) Axial image in a different patient demonstrates parallel orientation of ventricles in relation to the falx. (*C*) Coronal image demonstrates "steer horn" appearance of the frontal horns (*arrows*) due to their parallel orientation.

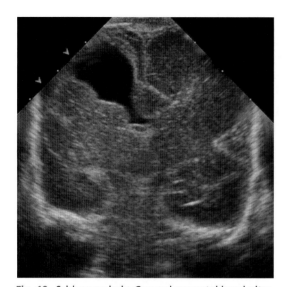

and involve a small or large portion of the cortex, making differentiation from porencephaly difficult. By definition, the cleft must be lined by gray matter, although this distinction can only be made with MR imaging. Mild ventriculomegaly may be seen and the CSP is frequently absent. Posterior fossa structures should be normal.

Holoprosencephaly (Dysgenesis)

The holoprosencephalies represent a spectrum of abnormalities that result from failure of normal separation of the midline intracranial structures (**Fig. 11**). The most commonly described types are alobar, semilobar, and lobar. The CSP is universally absent with all of the holoprosencephalies, and an absent CSP may often be the only notable sonographic finding seen on routine imaging with the lobar variant. The most severe form, alobar holoprosencephaly, may present with a large amount of CSF in the head, and assessment of the key structures described in **Table 3** is required to differentiate it from other causes. Typical sonographic findings with alobar holoprosencephaly include a large monoventricle, intact cortical mantle, absent falx and CSP, fusion of

Fig. 10. Schizencephaly. Coronal neonatal head ultrasound demonstrates a CSF-filled space extending from the ventricle to the calvarium. MR imaging verifies that the space is lined by cortical gray matter confirming open-lip schizencephaly. This appearance can mimic porencephalic change from prior insult and, thus, MR imaging may be necessary for confirmatory diagnosis.

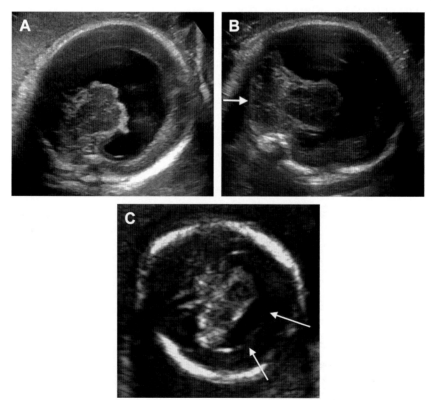

Fig. 11. Holoprosencephaly. (*A*) Coronal image at 36 weeks demonstrates a large smooth-walled monoventricle with intact cortical mantle and absent falx consistent with alobar holoprosencephaly. (*B*) Axial image in the same fetus demonstrates a normal posterior fossa (*arrow*). (*C*) Axial image in a different fetus at 18 weeks demonstrates a less prominent monoventricle (*arrows*) with intact cortex, absent falx, and fused thalami and choroid.

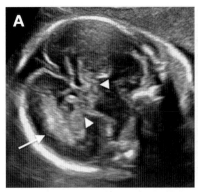
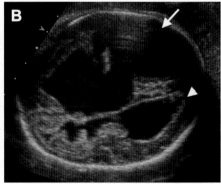

Fig. 12. Intracranial hemorrhage. (*A*) Coronal image at 20 weeks demonstrates bilateral germinal matrix hemorrhages (*arrowheads*) and increased echogenicity in the cerebral cortex (*arrow*) consistent with hemorrhage. (*B*) Follow-up in the same patient at 32 weeks shows bilateral asymmetric ventriculomegaly with a large area of porencephaly (*arrow*) that communicates with the ventricle and increased echogenicity and subtle nodularity of the ventricular wall (*arrowhead*).

the thalami and choroid, and a dorsal cyst. The posterior fossa is normal and numerous craniofacial abnormalities are frequently seen.

Intracranial Hemorrhage (Destructive)

Spontaneous intracranial hemorrhage is an uncommon prenatal occurrence that may be related to coagulopathy or trauma, although is more commonly idiopathic (**Fig. 12**). Typically it presents in the third trimester as an incidental finding following normal prior studies. The sonographic appearance is variable depending on the timing, location, and extent of the hemorrhagic event. The hemorrhage frequently includes both intraventricular and parenchymal components. Ventriculomegaly is frequently present, early on as obstructive hydrocephalus from the hemorrhage and later as a result of ex-vacuo dilatation or porencephalic change. The ventricular wall is often abnormally echogenic and in the setting of chronic

hemorrhage will appear nodular. If parenchymal hemorrhage is present, the cortex will show focally altered echogenicity that varies depending on the timing of the insult. Midline structures should be present and normal and the posterior fossa is normal.

Periventricular Leukomalacia (Destructive)

PVL results from an ischemic injury to the periventricular white matter, most commonly in the sensitive watershed areas of the peritrigonal region and frontal horns (**Fig. 13**). The cause is thought to be a reperfusion injury of ischemic white matter tracts resulting from a hypotensive episode or possibly infection. Although PVL is most commonly described in premature infants before 32 weeks, it can be seen on prenatal ultrasound. Early findings show increased periventricular echogenicity that eventually progresses to ventriculomegaly due to ex-vacuo dilatation from the loss of

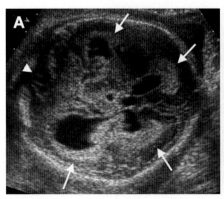
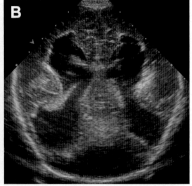

Fig. 13. Periventricular leukomalacia. (*A*) Oblique axial image at 26 weeks shows bilateral symmetric smooth-walled ventriculomegaly and increased echogenicity of the periventricular cortex diffusely (*arrows*). Midline structures are present and the posterior fossa is normal (*arrowhead*). (*B*) Neonatal coronal image demonstrates diffuse ventriculomegaly due to ex-vacuo dilatation from the periventricular ischemic insult.

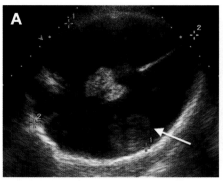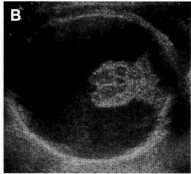

Fig. 14. Hydranencephaly. (*A*) Axial image shows a large amount of fluid in the head. A falx is present. Only a small globular area of cortical remnant is seen (*arrow*). (*B*) Axial image more inferiorly shows absence of cortex and preservation of thalami and posterior fossa.

periventricular white matter. More severe cases may manifest as multiple cysts in a periventricular location. The ventricular walls are smooth. Midline structures and posterior fossa should be normal in appearance.

Hydranencephaly (Destructive)

Hydranencephaly is the most extreme form of destructive insult that results in complete liquefaction of the cerebral hemispheres (**Fig. 14**). Various causes have been described including occlusion of the internal carotid arteries, massive hypoxia, infectious causes, and thromboembolic events. Depending on the timing of the insult, remnants of cerebral cortex may persist or the head may appear completely replaced with fluid. The classic appearance is complete absence of the cortical mantle. Differentiation from severe hydrocephalus is critical, because each diagnosis carries a significantly different prognosis for the fetus (see **Table 3**). The falx is present due to blood supply from the external carotid artery. Structures supplied by the posterior circulation including the thalami, choroid, brainstem, portions of occipital cortex, and posterior fossa are also preserved.

SUMMARY

As many CNS abnormalities can carry a poor neurologic prognosis for the fetus, accurate prenatal diagnosis is important for parental counseling and pregnancy management. A systematic approach to the fetal CNS starting with the size and appearance of the lateral ventricles will allow optimal diagnostic characterization of various abnormalities.

REFERENCES

1. American Institute of Ultrasound in Medicine. AIUM practice guideline for the performance of obstetric ultrasound examinations. J Ultrasound Med 2013; 32:1083–101.

2. Benacerraf B. The significance of the nuchal fold in the second trimester fetus. Prenat Diagn 2002;22: 798–801.

3. Cardoza JD, Goldstein RB, Filly RA. Exclusion of the fetal ventriculomegaly with a single measurement: the width of the lateral ventricular atrium. Radiology 1988;169:711–4.

4. Filly RA, Goldstein RB, Callen PW. Fetal ventricle: importance in routine obstetric sonography. Radiology 1991;181:1–7.

5. Heiserman J, Filly RA, Goldstein RB. Effect of measurement errors on sonographic evaluation of ventriculomegaly. J Ultrasound Med 1991;10:121–4.

6. Hertzberg BS, Kliewer MA, Bowie JD. Fetal ventriculomegaly: misidentification of the true medial boundary of the ventricle at US. Radiology 1997;205:813–6.

7. Laing FC, Frates MC, Brown DL, et al. Sonography of the fetal posterior fossa: false appearance of mega-cisterna magna and Dandy-Walker variant. Radiology 1994;192:247–51.

8. Bromley B, Nadel AS, Pauker S, et al. Closure of the cerebellar vermis: evaluation with second trimester US. Radiology 1994;193:761–3.

9. Filly RA, Cardoza JD, Goldstein RB, et al. Detection of fetal central nervous system anomalies: a practical level of effort for a routine sonogram. Radiology 1989;172:403–8.

10. Gaglioti P, Oberto M, Todros T. The significance of fetal ventriculomegaly: etiology, short- and long-term outcomes. Prenat Diagn 2009;29:381–8.

11. Oh K, Kennedy A, Frias A, et al. Fetal schizencephaly: pre-and postnatal imaging with a review of the clinical manifestations. Radiographics 2005;25:647–57.

12. Barkovich AJ, Norman D. Absence of the septum pellucidum: a useful sign in the diagnosis of congenital brain malformations. Am J Roentgenol 1989;152:353–60.

13. Falco P, Gabrielli S, Visentin A, et al. Transabdominal sonography of the cavum septum pellucidum in

normal fetuses in the second and third trimesters of pregnancy. Ultrasound Obstet Gynecol 2000;16: 549–53.

14. Bennett GL, Bromley B, Benacerraf BR. Agenesis of the corpus callosum: prenatal detection usually is not possible before 22 weeks of gestation. Radiology 1996;199:447–50.

15. Callen P, Callen A, Glenn O, et al. Columns of the fornix, not to be mistaken for the cavum septi pellucidi on prenatal sonography. J Ultrasound Med 2008;27:25–31.

16. Pilu G, Tani G, Carletti A, et al. Difficult early sonographic diagnosis of absence of the fetal septum pellucidum. Ultrasound Obstet Gynecol 2005;25: 70–2.

17. Ecker JL, Shipp TD, Bromley B, et al. The sonographic diagnosis of Dandy-Walker and Dandy-Walker variant: associated findings and outcomes. Prenat Diagn 2000;20(4):328–32.

18. Kolble N, Wisser J, Kurmanavicius J, et al. Dandy-Walker malformation: prenatal diagnosis and outcome. Prenat Diagn 2000;20:318–27.

Ultrasonography Evaluation of Scrotal Masses

Daniel Sommers, MD*, Thomas Winter, MD

KEYWORDS

- Scrotal ultrasonography • Intratesticular scrotal mass • Extratesticular scrotal mass

KEY POINTS

- Ultrasonography is the ideal modality for evaluating the scrotum.
- Normal scrotal anatomy and the sonographic assessment of intratesticular and extratesticular causes that may present as scrotal masses are discussed.

INTRODUCTION

This article reviews the anatomy and sonographic findings of scrotal masses. Normal anatomy, general imaging techniques, and assessment of intratesticular and extratesticular disorders will be discussed.

When a scrotal mass is palpated, the concern is for the presence of a testicular neoplasm. Ultrasonography (US) is an ideal modality for evaluating the scrotum in this scenario; it is readily available, inexpensive, and without ionizing radiation. US is nearly 100% sensitive for the detection of an intrascrotal mass.[1] Delineation between intratesticular and extratesticular processes is 98% to 100% accurate.[1–4]

NORMAL ANATOMY

The normal scrotal wall consists of epidermis, superficial dartos muscle and fascia, external spermatic fascia, cremasteric muscle and fascia, and internal spermatic fascia. The scrotum is a fibromuscular sac divided by a midline septum into a right and left hemiscrotum. Each hemiscrotum contains a testis, epididymis, spermatic cord, vascular network, and lymphatic network.

Separating the testis from the scrotal wall are the 2 layers of the tunica vaginalis; these form an isolated mesothelium-lined sac.[5,6] The parietal layer lines the scrotal wall and is separated from the visceral layer lining the tunica albuginea of the testis and covering the epididymis by a potential space that normally contains a small amount of fluid. The parietal and visceral layers of the tunica vaginalis join where the tunica attaches to the scrotal wall at the posterolateral aspect of the testis. The tunica albuginea covers the testis and epididymis with the exception of a small posteromedial area.[7]

The fibrous tunica albuginea covers the testis, protecting it from injury. Posteromedially, the tunica albuginea projects inward into the testes to form the mediastinum testis. Numerous fibrous septa extend from the mediastinum dividing the testis into 250 to 400 lobules. Each lobule consists of 1 to 3 seminiferous tubules that support the Sertoli cells and spermatocytes. The Leydig cells are adjacent to the tubules within the loose interstitial tissue and are responsible for testosterone secretion.

The seminiferous tubules converge to form larger tubuli recti, which open into the dilated

Disclosures: None.
Department of Radiology, University of Utah School of Medicine, 50 North Medical Drive #1A071, Salt Lake City, UT 84132, USA
* Corresponding author.
E-mail address: daniel.sommers@hsc.utah.edu

Radiol Clin N Am 52 (2014) 1265–1281
http://dx.doi.org/10.1016/j.rcl.2014.07.014
0033-8389/14/$ – see front matter © 2014 Elsevier Inc. All rights reserved.

spaces of the rete testis. The rete testis drains into the epididymal head (globus major) via 15 to 20 efferent ductules. The pyramid-shaped head of the epididymis is located at the superoposterior aspect of the testis and measures 5 to 12 mm in diameter. The narrow epididymal body (corpus) and tail (globus minor) are formed as the efferent ducts converge into a single duct. The curved tail of the epididymis courses inferolaterally and becomes the vas deferens, which continues superiorly into the spermatic cord.

The appendix testes and appendix epididymis are embryologic remnants of paramesonephric and mesonephric ducts, respectively, and consist of vascularized connective tissue.

Primary vascular supply to the testis is provided by the testicular artery, which arises from the aorta, just distal to the renal arteries. The testicular artery penetrates the tunica albuginea where it forms the capsular artery. The deferential artery, originating from the superior vesical artery, and the cremasteric artery, a branch of the inferior epigastric artery, both supply the epididymis, vas deferens, and peritesticular tissues.[7] Branches of the pudendal artery supply the wall of the scrotum. Venous drainage forms the pampiniform plexus around the upper half of the epididymis, which continues as the testicular vein through the deep inguinal ring. The spermatic cord contains the pampiniform plexus; vas deferens; testicular, cremasteric, and deferential arteries; genitofemoral nerve; and lymphatic vessels; and courses superior toward the superficial and deep inguinal rings.

US TECHNIQUE

Scrotal US examination is performed with the scrotum supported by a towel placed between the thighs with the patient in a supine position. Optimal results are obtained with a high-frequency (14–18 MHz) linear array transducer. The scrotum should be evaluated in both long and transverse axes.[8] The size and appearance of each testis and epididymis should be documented and compared with the contralateral side. Color and pulsed Doppler parameters are adjusted to evaluate for low flow velocities to show blood flow in the testes and surrounding structures. Transverse images that include portions of both testes should be acquired in both gray-scale and color Doppler modes to show symmetry. The structures within the scrotum, including the scrotal wall, should be examined thoroughly to evaluate for extratesticular masses or processes. Additional techniques such as Valsalva maneuver or upright positioning of the patient may be used to evaluate venous vascularity or for inguinal hernia as dictated by clinical concern.

US ANATOMY

The normal testis has a homogeneous, medium-level, granular echotexture (**Fig. 1**). Prepubertal testes are typically less echogenic than postpubertal testes secondary to incomplete maturation of the germ cell elements and tubules.[9] Although better visualized when the testis is surrounded by fluid, the tunica (visceral layer of tunica vaginalis and tunica albuginea) can often be seen as an echogenic outline of the testis. Where the tunica invaginates to form the mediastinum testis, it is visualized as an echogenic band that extends along the long axis of the testis (**Fig. 2**). The normal rete testis can be identified in about 20% of patients as a hypoechoic area near the mediastinum.[10] The space between the 2 leaves of the tunica vaginalis normally contains a small amount of anechoic fluid (see **Fig. 1**).

The epididymis is best visualized in a longitudinal view. The epididymal head is generally isoechoic or mildly hyperechoic to the testis, although its echotexture may be coarser.[11] The narrow body of the epididymis measures 2 to 4 mm and is often indistinguishable from the surrounding peritesticular tissues. The tail may be seen as a curved 2-mm to 5-mm structure at the inferior pole of the testis where is becomes the proximal vas deferens.[7]

Intratesticular flow can reliably be shown with color, power, and spectral Doppler.[9,12–14] Power Doppler may result in increased sensitivity for low-flow states.[15,16] The spectral waveforms of the intratesticular arteries, as well as the waveforms within the epididymis, typically have a low-resistance pattern.[12,14]

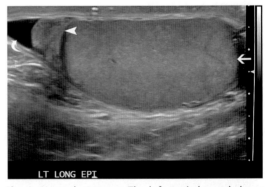

Fig. 1. Normal anatomy. The left testis (*arrow*) shows homogeneous, medium-level, granular echotexture. The epididymal head (*arrowhead*), well seen at the superior aspect of the testis, is generally isoechoic to mildly hyperechoic to the testis. A normal (physiologic) volume of fluid is present (*curved arrow*).

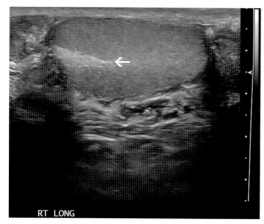

Fig. 2. Mediastinum testis. Long-axis view of the right testis shows the mediastinum testis (*arrow*), an invagination of the tunica albuginea, well seen as an echogenic band extending into the testis along its long axis.

US FINDINGS

When a palpable scrotal mass presents for US evaluation, the primary goals are localization of the mass (intratesticular vs extratesticular) and characterization of the mass. In general, intratesticular masses should be considered to be malignant.[17] If the mass is extratesticular and cystic, it is almost certainly benign, with the generally accepted prevalence of malignancy of extratesticular lesions being approximately 3% to 6%.[18–21]

INTRATESTICULAR SCROTAL MASSES

Testicular cancer typically manifests as a painless scrotal mass and represents the most common nonhematologic malignancy in men aged 15 to 49 years.[22,23] Other presenting symptoms include a sensation of heaviness or fullness in the pelvis or scrotum, testicular enlargement, and evidence of metastatic disease.[24] Approximately 10% to 15% of patients present with pain and a scrotal mass, which may be misdiagnosed as epididymo-orchitis,[25] or with pain and a scrotal mass following trauma to the scrotum.

Testicular tumors are subdivided into 2 major categories: germ cell tumors (GCTs) and stromal tumors. GCTs account for 90% to 95% of all testicular tumors. GCTs arise from primitive germ cells and are further subdivided into seminoma and nonseminomatous GCTs (NSGCTs). These tumors are almost uniformly malignant. Non–germ cell primary tumors of the testis derive from the sex cords (Sertoli cells) and the stroma (Leydig cells) and are typically malignant in 10% of cases. Nonprimary tumors including lymphoma, leukemia, and metastases can also present as intratesticular masses. Color Doppler imaging has limited ability to distinguish malignant from benign solid intratesticular masses.[24]

GCTs

Intratubular germ cell neoplasia is thought to be the precursor of most GCTs and is the equivalent of carcinoma in situ. The prevailing theory is that these abnormal cells develop along a unipotential line and form seminoma, or develop along a totipotential line and form nonseminomatous tumors.[26,27] Seminomas are radiosensitive tumors, whereas NSGCTs respond better to surgery and chemotherapy.[23]

- Seminomas account for 35% to 50% of all primary testicular neoplasms.[17,25] Seminoma is the most common primary neoplasm in cryptorchidism and the most common pure GCT. Seminomas are typically homogeneous, hypoechoic lesions that range from small, well-defined nodules to large, more heterogeneous masses that may replace and enlarge the testis (**Fig. 3**). Seminomas are usually confined by the tunica albuginea, rarely extending to peritesticular structures.[7] Bilateral tumors are rare, occurring in 2% to 3% of patients, and are typically asynchronous.[28,29]
- NSGCT is considered the most common primary testicular malignancy, accounting for up to 60% of cases.[17] Approximately 70% of NSGCTs produce hormonal markers: alpha-fetoprotein and human chorionic gonadotropin.[30] Between 32% and 60% of GCTs are mixed GCTs composed of at least 2 different cell types.[17,31] Pure NSGCTs are rare, but occur most often in the pediatric population.[17] The sonographic appearance of these tumors

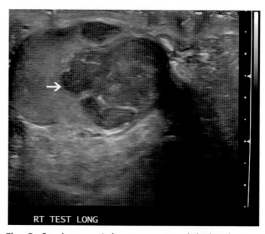

Fig. 3. Seminoma. A homogeneous, lobular, hypoechoic mass (*arrow*) is present that is beginning to replace and enlarge the right testis, although confined by the tunica.

depends on the relative proportions of each component, although as a group these tumors are more heterogeneous, showing irregular or ill-defined margins, echogenic foci, and cystic components (**Fig. 4**). Tunica invasion is common. NSGCTs include embryonal carcinoma, yolk-sac (endodermal sinus) tumors, teratoma, and choriocarcinoma.[17,32] Mixed GCTs that contain seminomatous components are treated as NSGCTs.[23]

- Regressed or burned-out GCTs are thought to occur secondary to the high metabolic rate of the tumor, causing it to outgrow its blood supply with subsequent tumor regression. The patient may present with widespread metastatic disease with involution of the primary tumor. These primary tumors are generally small, and can be hypoechoic, hyperechoic, or seen as a focal calcification or clustered macrocalcifications (**Fig. 5**). Histologic analysis may show a minimal amount of residual tumor or only fibrosis and scar tissue.[17]

Non-GCTs

Most non-GCTs are sex cord stromal tumors, accounting for 4% of testicular tumors, arising from cells that form the sex cords (Sertoli cells) and interstitial stroma (Leydig cells). Ninety percent of these tumors are benign. These tumors are typically small and discovered incidentally. Because there are no radiologic criteria allowing differentiation of these tumors from germ cell neoplasm, orchiectomy is typically performed.

- Leydig cell tumors are the most common sex cord stromal tumors and can occur in any age group (**Fig. 6**). Thirty percent of patients present with an endocrinopathy such as precocious puberty/virilization, gynecomastia, or decreased libido.
- Sertoli cell tumors are less common, and are less likely to be hormonally active. These tumors can be of 3 histologic types, including the subtype of large-cell calcifying Sertoli cell tumor (seen in the pediatric population), which can present with multiple and bilateral masses with large areas of calcification.[33]
- Other sex cord stromal tumors are less common and include granulosa cell tumors, fibroma-thecomas, and mixed sex cord stromal tumors (including gonadoblastoma).[28]

Other Malignant Tumors

- Lymphoma (almost exclusively non-Hodgkin B cell) accounts for 5% of testicular tumors. Testicular involvement occurs in only 1% to 3% of patients with lymphoma.[34] Lymphoma is the most common bilateral intratesticular tumor, and synchronous or metachronous involvement occurs, involving the contralateral testis in 38% of cases.[28] The epididymis and spermatic cord are often involved. Testicular lymphoma is the most common testicular neoplasm in men older than 60 years of age. Patients most commonly present with painless enlargement of the testis, although systemic symptoms such as weight loss, fever, and weakness have also been reported.[17] Testicular lymphoma may appear sonographically as single or multiple discrete hypoechoic lesions indistinguishable from GCTs, or it may diffusely infiltrate the entire testis and mimic orchitis or epididymo-orchitis (**Fig. 7**).[35–37]
- In acute leukemia the testes are a common site of infiltration. A blood-testis barrier limits the effect of chemotherapeutic agents in general, with this phenomenon commonly described in pediatric acute lymphoblastic leukemia, allowing persistence of leukemic cells in the testes after remission.[37] The sonographic appearance of testicular leukemia is varied; tumors may be unilateral or bilateral, diffuse, focal, hypoechoic, or hyperechoic.[37,38]
- Metastases to the testes are rare. The most common primary sources are prostate, lung, melanoma, colon, and renal, in descending prevalence (**Fig. 8**).[39]

Testicular Microlithiasis

Testicular microlithiasis (TM) is usually an incidental finding on a scrotal US (if associated with

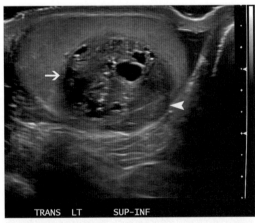

TRANS   LT   SUP-INF

Fig. 4. NSGCT. Large, intratesticular heterogeneous mass (*arrow*) with cystic and solid components proved to be a mixed GCT at orchiectomy. At the posterior margin (*arrowhead*), the mass is seen to expand the testis and invade the tunica.

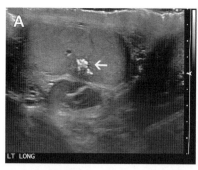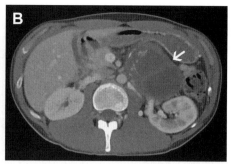

Fig. 5. Regressed, or burned-out GCT. (*A*) Left intratesticular lesion with small, clustered calcifications associated with a residual hypoechoic mass (*arrow*) consistent with a regressed NSGCT. (*B*) Heterogeneous left retroperitoneal mass (*arrow*) showing solid and cystic components with scattered calcifications, surgically proved to represent metastatic GCT.

a mass, the microcalcifications are irrelevant and management is driven by the mass). The small calcifications within the seminiferous tubules appear as punctate, nonshadowing, hyperechoic foci (greater than 5 in single field of view) (**Fig. 9**).[40] The microcalcifications are typically bilateral and scattered throughout the testis. TM has been correlated with testicular carcinoma.[41] The extent of the risk for subsequent development of neoplasm and the recommended surveillance in the setting of TM remain controversial,[40,42] with the most recent literature suggesting that there is no causal link and that follow-up should be determined by any other additional risk factors, not the microlithiasis.[43,44]

Benign Intratesticular Conditions

Nonneoplastic conditions that can present as testicular masses include orchitis, cysts, adrenal

rests, infarcts, hematomas, and benign vascular lesions.

- Orchitis most often represents an extension of epididymo-orchitis (**Fig. 10**) and may present as a focal hypoechoic, intratesticular mass, with diagnosis aided by clinical signs and symptoms. Orchitis may progress to a more serious infection that can lead to testicular ischemia, infarction, and intratesticular abscess (**Figs. 11** and **12**).[45]
- Cysts of the tunica albuginea range from 2 to 5 mm in size and often present as palpable masses (**Fig. 13**).
- Simple intratesticular cysts can occur within the testicular parenchyma, and range in size from 2 to 20 mm. These cysts are typically solitary. Careful examination is required to exclude solid or mural components (eg, cystic teratomas) (**Fig. 14**).
- Testicular adrenal rest tissue is typically seen in patients with congenital adrenal hyperplasia, and rarely in the setting of Cushing syndrome. Aberrant adrenal rests that were trapped in the developing gonad during fetal development may present as bilateral, eccentrically located, predominantly hypoechoic masses (**Fig. 15**).
- Epidermoid cysts are rare, benign, keratin-filled intratesticular masses.[28] One of the few benign intratesticular masses, they constitute 1% of testicular tumors and have no malignant potential. They are well circumscribed and may present as solid masses, have a target appearance, or have the classic appearance of a laminated or onion-skin pattern (**Fig. 16**). Doppler interrogation shows no flow within the cyst. Although the US appearance is characteristic, it is not pathognomonic because teratomas and other malignant tumors may have a similar

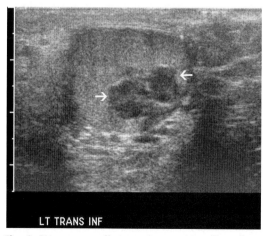

Fig. 6. Non–germ cell stromal tumor. Leydig cell tumor (*arrows*) seen as 2 adjacent hypoechoic, solid lesions within the testis that are sonographically indistinguishable from a germ cell neoplasm.

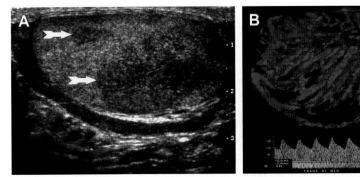

Fig. 7. Testicular lymphoma in a 42-year-old man who presented with bilateral painful intratesticular masses. (*A*) The left testis showed several hypoechoic masses (*arrows*), whereas the right testis (not shown) had a single large mass replacing most of the testis. (*B*) The intratesticular masses were hypervascular. The right testis showed marked hyperemia (on power Doppler; *top*) and low-resistance flow (on pulsed Doppler; *bottom*). Diagnosis was made with a core biopsy of a supraclavicular mass, and the left testis was normal at US following 2 months of chemotherapy.

appearance. However, the combination of US appearance, lack of vascularity, and negative tumor markers may suggest testis-sparing enucleation rather than orchiectomy.[46,47]

- Testicular hemangiomas are rare and may present as a hypoechoic mass with focal calcifications.[48]
- An intratesticular varicocele has a characteristic sonographic appearance of dilated tubular intratesticular veins near the mediastinum testis; Doppler examination should assist with the correct diagnosis (**Fig. 17**).[49]
- Segmental testicular infarct may present as a focal, wedge-shaped, or rounded area within the testis (**Figs. 18** and **19**). Segmental infarct may result from epididymo-orchitis,

autoimmune diseases, vasculitis, sickle cell disease, hypersensivity angiitis, trauma, and pelvic surgery (especially herniorrhaphy).[30]

- Intratesticular hematomas may occur as sequelae of scrotal trauma. They typically appear isoechoic or hyperechoic compared with the testis acutely, become smaller and more hypoechoic as they resolve, and lack vascularity on Doppler examination (**Fig. 20**). If surgical exploration is not performed, it is mandatory that these be followed to resolution to exclude the possibility of a testicular tumor mimicking a hematoma.
- Tubular ectasia of the rete testis may appear as a hypoechoic mass, although it represents

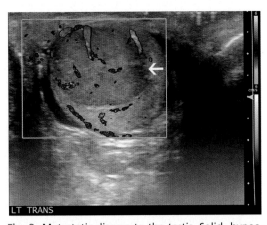

Fig. 8. Metastatic disease to the testis. Solid, hypoechoic, slightly heterogeneous, vascular intratesticular mass (*arrow*) identified at sonographic examination in patient with a history of metastatic melanoma. Metastatic disease was pathologically proved at orchiectomy.

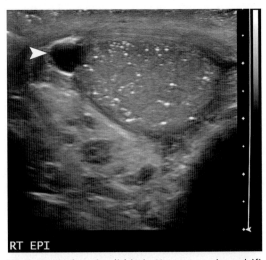

Fig. 9. Testicular microlithiasis. Numerous microcalcifications are seen as punctate, nonshadowing, hyperechoic foci (greater than 5 in a single field of view) within the right testis. Incidental note was made of an epididymal head cyst (*arrowhead*).

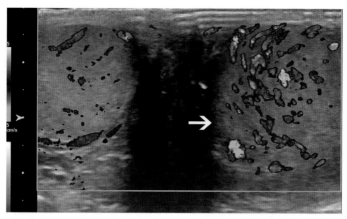

Fig. 10. Orchitis. Doppler image of the testes shows asymmetric hyperemia of the left testis (*arrow*) without a distinct intratesticular mass.

dilated tubules near the mediastinum and is a benign variant, occurring secondary to obstruction in the epididymis or efferent ductules and often associated with a spermatocele (**Fig. 21**).

EXTRATESTICULAR SCROTAL MASSES
Tunica Vaginalis

- Hydroceles are the most common cause of painless scrotal swelling.[50] Congenital hydroceles occur when there is incomplete closure of the processus vaginalis and peritoneal fluid accumulates in the sac; these patients are at increased risk for developing an indirect inguinal hernia. Acquired hydroceles form as a reaction to infection, trauma, testicular torsion, or tumors. Although typically anechoic, occasionally there are low-level echoes within the fluid secondary to protein or cholesterol content (**Fig. 22**).[51,52]
- Hematoceles are accumulations of blood within the tunica vaginalis, and may be acute or chronic. They typically have a more complex appearance than hydroceles, contain echogenic debris and septations, and may have mass effect on the adjacent testis (**Fig. 23**). Causes include trauma, surgery, and tumor. In the setting of an underlying

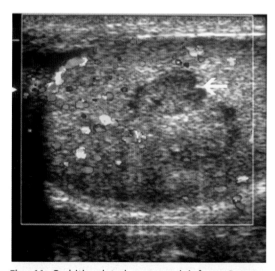

Fig. 11. Orchitis-related segmental infarct. Progression of orchitis to vascular compromise and intratesticular segmental infarct, presenting as an irregular, hypoechoic, nonvascular focus (*arrow*) within the testis. This focus was originally thought to represent a testicular tumor but intraoperative biopsy spared the patient an orchiectomy.

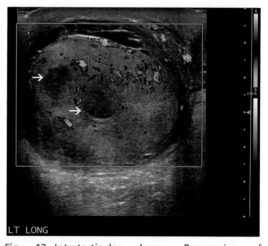

Fig. 12. Intratesticular abscess. Progression of epididymo-orchitis to the development of 2 separate hypodense avascular foci (*arrows*) not identified at initial scrotal sonogram, and consistent with intratesticular abscesses.

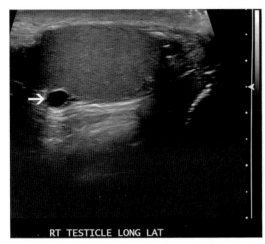

Fig. 13. Cyst of the tunica albuginea. Tunica cyst (*arrow*) is seen as a small peripheral, anechoic cystic lesion without internal features that involves the right tunica albuginea.

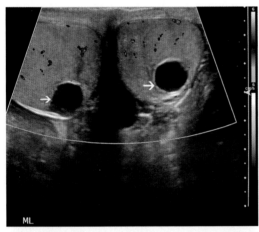

Fig. 14. Intratesticular cysts. Bilateral intratesticular cysts are shown (*arrows*) and seen as anechoic lesions without complicating features or internal vascularity.

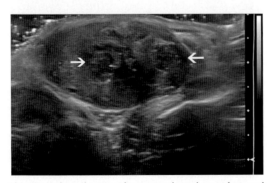

Fig. 15. Adrenal rests. Aberrant adrenal rests (*arrows*) presenting as bilateral, eccentrically located, hypoechoic masses in a patient with congenital adrenal hyperplasia.

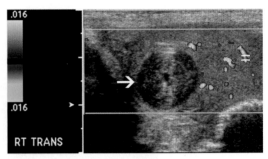

Fig. 16. Epidermoid cyst. Well-circumscribed, avascular intratesticular mass (*arrow*) with a classic laminated or onion-skin appearance.

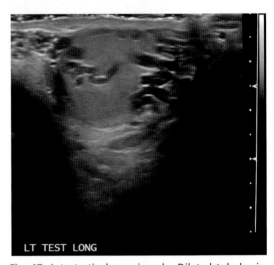

Fig. 17. Intratesticular varicocele. Dilated tubular intratesticular veins are present throughout the testis. Intratesticular varicoceles are often in close proximity to the mediastinum testis.

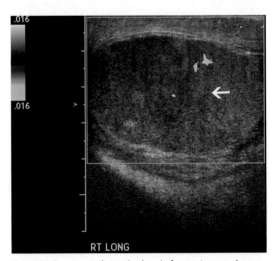

Fig. 18. Segmental testicular infarct. Large, hypoechoic area within the mid and superior aspect of the testis (*arrow*), without internal vascularity on Doppler interrogation. Segmental infarcts are more common in the superior and mid aspect of the testis.

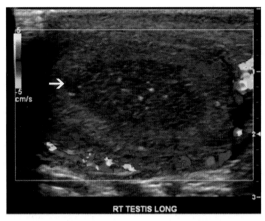

Fig. 19. Central testicular infarct. Central hypoechoic, avascular focus (*arrow*) following indirect inguinal herniorrhaphy initially suggesting a focal testicular infarct. Follow-up US showed a gradual reduction in size of the avascular focus consistent with progression of infarct.

varicocele, minor trauma may result in rupture of a dilated vein and development of a hematocele.

- A scrotal abscess (pyocele) most often results as a complication of epididymo-orchitis. An abscess appears heterogeneously echogenic, possibly containing gas manifesting as bright echogenic foci and shadowing (**Fig. 24**).
- Because the tunica vaginalis is lined by mesothelial cells, it can rarely become involved by

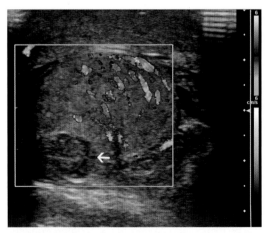

Fig. 20. Intratesticular hematoma. Posttraumatic hematoma (*arrow*) is seen as a peripheral, hypoechoic, intratesticular focus without internal vascularity. In the rare situation in which these are not immediately surgically explored, follow-up US is mandatory to ensure that the mass does not represent an occult tumor.

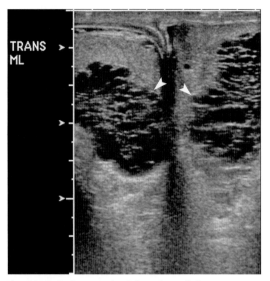

Fig. 21. Tubular ectasia. Dilatation of the rete testes (*arrowheads*) appears as hypoechoic masses within the mediastinum testis bilaterally in this patient with a history of prior vasectomy.

mesothelioma. A history of asbestos exposure is present in less than half of these patients.[45]

Paratesticular Masses

This category includes lesions that are extratesticular but within the tunica vaginalis, although they are not easily classified as arising from a particular paratesticular tissue.

- An indirect inguinal hernia can present as a scrotal mass, exiting the abdominal cavity via the inguinal ring and continuing along the inguinal canal into the scrotum. Sonographic

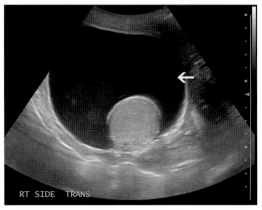

Fig. 22. Hydrocele. Simple hydrocele (*arrow*) presents as an anechoic collection within the space between the parietal and visceral layers of the tunica vaginalis.

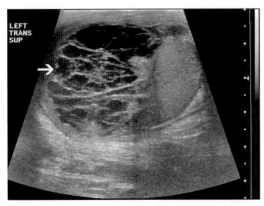

Fig. 23. Hematocele. Organizing collection (*arrow*) with echogenic septations and debris within the left tunica vaginalis consistent with hematocele. This hematocele shows mass effect on the left testis.

appearance of the hernia depends on its contents; typically omentum and/or bowel. Bowel is usually easy to identify (**Fig. 25**). Omentum-only hernias may be difficult to diagnosis because the echogenic appearance of the fat can overlap with lipomas and fat in the spermatic cord (**Fig. 26**). Following the spermatic cord in both directions and imaging

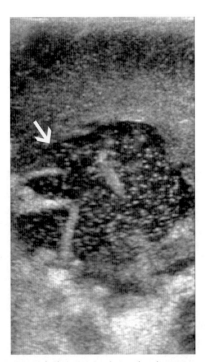

Fig. 24. Scrotal abscess. An irregular, heterogeneous, complex, extratesticular fluid collection (*arrow*) is present in this 24-year-old man with trisomy 21 who had a history of epididymo-orchitis.

during Valsalva may be helpful in making the diagnosis.

- Fibrous pseudotumor has many names, including fibroma, nodular fibropseudotumor, and scrotal mouse; it describes a benign fibroinflammatory reaction resulting in 1 or more nodules most commonly involving the tunica. US evaluation typically shows 1 or more solid, variably echogenic masses, attached to or closely associated with the testicular tunica (**Fig. 27**).
- Polyorchidism (supernumerary testis) is a rare condition, with 3 testes representing the most common form, although as many as 5 have been reported. The cause is an abnormal embryologic division of the genital ridge. Supernumerary testes are intrascrotal in approximately 75% of cases, with inguinal or retroperitoneal testes occurring progressively more infrequently (**Fig. 28**).[45]
- Scrotoliths, scrotal calculi, or scrotal pearls are free-floating calcified bodies within the tunica vaginalis. They may result from torsion of the appendix testes or appendix epididymis, or may represent inflammatory deposits that have formed along and separated from the tunica vaginalis.[53,54] On sonography they appear as mobile, echogenic foci with posterior acoustic shadowing (**Fig. 29**).

Epididymis

- Epididymitis is the most common cause of an acutely painful scrotum. It may be acute or chronic depending on the duration of disease and inciting organism. Infection usually occurs from direct extension of urinary tract pathogens in a retrograde fashion via the vas deferens from a lower urinary tract source of infection. In 20% to 40% of cases there is extension to the testis (epididymo-orchitis) that may lead to vascular compromise, ischemia, infarction, and intratesticular abscess.[7] Gray-scale findings of acute epididymitis include an enlarged, heterogeneous, often hypoechoic epididymis with hyperemia shown during color or power Doppler imaging (**Fig. 30**). Reactive hydrocele or pyocele with associated scrotal wall thickening may be present. Testicular involvement is suggested by testicular enlargement with heterogeneous echogenicity of the testicular parenchyma. Primary orchitis in isolation without epididymitis is rare and most commonly secondary to infection with the paramyxovirus causing mumps.[7] Chronic epididymitis is characterized at US by an enlarged epididymis with

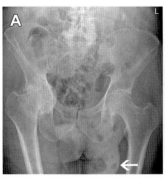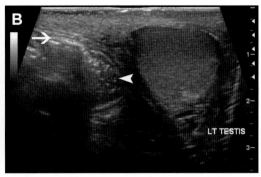

Fig. 25. Indirect inguinal hernia. (A) Abdominal radiograph shows bowel gas superimposed over the expected course of the left inguinal canal and the left hemiscrotum (*arrow*). (B) US examination of the left spermatic cord and left hemiscrotum in the same patient shows a small bowel loop extending into the superior left hemiscrotum with bowel wall (*arrow*), bowel contents (*arrowhead*) and shadowing from bowel gas present superior to the left testis.

increased heterogeneous echogenicity. Granulomatous epididymitis and granulomatous orchitis can be seen with tuberculosis, brucellosis, sarcoidosis, syphilis, and parasitic and fungal infections (**Fig. 31**).[45] Associated findings in chronic epididymitis include calcifications, hydroceles, scrotal wall thickening, and fistulas.[55–57] Testicular involvement is less common with these processes.

- The most common epididymal mass is a cyst, which is multiple in approximately 30% of men.[58] Spermatoceles and epididymal cysts are indistinguishable from one another; both appear as anechoic, well-defined masses (see **Fig. 9**). A spermatocele represents cystic dilatation of efferent ductules in the epididymal head.[59] Epididymal cysts contain clear serous fluid and can arise throughout the epididymis. Epididymal cysts were reported to be more common in the general population in a series by Holden and List,[60] although

spermatoceles were more common in patients after vasectomy.[60,61]

- Sperm granulomas can also occur in patients after vasectomy and represent a foreign body giant cell reaction to extravasated sperm. They typically present as well-defined, solid, subcentimeter, hypoechoic masses at US, although they range up to 4 cm and become more heterogeneous. Sperm granulomas most often occur at the transected ends of the vas deferens, can be multiple, and can be painful, although they are often asymptomatic.[60]
- Adenomatoid tumor is the most common epididymal tumor, accounting for 30% of paratesticular neoplasms. They are of mesothelial origin, may present as painless scrotal masses, and are universally benign, with no reports of recurrence or metastatic disease

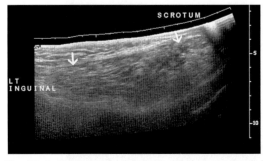

Fig. 26. Indirect inguinal hernia. US examination of the left spermatic cord shows a large heterogeneous mass (*arrows*) within the inguinal canal without bowel signature or bowel contents, consistent with a fat-containing indirect inguinal hernia.

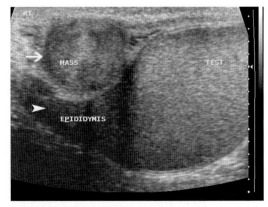

Fig. 27. Fibrous pseudotumor. Solid, heterogeneous mass (*arrow*) separate from the right testis and epididymis (*arrowhead*), but closely associated with the testicular tunica.

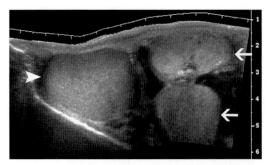

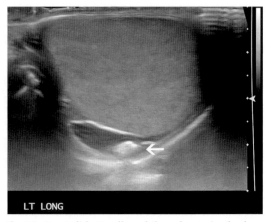

Fig. 28. Polyorchidism. Two left testes (*arrows*) separate from the right testis (*arrowhead*) are present, consistent with supernumerary testes or polyorchidism.

LT LONG

Fig. 29. Scrotolith. Small, mobile, echogenic, shadowing focus (*arrow*) present within the leaves of the left tunica vaginalis consistent with a scrotal pearl.

following excision.[62] These tumors are round, well-circumscribed masses ranging from a few millimeters up to 5 cm, and are more frequently found in the epididymal tail. On sonography, they typically appear hyperechoic and homogeneous, although great variability has been reported (**Fig. 32**).[19,63]

- Papillary cystadenoma of the epididymis is a rare tumor with a strong association with von Hippel-Lindau disease. Up to 40% of papillary cystadenomas are bilateral, an appearance that is virtually pathognomonic. A solid, palpable mass ranging from 1 to 5 cm (typically 1.5–2 cm) is the most frequent finding. At US, they typically present as echogenic, solid masses, although they may have distinct, small cystic spaces (**Fig. 33**).[64,65]
- Malignant epididymal masses. Most solid epididymal masses are benign. Malignant tumors of the epididymis are rare, and include sarcomas, metastases, and adenocarcinoma, with most representing metastases

from a primary tumor at another site. Genital tract lymphoma generally involves the testis, but can involve the epididymis in 60% of cases and the spermatic cord in 40%.[66] US features that increase the risk of malignancy in a well-defined epididymal mass include size greater than 1.5 cm and Doppler-detected vascularity.[20,66]

SPERMATIC CORD

The spermatic cord should be evaluated as part of every scrotal US examination.

- Hematomas, edema, and inflammation can present as diffuse cord abnormality. Hematomas of the cord can result from trauma or surgery, and can appear as elongated, echogenic masses involving the soft tissues of the cord (**Fig. 34**). Thickening of the cord

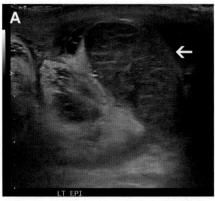

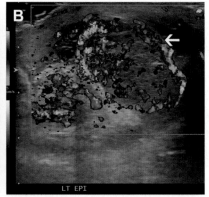

Fig. 30. Epididymitis. (*A*) Gray-scale US image shows an enlarged, heterogeneous, hypoechoic epididymal head (*arrow*) with thickening of the visualized spermatic cord structures. (*B*) Color Doppler image of the epididymal head shows significant hyperemia of the epididymis (*arrow*) and adjacent cord structures.

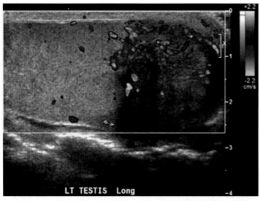

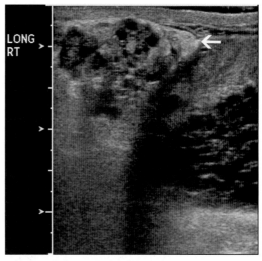

Fig. 31. Epididymal sarcoidosis. Color Doppler image shows hyperemia of a heterogeneous, enlarged epididymis that proved to be chronic granulomatous epididymal sarcoidosis in the setting of known sarcoidosis.

Fig. 33. Papillary cystadenoma. Enlarged, echogenic, right epididymis with multiple, distinct, small cystic spaces (*arrow*). Findings were present bilaterally in this patient with a history of von Hippel-Lindau disease.

may be present in epididymitis. Rotation or spiral twist of the spermatic cord, real-time whirlpool sign, has been reported to be a sensitive and specific sign for testicular torsion.[67]

- Varicoceles are present in approximately 15% of men, and up to 40% of men with infertility.[68,69] They are the most common mass of the spermatic cord, and represent abnormal dilatation of the veins of the pampiniform plexus, usually caused by incompetent valves of the internal spermatic vein. Normal vessels within the pampiniform plexus typically range up to 1.5 mm and may not be visualized. On gray-scale US, varicoceles present as multiple, anechoic, serpiginous, tubular structures of various sizes larger than 2 to 3 mm about the superior and lateral aspect of the testis. Color Doppler optimized for low flow velocities confirms venous pattern, with phasic variation and flow reversal during performance of the Valsalva maneuver.

- Lipomas are the most common extratesticular neoplasm, and most often originate from the spermatic cord. Lipomas are typically hyperechoic at US, although they contain varying amounts of fibrous, myxoid, or vascular tissue, making them more or less echogenic (**Fig. 35**).

- Additional less common benign tumors include leiomyomas, dermoid cysts, lymphangiomas, and adrenal rests. If lipomas are

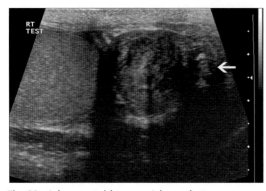

Fig. 32. Adenomatoid tumor. A large, heterogeneous, rounded, solid mass (*arrow*) arises from the right epididymal tail; it was surgically proved to be an adenomatoid tumor.

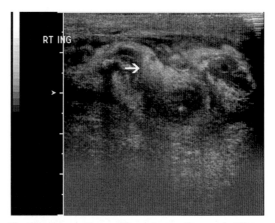

Fig. 34. Spermatic cord hematoma. Gray-scale US image shows a heterogeneous, echogenic, avascular collection (*arrow*) surrounding the spermatic cord structures and confined by the cord fascia in this patient who had blunt trauma to the right inguinal region.

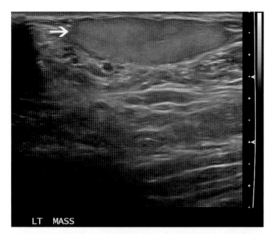

Fig. 35. Spermatic cord lipoma. A well-circumscribed, homogeneously echogenic mass (*arrow*) associated with the left spermatic cord is present superior to the left epididymis and left testis, consistent with a spermatic cord lipoma, which was proved at MR imaging.

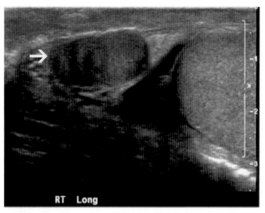

Fig. 36. Inflammatory pseudotumor. Well-circumscribed, mildly heterogeneous mass (*arrow*) associated with the inferior spermatic cord showed slow growth over the course of a 3-month follow-up and was found to represent an inflammatory pseudotumor on excision.

excluded, then 56% of spermatic cord masses are malignant, and most malignant masses are sarcomas, including rhabdomyosarcoma and liposarcoma.[18] The sonographic appearance of these tumors is variable, and therefore nonspecific (**Fig. 36**).[19,70]

SCROTAL WALL MASSES

- Noninflammatory causes of scrotal wall thickening include lymphedema, heart failure, liver failure, and venous obstruction. The thickened scrotal wall may appear hypoechoic, or alternating hypoechoic and hyperechoic.[71]
- Scrotal trauma may cause a scrotal wall hematoma, which may appear isoechoic to hyperechoic acutely, and become hypoechoic with maturation. Hematomas show no internal flow on Doppler interrogation and tend to decrease in size as they resolve.
- Cellulitis of the scrotal wall is most common in patients who are obese, diabetic, or immunocompromised. At US, the thickened scrotal wall is typically hypoechoic with increased blood flow at color Doppler US. Scrotal wall abscesses can develop in the setting of cellulitis.
- Fournier gangrene is a rare, polymicrobial necrotizing fasciitis of the scrotum that often extends to involve the perineum and lower abdominal wall. This condition constitutes a urologic emergency because of the high mortality. Although the diagnosis is based primarily on the clinical examination, imaging may have a role if clinical findings are ambiguous.

Crepitus has been reported in 18% to 62% of cases, with gas at US appearing as numerous, hyperechoic foci with reverberation artifact (**Fig. 37**).[72,73] Diffuse scrotal wall thickening is usually associated with a normal appearance of the testes and epididymides.

- Primary solid neoplasms of the scrotal wall are rare. Sporadic cases of metastatic disease have been reported, including melanoma, anal carcinoma, and lung carcinoma. These lesions are typically hypoechoic at US examination, although they have variable echogenicity.[74–76]

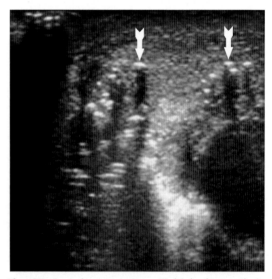

Fig. 37. Fournier gangrene. Multiple hyperechoic, shadowing foci (*arrows*) are seen throughout the scrotal wall in this 63-year-old diabetic who had crepitus on physical examination.

SUMMARY

Sonography is the ideal modality for evaluation and characterization of a scrotal mass. Extratesticular masses are usually benign, while intratesticular masses are generally malignant until proved otherwise. However, it is important to recognize the benign intratesticular conditions, thus possibly preventing orchiectomy when unwarranted, while appreciating the more significant findings of extratesticular masses that may warrant further intervention.

REFERENCES

1. Benson CB, Doubilet PM, Richie JP. Sonography of the male genital tract. AJR Am J Roentgenol 1989; 153(4):705–13.
2. Rifkin MD, Kurtz AB, Pasto ME, et al. The sonographic diagnosis of focal and diffuse infiltrating intrascrotal lesions. Urol Radiol 1984;6(1):20–6.
3. Rifkin MD, Kurtz AB, Pasto ME, et al. Diagnostic capabilities of high-resolution scrotal ultrasonography: prospective evaluation. J Ultrasound Med 1985;4(1):13–9.
4. Carroll BA, Gross DM. High-frequency scrotal sonography. AJR Am J Roentgenol 1983;140(3):511–5.
5. Larsen WJ. Human embryology. New York: Churchill Livingstone; 1993. p. 235–80.
6. Moore KL, Persaud TV. The developing human: clinically oriented embryology. 5th edition. Philadelphia: Saunders; 1993.
7. Dogra VS, Gottlieb RH, Oka M, et al. Sonography of the scrotum. Radiology 2003;227(1):18–36.
8. ACR-AIUM-SRU practice guideline for the performance of scrotal ultrasound examinations. Online publication. Available at: http://www.aium.org/resources/guidelines/scrotal.pdf.
9. Siegel MJ. The acute scrotum. Radiol Clin North Am 1997;35(4):959–76.
10. Thomas RD, Dewbury KC. Ultrasound appearances of the rete testis. Clin Radiol 1993;47(2):121–4.
11. Bree RL, Hoang DT. Scrotal ultrasound. Radiol Clin North Am 1996;34(6):1183–205.
12. Middleton WD, Thorne DA, Melson GL. Color Doppler ultrasound of the normal testis. AJR Am J Roentgenol 1989;152(2):293–7.
13. Lerner RM, Mevorach RA, Hulbert WC, et al. Color Doppler US in the evaluation of acute scrotal disease. Radiology 1990;176(2):355–8.
14. Keener TS, Winter TC, Nghiem HV, et al. Normal adult epididymis: evaluation with color Doppler US. Radiology 1997;202(3):712–4.
15. Hamper UM, DeJong MR, Caskey CI, et al. Power Doppler imaging: clinical experience and correlation with color Doppler US and other imaging modalities. Radiographics 1997;17(2):499–513.
16. Rubin JM, Bude RO, Carson PL, et al. Power Doppler US: a potentially useful alternative to mean frequency-based color Doppler US. Radiology 1994;190(3):853–6.
17. Woodward PJ, Sohaey R, O'Donoghue MJ, et al. From the archives of the AFIP: tumors and tumor-like lesions of the testis: radiologic-pathologic correlation. Radiographics 2002;22(1):189–216.
18. Beccia DJ, Krane RJ, Olsson CA. Clinical management of non-testicular intrascrotal tumors. J Urol 1976;116(4):476–9.
19. Frates MC, Benson CB, DiSalvo DN, et al. Solid extratesticular masses evaluated with sonography: pathologic correlation. Radiology 1997;204(1):43–6.
20. Alleman WG, Gorman B, King BF, et al. Benign and malignant epididymal masses evaluated with scrotal sonography: clinical and pathologic review of 85 patients. J Ultrasound Med 2008;27(8): 1195–202.
21. Kenney PJ. Solid extratesticular masses. Radiology 1998;206(1):290.
22. Siegel R, DeSantis C, Virgo K, et al. Cancer treatment and survivorship statistics, 2012. CA Cancer J Clin 2012;62(4):220–41.
23. Kreydin EI, Barrisford GW, Feldman AS, et al. Testicular cancer: what the radiologist needs to know. AJR Am J Roentgenol 2013;200(6):1215–25.
24. Winter TC. There is a mass in the scrotum–what does it mean?: Evaluation of the scrotal mass. Ultrasound Q 2009;25(4):195–205.
25. Horwich A. Testicular cancer: investigation and management. 2nd edition. London: Chapman and Hall Medical; 1996.
26. Cotran RS, Kumar V, Collins T. Pathologic basis of disease. 6th edition. Philadelphia: Saunders; 1999. p. 1011–34.
27. Heiken JP. Tumors of the testis and testicular adnexa. In: Pollack HM, McClennan BL, editors. Clinical urography. 2nd edition. Saunders; 2000. p. 1716–41.
28. Ulbright TM, Amin MB, Young RH. Tumors of the testis, adnexa, spermatic cord, and scrotum. In: Rosai J, Sobin LH, editors. Atlas of tumor pathology, fasc 25, ser 3. Washington, DC: Armed Forces Institute of Pathology; 1999. p. 1–366.
29. Walsh PC. Campbell's urology. 7th edition. Philadelphia: WB Saunders; 1998.
30. Akin EA, Khati NJ, Hill MC. Ultrasound of the scrotum. Ultrasound Q 2004;20(4):181–200.
31. Geraghty MJ, Lee FT Jr, Bernsten SA, et al. Sonography of testicular tumors and tumor-like conditions: a radiologic-pathologic correlation. Crit Rev Diagn Imaging 1998;39(1):1–63.
32. Sohaib SA, Koh DM, Husband JE. The role of imaging in the diagnosis, staging, and management of testicular cancer. AJR Am J Roentgenol 2008; 191(2):387–95.

33. Chang B, Borer JG, Tan PE, et al. Large-cell calcifying Sertoli cell tumor of the testis: case report and review of the literature. Urology 1998;52(3):520–2 [discussion: 522–3].

34. Duncan PR, Checa F, Gowing NF, et al. Extranodal non-Hodgkin's lymphoma presenting in the testicle: a clinical and pathologic study of 24 cases. Cancer 1980;45(7):1578–84.

35. Goodman JD, Carr L, Ostrovsky PD, et al. Testicular lymphoma: sonographic findings. Urol Radiol 1985;7(1):25–7.

36. Phillips G, Kumari-Subaiya S, Sawitsky A. Ultrasonic evaluation of the scrotum in lymphoproliferative disease. J Ultrasound Med 1987;6(4):169–75.

37. Mazzu D, Jeffrey RB Jr, Ralls PW. Lymphoma and leukemia involving the testicles: findings on gray-scale and color Doppler sonography. AJR Am J Roentgenol 1995;164(3):645–7.

38. Rayor RA, Scheible W, Brock WA, et al. High resolution ultrasonography in the diagnosis of testicular relapse in patients with acute lymphoblastic leukemia. J Urol 1982;128(3):602–3.

39. Richie JP. Neoplasms of the testis. In: Walsh PC, Retik AB, Vaughan ED, et al, editors. Campbell's urology. 7th edition. Philadelphia: Saunders; 1998. p. 2411–52.

40. Middleton WD, Teefey SA, Santillan CS. Testicular microlithiasis: prospective analysis of prevalence and associated tumor. Radiology 2002;224(2):425–8.

41. Backus ML, Mack LA, Middleton WD, et al. Testicular microlithiasis: imaging appearances and pathologic correlation. Radiology 1994;192(3):781–5.

42. Kim B, Winter TC 3rd, Ryu JA. Testicular microlithiasis: clinical significance and review of the literature. Eur Radiol 2003;13(12):2567–76.

43. Peterson AC, Bauman JM, Light DE, et al. The prevalence of testicular microlithiasis in an asymptomatic population of men 18 to 35 years old. J Urol 2001;166(6):2061–4.

44. Richenberg J, Brejt N. Testicular microlithiasis: is there a need for surveillance in the absence of other risk factors? Eur Radiol 2012;22(11):2540–6.

45. Woodward PJ, Schwab CM, Sesterhenn IA. From the archives of the AFIP: extratesticular scrotal masses: radiologic-pathologic correlation. Radiographics 2003;23(1):215–40.

46. Fu YT, Wang HH, Yang TH, et al. Epidermoid cysts of the testis: diagnosis by ultrasonography and magnetic resonance imaging resulting in organ-preserving surgery. Br J Urol 1996;78(1):116–8.

47. Eisenmenger M, Lang S, Donner G, et al. Epidermoid cysts of the testis: organ-preserving surgery following diagnosis by ultrasonography. Br J Urol 1993;72(6):955–7.

48. Venkatanarasimha N, McCormick F, Freeman SJ. Cavernous hemangioma of the testis. J Ultrasound Med 2010;29(5):859–60.

49. Das KM, Prasad K, Szmigielski W, et al. Intratesticular varicocele: evaluation using conventional and Doppler sonography. AJR Am J Roentgenol 1999;173(4):1079–83.

50. Micallef M, Torreggiani WC, Hurley M, et al. The ultrasound investigation of scrotal swelling. Int J STD AIDS 2000;11(5):297–302.

51. Gooding GA, Leonhardt WC, Marshall G, et al. Cholesterol crystals in hydroceles: sonographic detection and possible significance. AJR Am J Roentgenol 1997;169(2):527–9.

52. Collings C, Cronan JJ, Grusmark J. Diffuse echoes within a simple hydrocele: an imaging caveat. J Ultrasound Med 1994;13(6):439–42.

53. Linkowski GD, Avellone A, Gooding GA. Scrotal calculi: sonographic detection. Radiology 1985;156(2):484.

54. Dewbury KC. Scrotal ultrasonography: an update. BJU Int 2000;86(Suppl 1):143–52.

55. Chung JJ, Kim MJ, Lee T, et al. Sonographic findings in tuberculous epididymitis and epididymo-orchitis. J Clin Ultrasound 1997;25(7):390–4.

56. Salmeron I, Ramirez-Escobar MA, Puertas F, et al. Granulomatous epididymo-orchitis: sonographic features and clinical outcome in brucellosis, tuberculosis and idiopathic granulomatous epididymo-orchitis. J Urol 1998;159(6):1954–7.

57. Heaton ND, Hogan B, Michell M, et al. Tuberculous epididymo-orchitis: clinical and ultrasound observations. Br J Urol 1989;64(3):305–9.

58. Leung ML, Gooding GA, Williams RD. High-resolution sonography of scrotal contents in asymptomatic subjects. AJR Am J Roentgenol 1984;143(1):161–4.

59. Hricak H, Filly RA. Sonography of the scrotum. Invest Radiol 1983;18(2):112–21.

60. Holden A, List A. Extratesticular lesions: a radiological and pathological correlation. Australas Radiol 1994;38(2):99–105.

61. Jarvis LJ, Dubbins PA. Changes in the epididymis after vasectomy: sonographic findings. AJR Am J Roentgenol 1989;152(3):531–4.

62. Srigley JR, Hartwick RW. Tumors and cysts of the paratesticular region. Pathol Annu 1990;25(Pt 2):51–108.

63. Leonhardt WC, Gooding GA. Sonography of intrascrotal adenomatoid tumor. Urology 1992;39(1):90–2.

64. Choyke PL, Glenn GM, Walther MM, et al. Von Hippel-Lindau disease: genetic, clinical, and imaging features. Radiology 1995;194(3):629–42.

65. Alexander JA, Lichtman JB, Varma VA. Ultrasound demonstration of a papillary cystadenoma of the epididymis. J Clin Ultrasound 1991;19(7):442–5.

66. Bostwick D. Spermatic cord and testicular adnexa. In: Bostwick D, Eble JN, editors. Urologic surgical pathology. St Louis (MO): Mosby; 1997. p. 647–74.

67. Vijayaraghavan SB. Sonographic differential diagnosis of acute scrotum: real-time whirlpool sign, a key sign of torsion. J Ultrasound Med 2006;25(5): 563–74.

68. Meacham RB, Townsend RR, Rademacher D, et al. The incidence of varicoceles in the general population when evaluated by physical examination, gray scale sonography and color Doppler sonography. J Urol 1994;151(6):1535–8.

69. Kim ED, Lipshultz LI. Role of ultrasound in the assessment of male infertility. J Clin Ultrasound 1996;24(8):437–53.

70. Haller J, Tscholakoff D, Gundry C, et al. Sonography of unusual extratesticular lesions. Urol Radiol 1989;11(3):190–3.

71. Grainger AJ, Hide IG, Elliott ST. The ultrasound appearances of scrotal oedema. Eur J Ultrasound 1998;8(1):33–7.

72. Rajan DK, Scharer KA. Radiology of Fournier's gangrene. AJR Am J Roentgenol 1998;170(1):163–8.

73. Dogra VS, Smeltzer JS, Poblette J. Sonographic diagnosis of Fournier's gangrene. J Clin Ultrasound 1994;22(9):571–2.

74. Ferguson MA, White BA, Johnson DE, et al. Carcinoma en cuirasse of the scrotum: an unusual presentation of lung carcinoma metastatic to the scrotum. J Urol 1998;160(6 Pt 1):2154–5.

75. Nazzari G, Drago F, Malatto M, et al. Epidermoid anal canal carcinoma metastatic to the skin. A clinical mimic of prostate adenocarcinoma metastases. J Dermatol Surg Oncol 1994;20(11):765–6.

76. Siegal GP, Gaffey TA. Solitary leiomyomas arising from the tunica dartos scroti. J Urol 1976;116(1):69–71.

The Role of Sonography in Thyroid Cancer

Stephanie F. Coquia, MD*, Linda C. Chu, MD, Ulrike M. Hamper, MD, MBA

KEYWORDS

- Thyroid nodules • Thyroid cancer • Fine-needle aspiration biopsy
- Cervical lymph node metastases • Lateral neck compartment • Central neck compartment

KEY POINTS

- Thyroid nodules are commonly detected on ultrasound (US).
- Specific sonographic features are found in many malignant nodules and lymph nodes.
- Identification of cervical nodal metastasis is important for accurate staging and surgical management of de novo thyroid cancer.
- Pathologic diagnosis of a thyroid nodule requires fine-needle aspiration (FNA).
- US accurately provides imaging guidance for FNA of indeterminate or suspicious thyroid nodules and cervical lymph nodes.
- US is routinely used in the postoperative surveillance of the neck for tumor recurrence in the thyroid bed or nodal stations.

INTRODUCTION

According to the National Cancer Institute, an estimated 63,000 cases of thyroid cancer will be diagnosed in 2014.[1] When pathologically well differentiated and diagnosed early, the disease is highly treatable and can be curable. The 5-year relative survival rate of most types of stage I thyroid cancer approaches 100%.[2]

US is used routinely in the diagnosis and management of thyroid cancer, from initial detection and diagnosis to preoperative planning to postoperative surveillance. This review discusses the various roles of sonography in managing patients with thyroid cancer and reviews the sonographic appearance of thyroid cancer and nodal metastases.

NORMAL ANATOMY AND IMAGING TECHNIQUE

The thyroid gland is a bilobed gland that sits atop the trachea within the anterior-inferior neck (**Fig. 1**). The isthmus connects the right and left thyroid lobes. Each lobe measures approximately 4 to 6 cm in length and less than 2 cm in width and in the anterior-posterior dimension.[3] The normal isthmus measures less than 6 mm in the anterior-posterior dimension. The normal gland is homogeneous in echotexture and hyperechoic compared with the adjacent strap muscles (see **Fig. 1**).

After documentation of any thyroid lesion that has suspicious features for primary thyroid cancer, the cervical lymph nodes are imaged. A normal lymph node has an elongated shape (a 2:1 ratio between length and short-axis dimensions) and demonstrates an echogenic fatty hilum. Vascular flow is seen entering into the lymph node via the fatty hilum (**Fig. 2**) and the cortex is symmetrically hypoechoic.

The neck can be divided into nodal levels or stations by anatomic landmarks. The numeric classification system of the neck nodal stations is outlined in **Table 1** and depicted in **Fig. 3**.[4] Using this classification, the neck can be divided into

Russell H. Morgan Department of Radiology and Radiological Science, Johns Hopkins University School of Medicine, 601 North Caroline Street, Baltimore, MD 21287, USA
* Corresponding author. 601 North Caroline Street, JHOC 3142, Baltimore, MD 21287.
E-mail address: scoquia1@jhmi.edu

Radiol Clin N Am 52 (2014) 1283–1294
http://dx.doi.org/10.1016/j.rcl.2014.07.007
0033-8389/14/$ – see front matter © 2014 Elsevier Inc. All rights reserved.

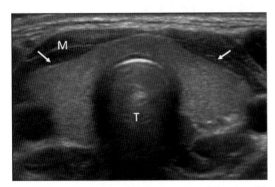

Fig. 1. Normal sonographic appearance of the thyroid. The thyroid (*arrows*) sits atop the trachea (T) and is a bilobed structure echogenic to the adjacent musculature (M).

central and lateral neck compartments. Stations I, VI, and VII are considered central neck compartments and stations II to V are considered lateral neck compartments. The medial edge of the common carotid artery serves as a landmark to divide the central from the lateral compartment. The distinction between the central and lateral neck compartments is important for the surgical management of thyroid cancer if nodal metastases are present (discussed later).

IMAGING PROTOCOLS
Thyroid

The thyroid gland is imaged with a linear high-frequency transducer (7–15 MHz). Occasionally, if the thyroid gland is enlarged, a curved, lower-frequency transducer may be used to fully image the thyroid.

The right and left thyroid lobes are imaged in the transverse and sagittal planes. Anterior-posterior dimension, width, and length are measured at the mid thyroid gland. The isthmus is measured in the anterior-posterior dimension. Nodules, if present, are measured in the transverse and sagittal planes in three dimensions and evaluated with color Doppler to document vascularity.

Cervical Lymph Nodes

The neck nodes are imaged with the same transducers as the thyroid: a high-frequency linear transducer for most of the nodal stations and occasionally a curved transducer for the lower and, therefore, deeper level IV and VI lymph nodes.

Each nodal station within the neck is evaluated to assess for the presence of normal or abnormal lymph nodes. Normal-appearing lymph nodes can be documented for each level, with the fatty hilum included in the image. Measurement of sonographically normal-appearing lymph nodes is not necessary. Abnormal lymph nodes (discussed later) should be imaged and measured in the transverse and sagittal planes. The nodes also should be interrogated with color Doppler US to assess for abnormal and disorganized blood flow.

General imaging protocols for the thyroid gland and cervical lymph nodes are summarized in **Table 2**.

IMAGING FINDINGS AND PATHOLOGY
Types of Thyroid Cancer

There are several types of primary thyroid cancer. Papillary thyroid carcinoma (PTC) is the most common, accounting for approximately 75% to 80% of thyroid cancers. PTC is multifocal in approximately 20% of cases and more common in females than males. PTC usually presents before age 40 years, often with cervical nodal metastases. It is also the most common thyroid malignancy in children. PTC has the best prognosis and highest survival rate of all thyroid cancers, reaching a 20-year survival rate of approximately 90% to 95%. Other types of thyroid carcinoma include follicular carcinoma (10%–20%), medullary carcinoma (5%–10%), and anaplastic carcinoma

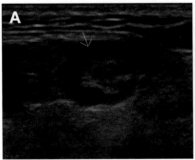
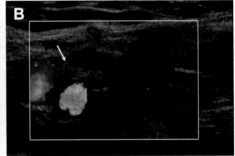

Fig. 2. Normal lymph nodes. (*A*) Lymph node with smooth, homogeneous, hypoechoic cortex (*arrow*), and central echogenic fatty hilum. (*B*) Another lymph node demonstrating normal central hilar flow (*arrow*).

Table 1
Cervical nodal stations: numeric classification

Nodal Station	Location
IA	Submental lymph nodes
IB	Submandibular lymph nodes

II	Internal jugular vein chain from base of skull to the inferior border of the hyoid bone
	    A: Anterior to the internal jugular vein
	    B: Posterior the internal jugular vein

III	Internal jugular vein chain from the inferior border of the hyoid bone to the inferior border of the cricoid cartilage
IV	Internal jugular vein chain from the inferior border of the cricoid cartilage to the supraclavicular fossa

V	Posterior triangle lymph nodes, posterior to the sternocleidomastoid muscle
	    A: From the skull base to the inferior border of the cricoid cartilage
	    B: From the inferior border of the cricoid cartilage to the clavicle

VI	Central compartment nodes from the hyoid bone to the suprasternal notch
VII	Central compartment nodes inferior to the suprasternal notch in the superior mediastinum

Note: The lateral compartments (II–V) are separated from the central compartments (I, VI, and VII) by the medial edge of the common carotid artery.
From Som PM, Curtin HD, Mancuso AA. An imaging-based classification for the cervical nodes designed as an adjunct to recent clinically based nodal classifications. Arch Otolaryngol Head Neck Surg 1999;125(4):391; with permission.

(1%–2%).[5] Follicular thyroid carcinoma most often affects women in the 6th decade of life and may present with metastatic lesions to bone, brain, lung, and liver via hematogenous spread. FNA biopsy (FNAB) cannot differentiate between follicular adenoma and carcinoma and surgical resection is required to make this distinction. Medullary thyroid carcinoma arises from the parafollicular cells (C cells) of the thyroid gland. It is often familial in origin (vs sporadic) and is associated with multiple endocrine neoplasia type 2 syndrome in 10% to 20% of cases. Patients present with

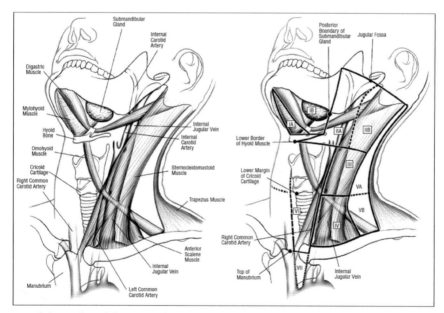

Fig. 3. Diagram of the neck nodal stations. (*From* Som PM, Curtin HD, Mancuso AA. An imaging-based classification for the cervical nodes designed as an adjunct to recent clinically based nodal classifications. Arch Otolaryngol Head Neck Surg 1999;125(4):394; with permission.)

Table 2	
Imaging protocols for thyroid and cervical lymph node examinations	
Thyroid imaging protocol	
Transducer	Linear 7–15 MHz (curved lower-frequency transducer as needed)
Gland measurements	Lobes: anterior-posterior dimension, width, longitudinal dimension Isthmus: anterior-posterior dimension
Nodules	Measurement of each nodule in three dimensions; color Doppler interrogation of nodule
Cervical lymph node imaging protocol	
Transducer	Linear 7–15 MHz (curved lower-frequency transducer as needed)
Nodes	Each nodal station evaluated on each side of the neck Documentation of abnormal lymph nodes: Size measured in three dimensions Color Doppler interrogation of node

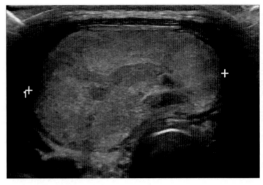

Fig. 4. PTC. This nodule measured 5.2 cm and was found in a 17-year-old girl who presented with neck swelling. The patient's age and the size of the nodule increased the probability of this nodule being malignant.

elevated calcitonin levels due to the secretion of calcitonin by the parafollicular cells. Anaplastic thyroid carcinoma is the rarest and most aggressive of the primary thyroid carcinomas, often fatal. Its dismal prognosis carries a 5-year survival rate of only 5%.[6] There is often local invasion of the adjacent soft tissues, trachea, and lymph nodes.

Risk factors for the development of thyroid carcinoma include a history of neck irradiation and a family history of thyroid cancer. Additional risk factors that increase the probability of cancer within a given thyroid nodule include age under 30 years or over 60 years and male gender.[7] Nodules greater than 2 cm also are reported to have an increased risk of cancer (**Fig. 4**).[8]

Lymphomatous involvement of the thyroid is rare, accounting for less than 5% of thyroid malignancies. It may present as a manifestation of generalized lymphoma or be primary to the thyroid gland, usually a non-Hodgkin lymphoma. Hashimoto thyroiditis is a risk factor for the development of thyroid lymphoma. Metastatic disease to the thyroid is also uncommon; primary malignancies include lung, breast, and renal cell carcinomas as well as melanoma.[6]

Thyroid Nodules

Thyroid nodules are common in the United States; it has been estimated that approximately 50% of the adult population has thyroid nodules, although less than 7% of these nodules prove malignant.[6] US features suspicious for malignancy are reviewed in this section. They are also summarized in **Table 3**.

Calcification

Calcification within the thyroid may be classified as microcalcification, coarse calcification, or peripheral rim calcification. Although calcification may be seen in both benign and malignant processes of the thyroid, it is the US feature most commonly associated with malignancy. Of these various types, microcalcifications are the most specific for thyroid malignancy, with a specificity of up to 95%.[6] Microcalcifications are most commonly found in PTC and appear as tiny punctate echogenic foci within the nodule (**Fig. 5**). Due to their small size, they usually do not demonstrate posterior acoustic shadowing. Colloid may also appear on US as tiny echogenic foci but tends to appear linear and demonstrates posterior ring-down or comet-tail artifact (**Fig. 6**).[9] Making this distinction can be difficult, however, and biopsy should be performed for indeterminate foci and for those foci lacking the comet-tail artifact. Furthermore, the presence of the ring-down artifact does not necessarily preclude contemplating biopsy; microcalcifications and colloid may coexist in the same nodule.

Coarse calcification and peripheral rimlike calcification may also be seen with thyroid malignancies; however, they also may be found in multinodular thyroids or goiters. Due to their larger size,

Table 3
Diagnostic criteria: sonographic features suggestive of malignancy

US Feature	Comment
Calcification	Micro-, macro-, coarse, peripheral (especially micro)
Solid hypoechoic nodule	Especially if very hypoechoic
Local invasion	More common in anaplastic and lymphoma
Edge refraction shadow	
Taller than wide	Nodule anterior-posterior dimension greater than width
Irregular margins	
Adjacent suspicious lymph nodes	
Size >2 cm	
Posterior acoustic shadowing	

these calcifications demonstrate posterior acoustic shadowing (**Fig. 7**). Coarse calcifications may be seen in PTC; however, they are more commonly associated with medullary thyroid carcinoma.[6] Nodules with coarse calcifications necessitate FNAB.

Solid hypoechoic nodule

Thyroid nodules may be completely cystic or solid or a combination of both. Likewise, thyroid nodules may be hyperechoic, isoechoic, or hypoechoic to the remainder of the thyroid parenchyma. Most PTCs are hypoechoic and nearly all medullary thyroid carcinomas are hypoechoic.[10] Some investigators believe the extremely hypoechoic nodule

confers a higher risk of malignancy. Benign nodules may also be hypoechoic; therefore, evaluation for additional suspicious features, such as calcification, should be performed. If no other suspicious features are present, these hypoechoic nodules can be biopsied when of sufficient size (discussed later).

Follicular neoplasms (adenoma and carcinoma) can also appear as solid, well-marginated, hypoechoic nodules with thin hypoechoic halos[10] and central linear hypoechoic striations or areas (**Fig. 8**). Because the distinction between follicular adenoma and carcinoma can only be made based on vascular and capsular invasion, the diagnosis can only be made by surgical resection. As such, once a nodule is diagnosed as a follicular neoplasm via FNAB, surgical management is the next step.

Local invasion

Anaplastic thyroid carcinoma and thyroid lymphoma may present as large, rapidly growing masses. The masses may be discrete or infiltrative. Extracapsular extension into the soft tissues is common with invasion into the trachea, neck vessels, and strap muscles. There is usually associated cervical lymphadenopathy.

Edge refraction shadow

Posterior acoustic shadowing from the edges of a solid nodule has also been associated with PTC. It is thought that the fibrotic reaction around the edge of the tumor is responsible for the edge refraction shadow.[10]

Other features suggesting malignancy in thyroid nodules

Additional suspicious features include nodules that are taller than they are wide,[11] have irregular shape or margins,[11] demonstrate posterior acoustic shadowing in the absence of edge refraction, or are accompanied by sonographically suspicious lymph nodes, such as lymph nodes with

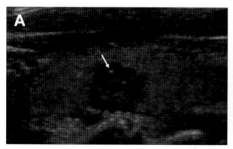 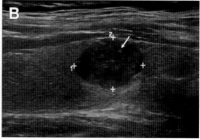

Fig. 5. (*A, B*) Examples of microcalcification. Multiple punctate echogenic foci (*arrows*) are seen within each of the hypoechoic nodules. Both of these nodules are markedly hypoechoic with irregular borders. These nodules were pathologically proved to be PTC.

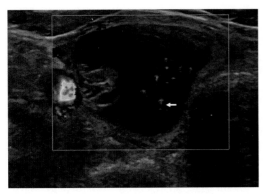

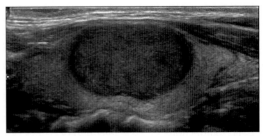

Fig. 8. Hypoechoic nodule. The nodule is well defined and homogeneously hypoechoic with a thin hypoechoic halo. FNA resulted in pathology of follicular neoplasm. The patient was scheduled for lobectomy for definitive diagnosis.

Fig. 6. Example of colloid within a predominately cystic thyroid nodule. The punctate echogenic foci demonstrate comet-tail artifact (*arrow*).

calcification, cystic change, or abnormally increased or disorganized blood flow. A more detailed discussion of the sonographic findings suspicious for cervical lymph node metastasis from thyroid carcinoma follows.

Although these features can be seen in thyroid malignancies, they are by no means pathognomonic; benign nodules may also demonstrate these features. The differential diagnosis of thyroid nodules is found in **Table 4**. Therefore, when nodules present with features suspicious or suggestive of malignancy, these should proceed to biopsy when of sufficient size.

Size criteria for biopsy

Multiple guidelines for FNAB of thyroid nodules exist because multiple medical specialties and

organizations are involved in the care of patients with thyroid nodules. These include recommendations from the American Thyroid Association (ATA), the Society of Radiologists in Ultrasound, and the American Association of Clinical Endocrinologists (AACE).[5,12,13] Regardless of the recommending body, the guidelines take into account the nodule's sonographic appearance as well as size. In addition, the ATA uses clinical risk stratification, providing differing guidelines for high-risk and low-risk patients. In general, for low-risk patients, the various guidelines recommend biopsy of solid nodules at sizes greater than 1 to 1.5 cm and mixed cystic and solid nodules at sizes greater than 1.5 to 2 cm. The ATA decreases its minimum size threshold to 5 mm in high-risk patients who have nodules with suspicious features or nodules accompanied by suspicious lymph nodes, whereas the AACE decreases its size threshold below 1.0 cm if there are suspicious sonographic features present.

Due to the multitude of guidelines available, it may be confusing as to which specific recommendations to follow. Each department or practice should meet with the referring endocrinologists and surgeons to decide which of the guidelines is to be used by all members of the clinical team to provide seamless care to patients.

Pitfalls of thyroid US in the detection of nodules

Parathyroid adenomas may be confused with thyroid nodules. Most parathyroid adenomas are extrathyroidal in location; evaluation for the echogenic thyroid capsule separating the adenoma from the thyroid tissue is helpful in making this distinction. Parathyroid adenomas are usually located posterior to the mid gland or inferior to the thyroid gland (**Fig. 9A**). Adenomas are quite vascular and obtain their vascular supply from the thyroid (see **Fig. 9B**).

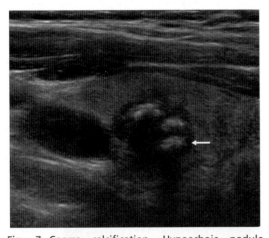

Fig. 7. Coarse calcification. Hypoechoic nodule with slightly indistinct and irregular border demonstrates a cluster of coarse echogenic calcifications demonstrating posterior acoustic shadowing (*arrow*). Pathology was PTC.

Table 4
Differential diagnosis of thyroid nodules

Diagnosis	Comment
Benign	
Adenomatoid nodule	
Follicular adenoma	Surgical excision is required to differentiate adenoma from carcinoma
Hashimoto thyroiditis	Lymphocytic thyroiditis can be used as alternative nomenclature
Parathyroid adenoma	Most are extrathyroidal in location; evaluate for capsule separating lesion from thyroid; correlate with parathyroid hormone level
Malignant	
PTC	
Follicular thyroid carcinoma	
Medullary thyroid carcinoma	
Anaplastic thyroid carcinoma	
Lymphoma	Treat with systemic therapy rather than thyroidectomy
Metastatic disease	

Note that benign and malignant nodules may have overlapping appearances and can only be differentiated by FNAB. Different pathology laboratories may use slightly different cytologic descriptions.

Hashimoto thyroiditis may also present with nodules. The nodules are usually subcentimeter in size (typically 2–3 mm and less than 6 mm) and numerous (termed *micronodulation* or *giraffe pattern*), however, causing diffuse heterogeneity of the gland. This diffuse heterogeneity may also create the appearance of larger nodules. The borders of these apparent lesions are indistinct, however. Moreover, because it is an autoimmune process, prominent reactive cervical lymph nodes, usually in level VI, may be present and could be confused as suspicious lymph nodes. These lymph nodes, however, usually have fatty hila and maintain the morphologic appearance of a benign lymph node. A truly discrete nodule, however, in a patient with Hashimoto thyroiditis should be viewed with concern because these patients are at increased risk for both lymphoma and PTC.

Management of multiple thyroid nodules
Patients sometimes present with multiple nodules, which may pose a dilemma regarding which nodules to biopsy. Regardless of the number of nodules present, the risk of thyroid cancer in a patient is unchanged.[5] Furthermore, it has been found that although a majority of cancers found in patients with multinodular thyroids are within the dominant nodule, approximately one-third of the cancers are found in the nondominant nodule.[5] Therefore, each nodule should be evaluated independently, evaluating for suspicious features and then triaging the nodules for biopsy in the order of most suspicious features and then by size.

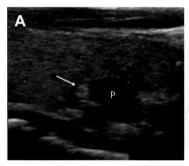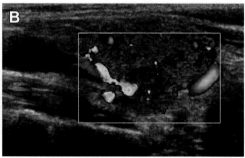

Fig. 9. Parathyroid adenoma. (*A*) The inferior parathyroid gland is typically located posterior and inferior to the thyroid. The echogenic thyroid capsule (*arrow*) separates the parathyroid adenoma (*P*) from the thyroid. (*B*) The parathyroid adenoma is quite vascular and receives its blood supply from the thyroid gland. Unlike the central hilar flow of a lymph node, the flow within a parathyroid adenoma is peripheral/polar in distribution.

Thyroid Nodule Fine-Needle Aspiration Biopsy

Biopsy and cytologic evaluation

Thyroid nodules can be sampled via US guidance or by palpation; however, in this day and age, they should be sampled with US guidance. After sterilization of the skin at the needle entrance site and administration of local anesthesia, FNA samples are obtained with small-gauge needles with a bevel tip, typically 25 or 26 gauge. Pathologic evaluation can be performed on site or the samples can be transported to a laboratory for off-site testing. The presence of at least 6 groups of benign follicular cells, with each group containing at least 10 cells, is required for a specimen to be considered adequate and benign, per the Bethesda System criteria.[14] Other alternative criteria for adequacy include the presence of abundant colloid (suggesting a benign macrofollicular nodule) or enough cells to suggest an alternative diagnosis, such as lymphocytic (or Hashimoto) thyroiditis or atypia. Aspirated thyroid nodules are classified as benign, atypia of undetermined significance/follicular lesion of undetermined significance (AUS/FLUS), follicular neoplasm, suspicious for malignancy, or malignant, per the Bethesda System classification.[14] Approximately 10% of thyroid FNAs from most laboratories are read, however, as nondiagnostic or inadequate.[14]

Management

Benign nodules are managed conservatively with clinical and imaging follow-up whereas nodules classified as follicular neoplasm, suspicious for malignancy, or malignant go on to surgical management. Nodules classified as AUS/FLUS fall into an indeterminate category, comprising between 3% and 6% of total diagnoses.[14] In these cases, repeat FNA is recommended. However, 20% of these nodules remain AUS after repeat biopsy. The risk of malignancy in these nodules is between 5% and 15%.[14]

To avoid diagnostic surgery for what may ultimately be a benign nodule, FNA samples can be sent for genomic testing. The Afirma Gene Expression Classifier (AGEC) from Veracyte (South San Francisco, California) classifies these cytologically indeterminate nodules as either benign or malignant, with a 95% negative predictive value.[15] To minimize the need for a third FNA specifically just to perform this test, additional FNA passes are obtained at the time of the second FNA for AGEC testing. This material is then reserved and analyzed in the event that the repeat (or second) FNA is also called indeterminate. A nodule classified as benign on AGEC is managed just as a nodule classified as benign on cytology, with

imaging and clinical follow-up.[15] A benign AGEC result, therefore, negates the necessity of performing surgery for diagnosis of cytologically indeterminate nodules. At one center, the number of diagnostic surgeries performed for these nodules dropped 10-fold after the implementation of AGEC testing, and 1 surgery was avoided for every 2 AGEC tests performed.[15] A suspicious for malignancy AGEC result correlates to a greater than 50% risk of malignancy for the nodule, and surgery should be performed for pathologic diagnosis.

Preoperative Evaluation for Cervical Nodal Metastases

Current best surgical practice in the United States recommends central lymph node dissection at the time of thyroidectomy as well as lateral neck dissection if there are confirmed metastatic cervical lymph nodes. Therefore, prior to thyroidectomy, the cervical lymph nodes should be evaluated for lymph node metastases both with palpation and US; if abnormal lymph nodes are suspected, FNA should be performed. Stulak and colleagues[16] in 2006 reported a sensitivity and specificity of 83.5% and 97.7% of preoperative US in the detection of lateral nodal metastasis in newly diagnosed thyroid cancer patients, respectively. Hence, a systematic sonographic evaluation of the neck nodes is performed bilaterally to identify suspicious nodes.

US features of suspicious nodes

Benign sonographic morphologic features of lymph nodes include the presence of an echogenic fatty hilum, central regular hilar vascular flow, and elongated shape. Deviations from this appearance should be considered abnormal.

A node demonstrating cystic change or the presence of calcification (mimicking the appearance of the primary tumor) has been shown to be 100% specific for metastatic disease.[17] Increased or eccentric irregular vascularity, round shape and/or loss of the normal elongated shape, hyperechogenicity of the node relative to the adjacent strap muscles, and loss of a fatty hilum are all features of abnormal lymph nodes. A summary of suspicious features is in **Box 1**, and examples of suspicious nodes are given in **Figs. 10–12**.

Metastatic disease from other primaries, however, such as squamous cell carcinoma, can produce cystic degeneration of a lymph node.

Management of suspicious nodes

Unlike the guidelines for thyroid nodule biopsy, no specific size criteria are commonly used in regard to lymph node biopsy. Some institutions may have

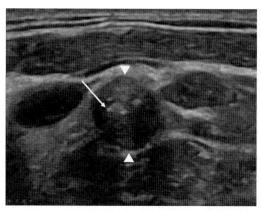

Fig. 11. Calcifications within a lymph node. Multiple echogenic foci (*arrow*) are seen within a lymph node (*arrowheads*), compatible with calcification. The lymph node is also round, another suspicious feature. The node was biopsied, with pathology of metastatic PTC.

their own size cutoff (ie, biopsy lymph nodes 8 mm or larger), formed by consensus between their surgeons, endocrinologists, and radiologists. For example, at the authors' institution, because of the high specificity of lymph nodes containing calcification or cystic areas in predicting metastatic disease, these are biopsied regardless of size. Those that are abnormal but do not contain these features are usually biopsied when 8 mm in size.

Lymph nodes that are homogeneously hypoechoic without an echogenic fatty hilum present and do not demonstrate any other suspicious features may be followed, with biopsy for those that demonstrate interval growth or interval

development of additional suspicious features. Again, this particular management step may be based on the consensus between the referring physicians and the radiologists.

Suspicious lymph nodes can be biopsied preoperatively to confirm the necessity for lateral neck dissection at the time of thyroidectomy. Because these nodes are usually not palpable, they are sampled under US guidance, using the same technique as described for FNA of thyroid nodules. If the lymph node is cystic, such that it yields insufficient cells for diagnosis, the fluid can be aspirated and sent for thyroglobulin.

Alternatively a surgeon may choose to proceed to surgery and remove the suspicious lymph nodes at the time of thyroidectomy. To help the surgeon find the nodes intraoperatively, preoperative

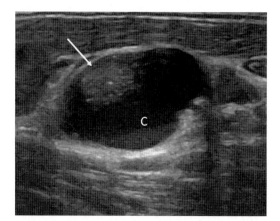

Fig. 10. Cystic replacement of a cervical lymph node. The lymph node is enlarged and has a large anechoic component, causing increased through transmission, compatible with cystic change (C). A small area of residual soft tissue is seen within the node (*arrow*). A punctate echogenic focus is seen within the soft tissue, compatible with calcification.

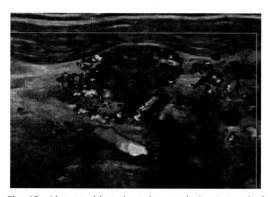

Fig. 12. Abnormal lymph node vascularity. Instead of central hilar flow, there is peripheral vascularity, which is increased. A fatty hilum is also not seen. This was biopsied with pathology of metastatic PTC.

US can be used to mark the suspicious nodes on the skin. In more complex cases, intraoperative US guidance can be provided.

Postoperative Surveillance

After thyroidectomy, in conjunction with laboratory follow-up and nuclear medicine radioiodine imaging, the neck is evaluated routinely with US for the development of nodal metastases. The initial US examination should be performed in the first 6 to 12 months and then periodically depending on a patient's risk for recurrence and thyroglobulin level.[12] The frequency and length of surveillance may also be dependent on the institution, endocrinologist, or surgeon. The risk of recurrence either within the thyroid bed or within the cervical lymph nodes in PTC has been reported to between 15% and 25%.[18]

The postoperative neck can be divided into lateral and central compartments (right lateral neck, right central neck, left lateral neck, and left central neck), discussed previously. Disease found in each separate compartment leads to its own separate neck dissection. Therefore, if multiple abnormal nodes are present in multiple compartments, a suspicious node from each compartment should be sampled to accurately plan surgical management and decrease the extent of the neck dissection.

Identification of thyroid cells within the lymph node is confirmatory for lymph node metastasis. In the event the lymph node sampling is nondiagnostic or indeterminate for metastatic disease, the lymph node can be aspirated and the sample sent for thyroglobulin assay. It is particularly helpful to aspirate and analyze the fluid within small cystic areas. A thyroglobulin level in a lymph node greater than the serum thyroglobulin level is diagnostic for metastatic disease.

Pitfalls in the postoperative surveillance period
In one study, approximately 34% of postoperative patients were found to have small thyroid bed nodules.[18] Of these nodules, only a small percentage (9%) increased in size during the median 3-year follow-up period, growing at a rate of 1.3 mm/y. Furthermore, only one-third of those proved malignant demonstrated interval growth. This behavior demonstrates the slow indolent nature of papillary thyroid cancer. Therefore, many small nodules in the thyroid bed without suspicious features can be observed over time.

In addition to recurrence, other masses can be seen in the surgical bed on postoperative examinations, such as residual thyroid tissue, scarring/fibrosis, and suture granulomas. Residual thyroid tissue may be focal and can be vascular, features that make it difficult to differentiate from recurrence by imaging. FNA can be performed to differentiate the mass as either malignant (compatible with recurrence) or benign (normal residual thyroid tissue). Scarring in the postsurgical bed can be nonspecific in appearance but typically is nonvascular and elongated, blending into the adjacent fat and muscle. These areas can also be observed over time for interval increase in size or development of suspicious features that prompt biopsy. Suture granulomas can present as focal masses within the thyroid bed. The sonographic appearance of suture granulomas has been described as a hypoechoic lesion with central echogenic lines or foci.[19] Although echogenic foci within a lesion may suggest microcalcification and, therefore, imply recurrence, features that support suture granuloma include centrality of the foci, paired foci, and foci larger than 1 mm.[19] Suture granulomas also tend to regress or resolve over time.[19]

Suture granulomas also may present within the neck, buried within the sternocleidomastoid muscle or subcutaneous tissue. Neuromas may also be seen within the neck, typically presenting as hypoechoic masses in close relation to the carotid artery. Traumatic neuromas may develop after neck dissection.[20]

Because many of these masses in the thyroid bed and neck can demonstrate either no growth or minimal growth over time, it is important to correlate with a patient's thyroglobulin level over time because this may indicate residual or progressive disease.

Alcohol ablation of lymph node metastases
As an alternative to surgical management, alcohol (ethanol) ablation can be performed in the treatment of cervical lymph node metastases, especially in patients who are either poor surgical candidates or those who wish to avoid surgery. The ethanol is administered through percutaneous injection under US guidance.[21]

SUMMARY

US plays a crucial role in the diagnosis and management of patients with thyroid cancer. Not only is it the best imaging modality for the detection of suspicious thyroid nodules and cervical nodal metastases but also the imaging modality of choice to provide guidance during the performance of thyroid and nodal biopsies. Knowledge of the sonographic anatomy of the thyroid gland and nodal stations as well as features commonly seen in malignant thyroid nodules and nodal metastases and experience with the use of the latest state-of the art high-resolution US equipment is imperative to its effective use in the evaluation of thyroid cancer patients. A summary of the pearls, pitfalls, and variants and what radiologists need to know is found in **Boxes 2** and **3**.

Many groups of physicians (radiologists, surgeons, and endocrinologists) are involved in the care of patients with thyroid cancer and the recommendations and management steps discussed in this article may vary by institution. Therefore, multidepartmental collaboration and meetings are essential to keeping a practice up to date to ensure satisfaction of the referring physicians and providing optimal patient care.

Box 2
Pearls, pitfalls, and variants

- Hashimoto thyroiditis can present with diffuse small nodules (<6 mm) or diffuse heterogeneity that can appear like nodules.

- Parathyroid adenomas may be confused with thyroid nodules or lymph nodes due to their location:

  - Evaluate for an echogenic line denoting the thyroid capsule to place the lesion as extrathyroidal in location.

  - Parathyroid adenomas are usually located posterior to the mid gland and inferior to the inferior pole of the thyroid.

  - Parathyroid adenomas demonstrate polar/peripheral vascular flow from the thyroid rather than central hilar vascular flow on color Doppler.

- Microcalcifications within thyroid nodules may not demonstrate posterior acoustic shadowing.

- Colloid can be confused with microcalcification: evaluate for comet-tail artifact.

- Rapid growth and invasion of adjacent structures can be seen in anaplastic thyroid carcinoma and lymphoma.

- The presence of cystic change and calcification in cervical lymph nodes is 100% specific for metastatic thyroid cancer. Occasionally, metastases from other primaries, most commonly squamous cell head and neck cancer, sometimes cause cystic degeneration in cervical lymph nodes.

- The differential diagnosis of thyroid bed and neck masses seen postoperatively other than recurrence includes residual thyroid tissue, scarring/fibrosis, scar granuloma, and neuromas.

Box 3
What the radiologist needs to know

- In the adult population, 50% have thyroid nodules, but only 7% are malignant.

- Microcalcification has the highest specificity for thyroid carcinoma.

- Most malignant nodules are hypoechoic.

- A thyroid nodule biopsy returning a diagnosis of AUS/FLUS should be repeated with additional samples reserved for AGEC gene testing.

- Preoperative US of the neck is performed to evaluate the need for lateral neck dissection.

- The location and number of lymph node biopsies to be performed are determined by the number of neck compartments showing suspicious lymph nodes (right and left lateral neck, central neck—if postoperative). At least 1 biopsy in each compartment should be performed to definitively diagnose metastatic involvement prior to surgery.

- In the post-thyroidectomy patient, indeterminate or nondiagnostic lymph node biopsies, especially with cystic areas, should be tested for thyroglobulin.

- Thryoid bed masses may be stable in size or show minimal growth over time; correlation with thyroglobulin levels is imperative to assessing the risk of recurrence when the sonographic appearance is indeterminate.

REFERENCES

1. General information about thyroid cancer. In: thyroid cancer treatment PDQ. 2014. Available at: http://www.cancer.gov/cancertopics/pdq/treatment/thyroid/HealthProfessional. Accessed March 3, 2014.

2. Thyroid cancer survival by type and stage. In: thyroid cancer. 2014. Available at: http://www.cancer.org/cancer/thyroidcancer/detailedguide/thyroid-cancer-survival-rates. Accessed March 3, 2014.

3. Middleton WD, Kurtz AB, Hertzberg BS. Neck and chest. In: Ultrasound: The Requisites. St Louis (MO): Mosby; 2004. p. 244–77.

4. Som PM, Curtin HD, Mancuso AA. An imaging-based classification for the cervical nodes designed as an adjunct to recent clinically based nodal classifications. Arch Otolaryngol Head Neck Surg 1999; 125(4):388–96.

5. Frates MC, Benson CB, Chrboneau JW, et al. Management of thyroid nodules detect at US: Society of Radiologists in ultrasound consensus conference statement. Ultrasound Q 2006;22(4):231–8.

6. Hoang JK, Lee WK, Lee M, et al. US features of thyroid malignancy: pearls and pitfalls. Radiographics 2007;27(3):847–61.

7. Polyzos SA, Kita M, Avramidis A. Thyroid nodules – Stepwise diagnosis and management. Hormones 2007;6(2):101–19.

8. Kamran SC, Marqusee E, Kim MI, et al. Thyroid nodule size and prediction of cancer. J Clin Endocrinol Metab 2013;98(2):564–70.

9. Beland MD, Kwon L, Delellis RA, et al. Nonshadowing echogenic foci in thyroid nodules. J Ultrasound Med 2011;30(6):753–60.

10. Reading CC, Charboneau JW, Hay ID, et al. Sonography of thyroid nodules: a "classic pattern" diagnostic approach. Ultrasound Q 2006;21(3):157–65.

11. Kim JY, Lee CH, Kim SY, et al. Radiologic and pathologic findings of nonpalpable thyroid carcinomas detected by ultrasonography in a Medical Screening Center. J Ultrasound Med 2008;27(2):215–23.

12. Cooper DS, Doherty GM, Haugen BR, et al. Revised American Thyroid Association Management Guidelines for patients with thyroid nodules and differentiated thyroid cancer. Thyroid 2009;19(11):1167–217.

13. Gharib H, Papini E, Valcavi R, et al. American Association of Clinical Endocrinologists and Associazione Medici Endocrinologi medical guidelines for clinical practice for the diagnosis and management of thyroid nodules. Endocr Pract 2006;12(1):63–102.

14. Cibas ES, Ali SZ. The Bethesda system for reporting thyroid cytopathology. Am J Clin Pathol 2009;132:658–65.

15. Duick DS, Klopper JP, Diggans JC, et al. The impact of benign gene expression classifier test results on the endocrinologist – patient decision to operate on patients with thyroid nodules with indeterminate fine-needle aspiration cytopathology. Thyroid 2012;22(10):996–1001.

16. Stulak JM, Grant CS, Farley DR, et al. Value of preoperative ultrasonography in the surgical management of initial and preoperative papillary thyroid cancer. Arch Surg 2006;141:489–96.

17. Shin LK, Olcott EW, Jeffrey RB, et al. Sonographic evaluation of cervical lymph nodes in papillary thyroid cancer. Ultrasound Q 2013;29:25–32.

18. Rondeau G, Fish S, Hann LE, et al. Ultrasonographically detected small thyroid bed nodules identified after total thyroidectomy for differentiated thyroid cancer seldom show clinically significant structural progression. Thyroid 2011;21(8):845–53.

19. Kim JH, Lee JH, Shong YK, et al. Ultrasound features of suture granulomas in the thyroid bed after thyroidectomy for papillary thyroid carcinoma with an emphasis on their differentiation from locally recurrent thyroid carcinomas. Ultrasound Med Biol 2009;35(9):1452–7.

20. Huang LF, Weissman JL, Fan C. Traumatic neuroma after neck dissection: CT characterstics in four cases. AJNR Am J Neuroradiol 2000;21:1676–80.

21. Lewis BD, Hay ID, Charboneau JW, et al. Percutaneous ethanol injection for treatment of cervical lymph node metastases in patient with papillary thyroid carcinoma. AJNR Am J Neuroradiol 2002;178:699–704.

Sonographic Evaluation of Palpable Superficial Masses

Paul DiDomenico, MD*, William Middleton, MD

KEYWORDS

- Ultrasound • Superficial soft tissue masses • Lipoma • Solid and cystic masses
- Soft tissue malignancy

KEY POINTS

- Palpable soft tissue masses are common and ultrasonography is a first-step imaging modality in their evaluation.
- Most soft tissue masses are benign, and ultrasonography has high sensitivity and specificity for many common diagnoses.
- Knowledge of proper scanning technique as well as the sonographic appearance of specific disease entities is key to generating and refining a differential diagnosis.

INTRODUCTION

Superficial soft tissue lesions are commonly encountered in clinical practice, and often manifest as palpable masses. With an incidence of approximately 3 per 1000 people per year, 99% of these lesions prove to be benign.[1] Ultrasonography is an attractive way to image these lesions because it is inexpensive, readily available, and does not rely on ionizing radiation. With proper scanning technique, ultrasonography can readily confirm the presence of a mass, differentiate solid from cystic lesions, define the anatomic extent of the lesion, and detect vascular lesions with high sensitivity. In most cases, ultrasonography can accurately characterize the lesion, obviating biopsy and reducing unnecessary further work-up.[1] When needed, ultrasonography can also provide guidance for percutaneous biopsy. This article reviews the capabilities of ultrasonography in evaluating superficial soft tissue lesions and the sonographic appearance of common and uncommon disease entities.

APPROACH TO SONOGRAPHIC EVALUATION

Unlike many ultrasonography examinations that involve screening entire organs in search of an abnormality, often a superficial soft tissue lesion is directly palpable, aiding the radiologist or technologist in performing a focused sonographic examination. Once a brief visual inspection and physical examination have been performed, selection of the appropriate ultrasonography probe should be made in consideration of the potential depth of the lesion and the tissue penetration required. Good sonographic technique includes adjustment of the field of view to the appropriate depth, with concomitant adjustment of the focal zone to center on the suspected area of abnormality (Fig. 1). Superficial lesions are best evaluated with high-frequency transducers, whereas lower frequency transducers are necessary for deeper lesions. For very superficial lesions, a thick layer of gel should be used to provide some separation between the probe and the lesion and thus avoid near-field reverberation artifacts (Fig. 2).

Disclosure: The authors have nothing to disclose.
Mallinckrodt Institute of Radiology, Washington University School of Medicine, 510 South Kingshighway Boulevard, St Louis, MO 63110, USA
* Corresponding author.
E-mail address: paul.didomenico2@va.gov

Radiol Clin N Am 52 (2014) 1295–1305
http://dx.doi.org/10.1016/j.rcl.2014.07.011

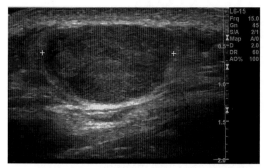

Fig. 1. Solitary fibrous tumor. Proper selection of ultrasound transducer and correct adjustment of depth and focal zone enable visualization of a superficial soft tissue mass (*cursors*) in the soft tissues of the base of the neck. The technical parameters at the right aspect of the image show that a linear 6-MHz to 15-MHz transducer was used, set at a transmit frequency of 15 MHz (optimal for superficial imaging), and penetrating to a depth of 2.0 cm. The small hourglass shapes at the right edge of the image show the focal zones corresponding with the depth of the mass.

Because some palpable abnormalities are caused by conditions other than masses, the first priority of a sonographic examination is to identify the mass. If no mass is seen, determination of alternate causes of the palpable abnormality is important. For instance, hernias can present as a mass in the abdominal wall and muscle hernias can produce palpable abnormalities in the extremities. In both situations, the dynamic nature of sonography allows real-time imaging during various maneuvers, such as real-time compression of a mass, Valsalva maneuver, or muscular contraction (**Fig. 3**).

Once identified, the next step in evaluating a superficial soft tissue lesion should be to determine whether it is solid, cystic, or mixed (**Fig. 4**). Solid lesions have an internal echotexture of variable echogenicity relative to surrounding normal tissues. Cystic lesions and fluid collections are either anechoic or very hypoechoic and can produce increased through-transmission of the ultrasound beam manifested as increased echogenicity seen posterior to the lesion. More complex cysts or fluid collections may have varying degrees of internal echoes and/or thick walls. This descriptive information should be documented because it should correlate with the suggested differential diagnosis.

The next consideration should be to determine the site of origin of the lesion, its relationship to adjacent structures, and whether it is mobile or fixed (**Fig. 5**). The margin, shape, and size have been shown to correlate with the presence or absence of malignancy. Of these criteria, tumor size of greater than 5 cm and infiltrative or lobular margins have been shown to be highly suggestive of malignancy.[2]

A particular strength of ultrasonography is its ability to detect blood flow within a lesion. Color or power Doppler evaluation (**Fig. 6**) can provide crucial information as to the presence and extent of vascular flow to a lesion, and this information can aid in generating and/or narrowing the differential diagnosis. In general, the presence of internal vascularity indicates at least the possibility that the lesion is neoplastic, either benign or malignant (**Fig. 7**). Therefore, it is crucial to optimize technical factors so that Doppler sensitivity is maximized. For superficial lesions, using a high Doppler transmit frequency is beneficial. It is also important to avoid putting pressure on the lesion with the transducer. For deeper lesions, lower Doppler transmit frequencies are needed to maximize sensitivity. It is often necessary to try various transmit frequencies to determine which is optimal. Color Doppler can detect the relative speed and direction of blood flow, whereas power Doppler is slightly more sensitive for detecting the presence or absence of flow.

A unique aspect of ultrasonography as an imaging modality is that clinicians can assess the compressibility of a mass by applying pressure

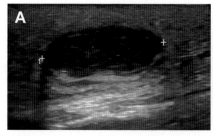
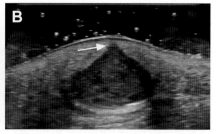

Fig. 2. Epidermal inclusion cyst. (*A*) A superficial mass (*cursors*) is shown to be hypoechoic and well circumscribed, with increased through-transmission of the ultrasound beam. (*B*) Using a thick layer of overlying gel allows better visualization and reveals a tract leading to the skin surface, consistent with an epidermal inclusion cyst (*arrow*). Small air bubbles in the gel layer cause hyperechoic reflectors.

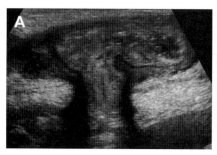
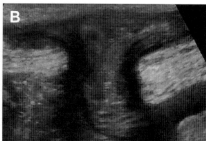

Fig. 3. Abdominal wall hernia. Real-time gray-scale sonography shows heterogeneously hyperechoic bowel and fat herniating through a defect in the echogenic abdominal wall (*A*) and reducing through the defect with compression (*B*).

with the probe during the real-time scan. Elastography is a newer sonographic technique that can evaluate tissue elasticity under mechanical pressure, or in response to externally applied energy, in order to distinguish soft and hard masses. This information can provide another clue as to the potentially benign or malignant nature of a mass (**Fig. 8**).[3]

BENIGN SOLID MASSES
Lipoma

Lipomas are common and clinicians often refer patients with a strong clinical suspicion of the diagnosis based on history and physical examination alone. Lipomas are soft masses composed of encapsulated mature adipose cells. Eighty percent of lipomas occur in adults, and the typical

presentation is of a slow-growing palpable mass in middle-aged patients.[4] In one case series, 54% of all superficial masses referred for sonographic evaluation over a 3-year period were lipomas.[1] The sonographic appearance is typically of a well-circumscribed mass that can have variable echogenicity compared with the surrounding soft tissues. In the case series previously referred to, 59% of masses were isoechoic (**Fig. 9A**), 26% were hyperechoic (see **Fig. 9B**), and 15% were hypoechoic to adjacent fat.[1] Additional common features include curved echogenic lines within the mass, minimal or no acoustic shadowing, and minimal or no internal blood flow. When referred for sonographic evaluation, ultrasonography has been shown to have variable accuracy, reportedly as high as 96% sensitivity, 97% specificity, and overall accuracy of 96% for the

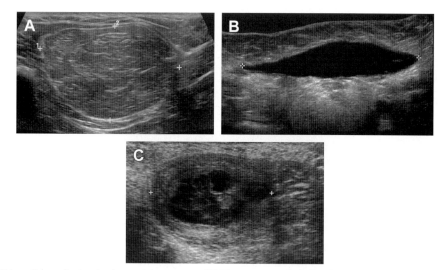

Fig. 4. Solid, cystic, and mixed echogenicity masses. (*A*) Lipoma. A well-defined, solid, soft tissue mass (*cursors*) in the left upper extremity that is isoechoic to surrounding tissues with internal curved echogenic lines. (*B*) Postoperative abdominal wall seroma. A fluid collection (*cursors*) within the abdominal wall is anechoic and has imperceptible walls separating it from the surrounding soft tissues. (*C*) Abscess. A complex cystic mass (*cursors*) in the posterior knee, with some internal septae evident, as well as increased through-transmission of the ultrasound beam caused by fluid content.

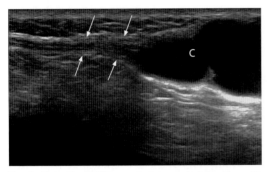

Fig. 5. Neural ganglion cyst. An anechoic lesion with increased through-transmission of the ultrasonography beam is consistent with a cyst (C). Careful inspection of adjacent structures showed that it arose from the sural nerve (*arrows*).

diagnosis of lipoma.[1] However, other investigators have reported lower numbers, ranging from 49% to 86% in overall accuracy.[4] In most cases, typical sonographic findings of a lipoma require no further evaluation other than periodic clinical follow-up. If the lesion is large, growing rapidly, has a heterogeneous echotexture, or moderate internal vascularity, then another cause such as a liposarcoma is possible and magnetic resonance imaging should be considered for further evaluation.

Giant Cell Tumor of the Tendon Sheath

Giant cell tumor of the tendon sheath (GCTTS) is a benign tumor that is histologically identical to pigmented villonodular synovitis. Giant cell tumors arise from the tendon sheath, and may wrap

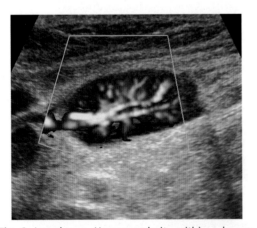

Fig. 6. Lymphoma. Hypervascularity within a hypoechoic lymph node in the right groin is well shown by power Doppler imaging. This degree of vascularity is abnormal and indicates either inflammation or neoplastic involvement. The normal distribution of vessels is more consistent with lymphoma than metastatic disease.

around the tendon. GCTTS is the most common solid mass in the hand, and after ganglion cysts is the second most common palpable mass lesion along the flexor tendons of the fingers.[5] GCTTS can be seen in other joints as well, and accounts for approximately 4% of all soft tissue tumors.[6] In the hand, the lesion typically presents as a focal palpable nodule on the volar surface of the fingers. The classic sonographic appearance is a solid, homogeneous, hypoechoic mass that has detectable internal blood flow and may be hypervascular (Fig. 10).[5] Because a GCTTS does not arise from the tendon, it does not move with the tendon during flexion and extension of the fingers and this can be confirmed at real-time sonography. Given their characteristic location and clinical features, an estimated 70% to 90% of these lesions can be diagnosed through clinical and imaging features and are resected without prior biopsy.[7]

Neural Masses

Peripheral nerve masses are another common type of mass referred for sonographic examination. Traumatic neuromas may result from acute or repetitive trauma and are a nonneoplastic response to damage to a nerve. They are usually small and may present with pain, but not as a palpable mass. In contrast, schwannomas are benign neoplasms arising from the Schwann cells supplying myelin to a peripheral nerve, and commonly arise in the head and neck, flexor surfaces of the extremities, and along the vertebral column, most commonly in adults between the ages of 20 and 50 years. They can occur sporadically or in the setting of neurofibromatosis type 2 in 2% to 3% of cases.[8] A neurofibroma is a more complex benign neoplasm composed of fibroblasts and other cell types in addition to Schwann cells. They are typically seen in adults aged 20 to 30 years and may occur in isolation or in conjunction with neurofibromatosis type 1. Thus, the clinical history and location of the neural mass are helpful in making the diagnosis. Schwannomas and neurofibromas each account for 5% of all soft tissue tumors.[6] Tenderness and/or numbness may be presenting clinical symptoms. On sonography, neural tumors are solid hypoechoic masses that often show increased through-transmission and are typically hypervascular on color Doppler imaging (Fig. 11). When they arise from larger peripheral nerves, the continuity of the mass and the nerve is evident on sonography. Lesions that are in the middle of the nerve tend to be neurofibromas, whereas lesions that are eccentric tend to be schwannomas. Although most of these lesions

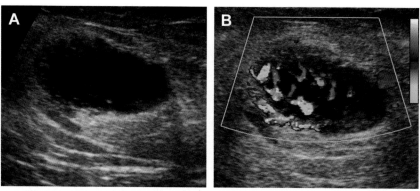

Fig. 7. Lymphoma. (A) A nearly anechoic lesion in the left upper thigh simulates a fluid collection. (B) Color Doppler reveals extensive internal vascularity indicating vascularized soft tissue as opposed to fluid. This finding makes neoplasm more likely and this is a well-recognized appearance for lymphoma.

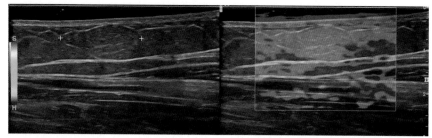

Fig. 8. Lipoma. A palpable mass in the left forearm appears isoechoic to surrounding subcutaneous fat on gray-scale imaging (cursors) and is difficult to identify. Elastography shows that this nodule is predominantly green, whereas adjacent fat is red and yellow, indicating that the nodule is slightly firmer than adjacent fat. This finding helps to confirm that the subtle lesion seen on gray-scale imaging corresponds with the palpable abnormality.

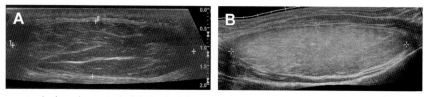

Fig. 9. Lipomas, typical and atypical. (A) Typical lipoma. An encapsulated, isoechoic soft tissue mass (cursors) within the scalp, with curved echogenic lines within the mass, as are often seen in lipomas. (B) Atypical lipoma. An encapsulated, homogeneously hyperechoic mass (cursors) overlying the right triceps, appearing more echogenic than a typical lipoma.

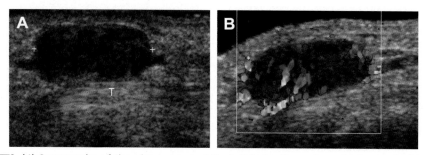

Fig. 10. GCTTS. (A) Sonography of the ulnar aspect of the left index finger to evaluate a palpable mass at the level of the proximal interphalangeal joint reveals an ovoid hypoechoic nodule (cursors) located immediately adjacent to the flexor tendon (T). (B) Color Doppler revealed increased internal vascularity. With passive flexion of the finger, the nodule did not move with the underlying tendon.

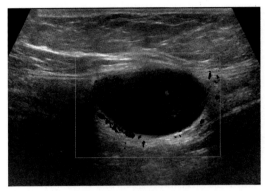

Fig. 11. Schwannoma. A well-circumscribed hypoe-choic mass in the anterior abdominal wall, with poste-rior acoustic enhancement and internal vascular flow on color Doppler imaging.

are benign, tumor size of greater than 5 to 10 cm is concerning for malignancy.[8]

Fat Necrosis

Fat necrosis is commonly encountered in breast imaging and may occur following direct trauma, although many potential causes exist, including thermal injuries, instrumentation, vasculitis, or autoimmune disorders. Vascular impairment with lipase-mediated saponification of fat results in a focal area of necrosis that often presents as a palpable subcutaneous mass. Fat necrosis in the extremities has a variable sonographic appear-ance, but it rarely appears as a well-defined mass. Sonographic appearances have been described ranging from a hypoechoic mass, to an isoechoic mass with a hypoechoic halo, or to a poorly defined hyperechoic region in the subcu-taneous fat. Fat necrosis should be considered when masses that do not have a typical appear-ance for anything else are encountered (Fig. 12).[9,10] Given this variable appearance, consideration should be given to a potential differ-ential diagnosis of a lipoma, which should have a

more oblong appearance and is normally well defined, and an epidermal inclusion cyst, which may show increased through-transmission of the ultrasound beam and/or a linear connection to the skin surface.[9]

Epidermal and Dermal Masses

Skin appendage masses arise from the epidermis and dermis and are classified as proliferations of follicular lineage or eccrine-apocrine differentia-tion.[11] A variety of benign cutaneous nodules arising from hair follicles or sweat glands may be seen, often occurring on the head, neck, or ex-tremities. The most common of these lesions is the epidermal inclusion cyst, which is a benign proliferation of squamous epithelium lined by true epidermis. They can be congenital or acquired, and may arise following trauma or occlusion of the pilosebaceous unit. These lesions can present as a palpable bump, most commonly on the scalp, face, neck, and back. The superficial location and typically small size of these lesions favors sono-graphic evaluation with a high-frequency probe. They appear as small, round or oval, homoge-neous, hypoechoic masses in the superficial soft tissues. They may have swirling echogenic lines and they appear more heterogeneous as they become larger (Fig. 13). A characteristic pseudo-testis sign of an oval homogeneous mass with low to medium echogenicity, simulating a testicle, has been described in 62% of epidermal inclusion cysts.[12] Although infrequently seen, a narrow tract leading from the mass to the skin surface can help to confirm the diagnosis.

Palmar Fibromatosis (Dupuytren Contracture)

The fibromatoses are a large group of soft tissue masses along the superficial fascia and have various eponyms depending on the location of the lesion. These are common, benign, fibroblastic

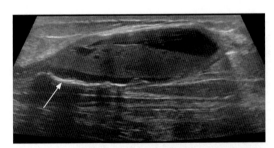

Fig. 12. Fat necrosis. A well-circumscribed, heteroge-neous solid and cystic mass with posterior calcification (arrow) in a patient with a palpable area of swelling in the soft tissues of the anterior right thigh with increasing pain.

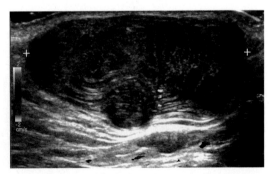

Fig. 13. Epidermal inclusion cyst. An oval subcutane-ous mass (cursors) in the right neck, with swirling internal echogenic lines, no detectable vascularity and posterior acoustic enhancement.

proliferations that can occur in the superficial or deep tissues, and as a group comprise approximately 8% of all superficial masses. Palmar fibromatosis, also known as Dupuytren contracture, is the most common type of fibromatosis.[6] It is a nodular fibroblastic proliferation occurring on the volar surface of the hand in adults, and ultimately can result in a flexion contracture of the fingers, requiring surgical treatment. About 1% to 2% of the general population is affected, and up to 20% of adults are affected by the age of 65 years. The disease occurs about 3 to 4 times more commonly in men than in women. Fifty percent of cases occur bilaterally and 5% to 20% in conjunction with plantar fibromatosis.[6,13] The typical presentation is the insidious onset of a painless, subcutaneous, firm nodule in the palmar surface of the hand, usually overlying the fourth or fifth metacarpal bone. Ultrasonography typically shows poorly marginated, flat hypoechoic nodules in the palmar subcutaneous tissues, superficial to the flexor tendons (**Fig. 14**).

Desmoid Tumor

Another fibromatosis lesion, desmoid tumors (or desmoid-type fibromatosis[13]) are uncommon benign fibroblastic tumors. They arise from the connective tissue of muscle and overlying fascia. The peak incidence is from age 20 to 40 years with a 2:1 female/male predilection.[6] These tumors can occur sporadically or in conjunction with familial adenomatous polyposis (Gardner) syndrome. The mass is usually painless, grows insidiously, and can occur anywhere on the body; most commonly the shoulder or upper arm, followed by the chest wall or back, and thigh.[13] On sonography, desmoid tumors appear as solid, hypoechoic masses with variable borders and usually with increased vascularity (**Fig. 15**).

MALIGNANT MASSES

The possibility that a superficial soft tissue lesion may be malignant should always be considered,

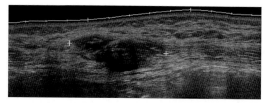

Fig. 15. Desmoid tumor. A poorly defined hypoechoic solid mass (*cursors*) in the periumbilical abdominal wall musculature.

although only 1% of all superficial masses are malignant. Because most benign soft tissue masses have typical ultrasonography appearances, any soft tissue mass that cannot confidently be characterized as benign should be viewed with suspicion. Sonographic features suspicious for malignancy include large size at presentation (>5 cm), infiltrative or lobular margins, rapid growth over time, deep location, and increased blood flow on color Doppler.[2,14] Also, a superficial lesion that extends through deep fascial layers is more likely to be malignant (**Box 1**).[2,11]

The most common primary soft tissue malignancies tend to occur in adults more than 50 years of age. Pleomorphic sarcoma, liposarcoma, and leiomyosarcoma, are the most common malignancies, accounting for approximately 24%, 16% to 18%, and 5% to 10% of all soft tissue sarcomas respectively.[11] Pleomorphic sarcoma (formerly called malignant fibrous histiocytoma) has both superficial and pleomorphic forms. The superficial (cutaneous) form is termed atypical fibroxanthoma, which usually has a benign course and most commonly occurs on the head and neck. The more aggressive pleomorphic form most commonly occurs in the lower extremities (**Fig. 16**).[6] Liposarcomas are more often encountered in the extremities and are often seen in the thigh (**Fig. 17**). Leiomyosarcoma is a highly vascular lesion, occurring in older adults, with a close association with underlying blood vessels.

Between 5% and 10% of all patients with cancer develop soft tissue metastases.[11] Any malignancy

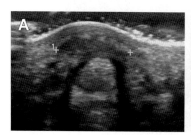
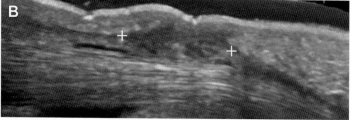

Fig. 14. Dupuytren contracture. (*A*) An oval hypoechoic nodule (*cursors*) in the palmar subcutaneous tissues, in a classic location superficial to the flexor tendon of the fourth metacarpal (transverse image). (*B*) Longitudinal panoramic image.

can metastasize to the soft tissues, but in women breast cancer is the most common, whereas malignant melanoma and lung cancer are most common in men (**Fig. 18**).[11] Extranodal lymphoma can also occur in the soft tissues and this usually occurs in advanced non-Hodgkin disease (**Fig. 19**).

CYSTIC MASSES
Ganglion Cyst

Ganglion cysts are the most common palpable lesions found in the hand or wrist.[15] They consist of a mucin-filled cyst arising from a joint or tendon sheath, and may be related to antecedent trauma, although the precise pathogenesis is unclear. Up to 70% arise from the scapholunate joint on the dorsal surface of the wrist, whereas another 20% originate on the volar side of the wrist between the flexor carpi radialis tendon and radial artery. The remainder arise from the flexor tendon sheaths or interphalangeal joints. These lesions typically present as firm, palpable, periarticular nodules. Because these cysts are filled with thick mucinous fluid, the sonographic appearance is classically that of an anechoic cyst with well-defined thick walls, posterior acoustic enhancement, and occasionally internal echoes or locules (**Fig. 20**). A neck can be seen connecting the cyst to the joint of origin in approximately 25% of cases.[15] Ultrasonography has an accuracy of up to 87% for diagnosing these lesions.[7] Other lesions that can be mistaken for a ganglion cyst

(either clinically or sonographically) are joint and tendon sheath effusion, bony protuberances, synovitis, and foreign bodies. Collapsed ganglion cysts can simulate solid or complex masses.

Baker Cyst

A Baker cyst is a common cause of pain posterior to the knee and may or may not be palpable. The cyst is formed by a distended bursa lined with synovium arising between the gastrocnemius and semimembranosus tendons and that communicates with the knee joint.[16] The cyst may contain internal debris or blood and may have septations and solid components. The cysts can rupture, with leakage of contents into the surrounding soft tissues. Ultrasonography shows an anechoic or hypoechoic fluid collection medially in the popliteal fossa that wraps around the medial aspect of the medial head of the gastrocnemius muscle with a beaklike neck directed toward the joint (**Fig. 21**). Dissection or rupture into the calf typically occurs superficial to the gastrocnemius muscle. Ultrasonography has high accuracy for the diagnosis of Baker cysts. In one case series of 23 soft tissue masses located posterior to the knee, which included 21 proven Baker cysts, all 21 were correctly identified sonographically.[16]

VASCULAR MASSES
Hemangioma

Many benign vascular lesions occur within the soft tissues and definitive diagnosis may require excision before they can be classified as hemangioma, lymphangioma, or other specific entities. Hemangiomas are common and may arise within the soft tissues as well as within muscles and can occur sporadically or in conjunction with syndromes such as von Hippel-Lindau and Klippel-Trénaunay syndrome. They are classified according to the predominant type of vessel from which they arise, with the capillary and arteriovenous forms likely to be superficial, whereas the venous and cavernous forms are more likely to

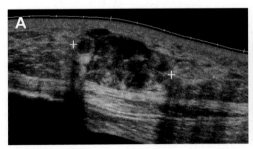
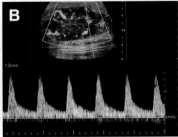

Fig. 16. Undifferentiated pleomorphic sarcoma, also known as malignant fibrous histiocytoma. (*A*) A hypoechoic mass (*cursors*) in the soft tissues of the left thigh with irregular, lobulated margins (sagittal panoramic gray-scale view). (*B*) Color Doppler image shows marked internal vascularity.

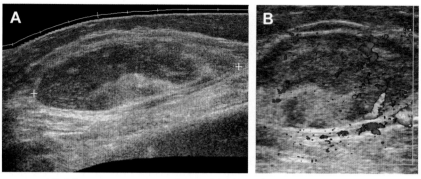

Fig. 17. Liposarcoma. (*A*) A heterogeneous mass (*cursors*) in the soft tissues of the left forearm with hyperechoic components (sagittal panoramic gray-scale view). (*B*) Transverse color Doppler image showing increased vascular flow. Unlike benign lipomas, liposarcomas usually have readily detectable internal blood flow.

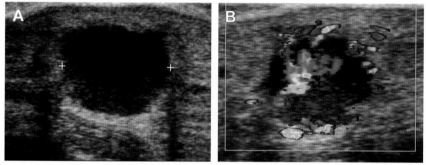

Fig. 18. Metastatic melanoma. (*A*) A very hypoechoic subcutaneous nodule (*cursors*) with (*B*) intense central hypervascularity in the soft tissues of the right leg.

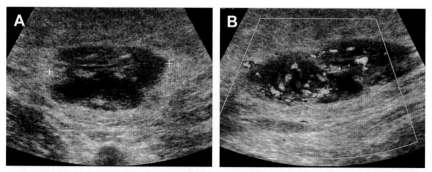

Fig. 19. Extranodal lymphoma. (*A*) A heterogeneous but predominantly hypoechoic nodule (*cursors*) with irregular margins in the soft tissues of the left thigh (transverse gray-scale view). (*B*) Sagittal color Doppler image shows increased vascularity.

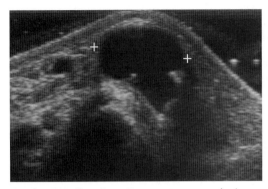

Fig. 20. Ganglion cyst. Transverse gray-scale image showing an anechoic cyst (*cursors*) in the volar soft tissues of the right wrist.

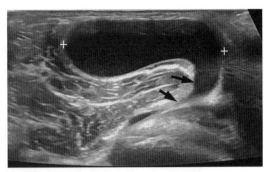

Fig. 21. Baker cyst. A well-circumscribed fluid collection (*cursors*) posterior to the left knee, extending between the semimembranosus and medial gastrocnemius tendons. The neck of the cyst wraps around the medial head of the gastrocnemius muscle (*black arrows*).

be intramuscular.[17] Overall, hemangiomas comprise approximately 8% of all soft tissue tumors.[6] These lesions may be seen superficially from early in life, following a course of proliferation and subsequent gradual involution, or may occur in adults as a deeper soft tissue mass with an auscultatory bruit. Venous hemangiomas may contain calcified phleboliths that are visible on plain radiographs. When superficial, ultrasonography can confirm the presence of vascularity within a mixed echogenicity mass in the subcutaneous tissues. Power Doppler may be helpful in detecting slow flow or flow in small vessels (**Fig. 22**). A dominant vessel supplying the mass may be identified. Defining the presence of a soft tissue mass is important in distinguishing hemangiomas from arteriovenous malformations, because these are abnormal communications between arteries and veins without a defined soft tissue mass. Because both lesions can have variable degrees of vessel density, peak arterial and venous velocities, and resistive indices, the presence of a soft tissue mass in the case of hemangioma is considered the most reliable differentiating feature.[18] In contrast, lymphangiomas or lymphatic malformations are more commonly found on the head and neck in the pediatric population and consist of cystic spaces with multiple internal septations, with minimal or no internal vascularity.

Glomus Tumor

A glomus tumor (glomangioma) is a benign hamartomatous vascular tumor that is histologically similar to the glomus body, a component of the dermis layer of the skin involved in body temperature regulation and most prevalent in the fingers and toes. The glomus body is an arteriovenous shunt surrounded by a connective tissue capsule. Glomus tumors are soft tissue nodules that characteristically occur in the extremities, and are uncommon, comprising approximately 1% of all soft tissue tumors.[6] Seventy-five percent occur in the distal hand or foot, with 65% classically presenting within the nail bed as a painful mass.[17] At sonography the appearance is that of a small hypoechoic mass that may show bony erosion, and with marked hypervascularity (**Fig. 23**). The sonographic features in the appropriate clinical setting have been shown to have high accuracy for diagnosis of these lesions before resection, with 11 of 12 lesions correctly identified before surgery in one case series.[19]

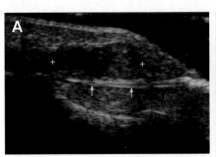
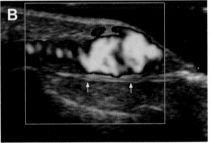

Fig. 22. Hemangioma. (*A*) A solid, hypoechoic mass (*cursors*) superficial to the finger nail (*arrows*) seen on longitudinal gray-scale view and (*B*) intense hypervascularity with a feeding vessel seen on power Doppler imaging.

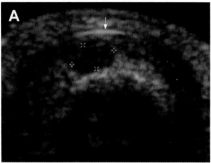
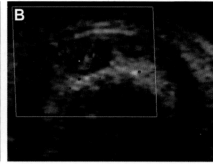

Fig. 23. Subungual glomus tumor. (A) A small hypoechoic hypervascular mass (cursors) seen in the subungual soft tissues of the finger on transverse gray-scale view. The finger nail (arrow) is seen immediately superficial to the mass. (B) Transverse color Doppler image shows increased blood flow. The patient presented with pain located at the base of the distal phalanx on the dorsal surface of the left third digit.

SUMMARY

Ultrasonography is an excellent first-line imaging modality for evaluating superficial soft tissue masses, offering advantages of speed, lower cost, availability, and avoiding the use of ionizing radiation. Knowledge of the typical imaging appearance of specific disease entities can allow an accurate diagnosis of most benign lesions, and, if malignancy is suspected, ultrasonography can provide guidance for percutaneous biopsy.

REFERENCES

1. Wagner JM, Lee KS, Rosas H, et al. Accuracy of sonographic diagnosis of superficial masses. J Ultrasound Med 2013;32(8):1443–50.

2. Chiou HJ, Chou YH, Chiu SY, et al. Differentiation of benign and malignant superficial soft-tissue masses using grayscale and color Doppler ultrasonography. J Chin Med Assoc 2009;72(6):307–15.

3. Dewall RJ. Ultrasound elastography: principles, techniques, and clinical applications. Crit Rev Biomed Eng 2013;41(1):1–19.

4. Inampudi P, Jacobson JA, Fessell DP, et al. Soft-tissue lipomas: accuracy of sonography in diagnosis with pathologic correlation. Radiology 2004;233(3):763–7.

5. Middleton WD, Patel V, Teefey SA, et al. Giant cell tumors of the tendon sheath: analysis of sonographic findings. AJR Am J Roentgenol 2004;183(2):337–9.

6. Goldblum J, Weiss S, Folpe A. Enzinger and Weiss's soft tissue tumors. Philadelphia: Saunders; 2013.

7. Teefey SA, Middleton WD, Patel V, et al. The accuracy of high-resolution ultrasound for evaluating focal lesions of the hand and wrist. J Hand Surg Am 2004;29(3):393–9.

8. Bancroft LW, Pettis C, Wasyliw C. Imaging of benign soft tissue tumors. Semin Musculoskelet Radiol 2013;17(2):156–67.

9. Walsh M, Jacobson JA, Kim SM, et al. Sonography of fat necrosis involving the extremity and torso with magnetic resonance imaging and histologic correlation. J Ultrasound Med 2008;27(12): 1751–7.

10. Fernando RA, Somers S, Edmonson RD, et al. Subcutaneous fat necrosis: hypoechoic appearance on sonography. J Ultrasound Med 2003;22:1387–90.

11. Beaman FD, Kransdorf MJ, Andrews TR, et al. Superficial soft-tissue masses: analysis, diagnosis, and differential considerations. Radiographics 2007;27(2):509–23.

12. Huang CC, Ko SF, Huang HY, et al. Epidermal cysts in the superficial soft tissue: sonographic features with an emphasis on the pseudotestis pattern. J Ultrasound Med 2011;30(1):11–7.

13. Murphey MD, Ruble CM, Tyszko SM, et al. From the archives of the AFIP: musculoskeletal fibromatoses: radiologic-pathologic correlation. Radiographics 2009;29(7):2143–73.

14. Hung EH, Griffith JF. Pitfalls in ultrasonography of soft tissue tumors. Semin Musculoskelet Radiol 2014;18(1):79–85.

15. Teefey SA, Dahiya N, Middleton WD, et al. Ganglia of the hand and wrist: a sonographic analysis. AJR Am J Roentgenol 2008;191(3):716–20.

16. Ward EE, Jacobson JA, Fessell DP, et al. Sonographic detection of Baker's cysts: comparison with MR imaging. AJR Am J Roentgenol 2001; 176(2):373–80.

17. Blacksin MF, Ha DH, Hameed M, et al. Superficial soft-tissue masses of the extremities. Radiographics 2006;26(5):1289–304.

18. Paltiel HJ, Burrows PE, Kozakewich HP, et al. Soft-tissue vascular anomalies: utility of US for diagnosis. Radiology 2000;214(3):747–54.

19. Marchadier A, Cohen M, Legre R. Subungual glomus tumors of the fingers: ultrasound diagnosis. Chir Main 2006;25(1):16–21 [in French].

Ultrasonographic Evaluation of the Renal Transplant

Shuchi K. Rodgers, MD*, Christopher P. Sereni, MD,
Mindy M. Horrow, MD, FACR

KEYWORDS

- Ultrasonography • Renal transplant • Vascular • Doppler • Renal artery stenosis • Rejection

KEY POINTS

- Categorization of transplant complications by time of occurrence is helpful for formulating appropriate differential diagnoses.
- Renal transplant complications may arise in the perinephric space, renal vasculature, renal parenchyma or collecting system.
- The combination of gray-scale ultrasound with color and spectral Doppler is necessary for complete renal transplant evaluation.

INTRODUCTION

Renal transplantation is a mainstay treatment of end-stage renal disease. Ultrasonography is an excellent tool for transplant evaluation in the immediate postoperative period and for long-term follow-up. Advances in imaging, surgical technique, and medical management have increased graft survival rates. Complications can be categorized based on timing of occurrence, but can also be divided by location into perinephric, vascular, parenchymal, and collecting system abnormalities (**Table 1**).[1] **Box 1** lists common indications for kidney transplant imaging.

SURGICAL TECHNIQUE

In adults, the transplant kidney is typically placed in an extraperitoneal location in either iliac fossa, usually the right because of the straighter course of the right iliac vein. The superficial location of the external iliac vessels facilitates surgical dissection and creation of vascular anastomoses. In deceased donor transplants, the donor renal artery is harvested with a small oval-shaped patch of aorta termed a Carrel patch, which is used for anastomosis to the external iliac artery. In living donor renal transplants, the main renal artery is typically harvested in isolation and anastomosed directly end-to-side with the external iliac artery or end-to-end with the internal iliac artery. An end-to-side anastomosis is made between the donor renal vein and the external iliac vein. A ureteroneocystostomy is created by implanting the donor ureter into the dome of the urinary bladder.

Multiple surgical variations exist; therefore, discussion with the transplant surgeon or correlation with the operative report is helpful. Common variations include intraperitoneal placement of the renal transplant (more common in children), ureteral implantation into an interposed bowel segment, and creation of a ureteroureterostomy

Disclosures: None.
Department of Radiology, Sidney Kimmel Medical College at Thomas Jefferson University, Einstein Medical Center, 5501 Old York Road, Philadelphia, PA 19141, USA
* Corresponding author.
E-mail address: rodgerss@einstein.edu

Radiol Clin N Am 52 (2014) 1307–1324
http://dx.doi.org/10.1016/j.rcl.2014.07.009
0033-8389/14/$ – see front matter © 2014 Elsevier Inc. All rights reserved.

radiologic.theclinics.com

Table 1	
Time of occurrence of renal transplant complications	
Immediate (<1 wk following transplantation)	Acute tubular necrosis Acute rejection Renal artery thrombosis Renal vein thrombosis Perinephric hematoma Graft infection and abscess Compartment syndrome
Early (1 wk to 1 mo following transplantation)	Acute rejection Urinary tract obstruction Urine leak Urinoma Renal vein thrombosis
Late (>1 mo following transplantation)	Chronic rejection Medication toxicity Ureteral stricture Vesicoureteral reflux Renal artery stenosis Arteriovenous fistula and pseudoaneurysm Lymphocele Seroma Renal masses and posttransplant lymphoproliferative disorder Renal calculi Medullary nephrocalcinosis
Occur at any time	Torsion of the transplant kidney Pyelonephritis Segmental infarct

---

Box 1
Indications for kidney transplant imaging

- Immediate postoperative evaluation
- Routine surveillance imaging
- Follow peritransplant collections
- Elevated or rising creatinine
- Pain in region of transplant
- Decreased urine output
- Fevers and chills
- Severe hypertension refractory to medical therapy
- Hypertension and unexplained graft dysfunction

---

or pyeloureterostomy. In pediatric deceased donors, both kidneys and the accompanying aorta and inferior vena cava can be transplanted into a single adult recipient.

NORMAL RENAL TRANSPLANT ULTRASONOGRAPHY FINDINGS

The normal transplant kidney demonstrates the same features as a normal native kidney. However, corticomedullary differentiation in a transplanted kidney is usually more pronounced, owing to its more superficial location. The ability to scan with a higher-frequency transducer also allows for better appreciation of the renal echotexture and shape of the individual cortical segments. Often the collecting system is slightly dilated because of the expected reflux at the ureterovesical anastomosis in addition to autonomic denervation, and typically is limited to the renal pelvis. The fluid in the renal pelvis allows visualization of the urothelium, which should be thin. After 2 months, the normal transplant kidney usually hypertrophies and can elongate by 2 to 3 cm.

On color Doppler imaging, arterial and venous flow should extend to within a few millimeters of the capsule throughout all renal segments, although this depends on depth of the transplant kidney, transducer frequency, and sensitivity of the color Doppler settings. Occasionally flow will appear to be decreased or absent in deeper portions of the kidney, which should prompt evaluation with power Doppler, as it is more sensitive than color Doppler.

Spectral Doppler interrogation of the arterial waveforms should show brisk systolic upstrokes. Intralobular or arcuate artery resistive indices (RIs) of greater than 0.80 are often used as a nonspecific parameter for transplant dysfunction.[2] Peak systolic velocity (PSV) of the main renal artery should be less than 250 to 300 cm/s. Normal triphasic high-resistance waveforms should be observed in the ipsilateral external iliac artery. The normal PSV ratio of the renal artery to the ipsilateral external iliac artery has been described to be less than 1.8 to 3.5.[3,4] The main renal vein should have monophasic to mildly pulsatile flow, depending on the cardiac status, with similar findings in the ipsilateral external iliac vein. Normal ultrasonography findings are shown in **Fig. 1**, and a summary of the technique is given in **Box 2**.

VASCULAR ABNORMALITIES
Renal Artery Stenosis

Vascular complications occur in fewer than 10% of renal transplants.[5] Renal artery stenosis (RAS) is

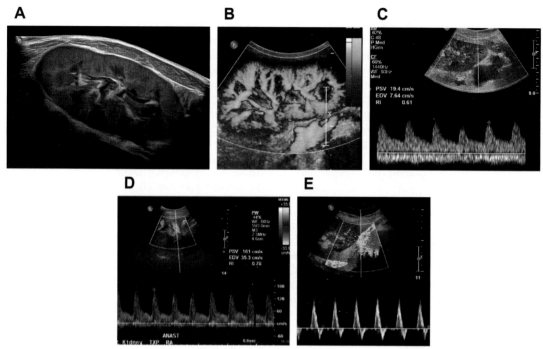

Fig. 1. Normal renal transplant ultrasonography. (*A*) Gray-scale sagittal image of the transplant kidney using a linear 12-MHz transducer shows normal corticomedullary differentiation with a slightly echogenic cortex and hypoechoic medullary pyramids. (*B*) Power Doppler ultrasonography shows normal perfusion, which extends to a few millimeters from the renal capsule. (*C*) Arcuate artery spectral Doppler tracing shows a normal brisk systolic upstroke and normal resistive index of 0.61. (*D*) Main renal artery spectral Doppler tracing shows a brisk systolic upstroke and normal diastolic flow throughout the cardiac cycle, and a normal angle corrected peak systolic velocity. (*E*) External iliac artery spectral Doppler tracing shows a normal high-resistance triphasic waveform.

Box 2
Imaging technique

- Curved 5- or 9-MHz transducer, with higher frequency transducers used if possible

- Gray-scale assessment for size, echogenicity, corticomedullary differentiation, masses, scarring, calcifications, perinephric collections, hydronephrosis, and urothelial thickening

- Urinary bladder assessed for debris, blood, distal portion of urinary stent, and urine volume

- Qualitative assessment of transplant perfusion using color or power Doppler

- Spectral Doppler of upper-pole, mid, and lower-pole intralobular or arcuate arteries with measurement of the peak systolic velocity, end-diastolic velocity, and resistive index

- Spectral Doppler of the transplant renal artery and vein at the anastomosis, the mid-portion, and hilum

- Spectral Doppler of the ipsilateral external iliac vessels performed proximally, distally, and at the level of the anastomosis

the most common vascular complication, typically occurring within the first year, and usually in the first 3 months after transplantation. However, RAS may occur in the allograft at any time. Most renal artery stenoses occur at the anastomosis, with increased risk in end-to-end anastomoses over end-to-side anastomoses.[6] The most common causes of RAS with respect to location are detailed in **Table 2**.

Findings on color Doppler include turbulent flow with color aliasing at the stenosis, with parvus-tardus waveforms in the downstream renal artery

Table 2
Most common causes of renal artery stenosis (RAS) with respect to location

Location of RAS	Cause
At the anastomosis	Vessel perfusion injury, faulty surgical technique, reaction to suture material
Distal to the anastomosis	Injury during clamping, rejection, turbulent flow from kidney malposition, artery kink/twisting, external compression

and renal parenchymal arteries. PSV in the renal artery should exceed 250 to 300 cm/s with a ratio of PSV at the RAS to the ipsilateral external iliac artery of greater than 1.8 to 3.5 (**Fig. 2, Table 3**).

Most patients with end-stage renal disease are hypertensive and, after renal transplantation, most will have a reduction in hypertension. The following situations should prompt a search for transplant RAS: severe or worsening hypertension refractory to medical therapy; hypertension and concomitant audible bruit over the graft; and hypertension and unexplained graft dysfunction.

External Iliac Artery Stenosis

Rarely parvus-tardus waveforms in the main renal artery and intrarenal arteries may be caused by a stenosis in the ipsilateral common or external iliac artery. Spectral Doppler may show elevated velocities at the stenosis and downstream parvus-tardus waveforms, including the femoral or popliteal arteries (**Fig. 3**).

Renal Artery Thrombosis

Renal artery thrombosis (RAT) is a rare complication occurring in fewer than 1% of cases.[5] RAT typically occurs in the early postoperative period, and may result in transplant loss unless addressed immediately. RAT is usually a result of surgical

technique, and the most common causes include kinking or torsion of the renal artery and dissection of the arterial wall. Other causes include acute or hyperacute rejection, acute tubular necrosis, and hypercoagulable state. Patients typically present with absent urinary output, renal failure, and swelling and tenderness over the graft.

Doppler ultrasonography demonstrates absent arterial and venous flow distal to the thrombosed segment of the renal artery. Color and power Doppler parameters must be made sensitive to avoid a false-positive Doppler result. RAT must be treated immediately, usually with surgery or catheter-directed thrombolytic therapy (**Table 4**).

Segmental Infarction

Segmental infarction may occur at any time throughout the life of a renal transplant. Infarcts may be single or multifocal, and potential causes include vascular thrombosis, ligation of accessory renal arteries at the time of transplantation, transplant rejection, or severe pyelonephritis.

On gray-scale ultrasonography, the acutely infarcted kidney may be enlarged and wedge-shaped, and the renal parenchyma is often hypoechoic. The infarcted parenchyma regresses in size over time. Flow is not visualized in the affected parenchyma on color or power Doppler imaging (**Fig. 4, Table 5**).

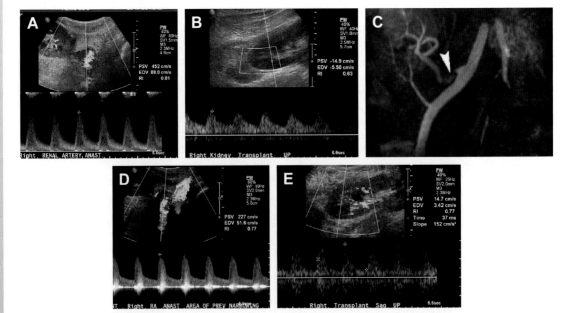

Fig. 2. Transplant renal artery stenosis. (*A*) Spectral Doppler of main renal artery just beyond anastomosis shows aliasing and markedly elevated angle corrected peak systolic velocity of 452 cm/s. (*B*) Spectral Doppler of downstream arcuate artery shows a delayed systolic upstroke (parvus-tardus waveform). (*C*) Noncontrast magnetic resonance angiography shows a short-segment high-grade stenosis (*arrowhead*) of the proximal transplant renal artery. (*D*) Spectral Doppler of main renal artery after angioplasty and stenting shows normal velocity at the anastomosis. (*E*) Spectral Doppler image of arcuate artery shows a normal systolic upstroke.

Table 3	
Ultrasonography of transplant renal artery stenosis	
Timing	Usually occurs in first 3 mo posttransplantation
Ultrasonography findings	Elevated peak systolic velocities typically >250–300 cm/s at stenosis with parvus-tardus waveforms in the parenchymal arteries
	Ratio of peak systolic velocities in renal artery to external iliac artery >1.8–3.5
Pitfall	High main renal artery velocities with normal parenchymal color Doppler flow may be secondary to angle of takeoff or edema at anastomosis; this can be normal in the immediate posttransplant period
	Parvus-tardus waveforms in the main renal artery secondary to a stenosis in the common or external iliac artery

Renal Vein Thrombosis

Renal vein thrombosis (RVT), which most frequently occurs in the first postoperative week, is a rare complication that occurs in fewer than 5% of cases. Clinical presentation includes elevated creatinine, abrupt anuria, and swelling or pain over the transplant. Causes include surgical technique (dysfunctional anastomosis), venous compression from adjacent collection, hypercoagulable states, acute rejection, and hypovolemia. Renal transplants in the left lower quadrant have an increased incidence of RVT secondary to compression of the left iliac vein by the left common iliac artery (iliac artery compression syndrome).[7]

Ultrasonography findings include an enlarged kidney with absent or diminished venous flow in the main renal vein (**Fig. 5, Table 6**). The classic spectral Doppler finding is complete reversal of diastolic flow in the main renal artery and intrarenal arterial branches. Reversal of diastolic flow can also occur in acute rejection, severe acute tubular necrosis (ATN), or Page kidney. Different causes of reversed diastolic flow cannot be distinguished by waveform morphology.[8] Early recognition of RVT is imperative to salvage the graft, which can be achieved by intraoperative thrombectomy or catheter-directed thrombolysis.

Occasionally RVT may occur from proximal extension of an ipsilateral external iliac deep

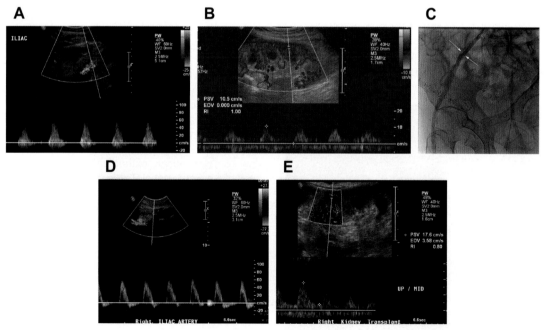

Fig. 3. External iliac artery (EIA) stenosis. (*A*) Color and spectral Doppler of right EIA shows a delayed systolic upstroke (parvus-tardus waveform). (*B*) Arcuate artery spectral Doppler shows a delayed systolic upstroke. The resistive index is 1.0 secondary to ATN. (*C*) Conventional angiogram with catheter tip in proximal right external iliac artery shows a focal EIA stenosis (*arrows*). (*D, E*) Color and spectral Doppler of EIA and arcuate artery after angioplasty and stenting of the right EIA stenosis shows a normalized systolic upstroke in both arteries.

Table 4	
Ultrasonography of transplant renal artery thrombosis	
Timing	Immediate: less than 1 wk posttransplant
Ultrasonography findings	Absent renal arterial and venous flow distal to the thrombosed segment
Pitfall	Color and power Doppler parameters must be made sensitive to avoid a false-positive result

Table 5	
Ultrasonography of renal transplant segmental infarction	
Timing	Can occur at any time
Ultrasonography findings	May be single or multifocal Color or power Doppler flow is not visualized in the affected parenchyma

venous thrombosis (DVT) (**Fig. 6**). Therefore, kidney transplant patients with a lower extremity DVT on the same side as the allograft should also undergo imaging of the ipsilateral external iliac and transplant renal veins.

Renal Vein Stenosis

Clinically significant transplant renal vein stenosis is exceedingly rare and may present as a slow deterioration in graft function. Underlying causes include infection, scar or fibrosis at the anastomosis, graft rejection, high-pressure turbulent flow in the setting of arteriovenous fistula, or, most commonly, compression by an adjacent collection.[9–11] Ultrasonography findings include elevated velocities in the narrowed segment of the renal vein, but care must be taken to avoid inadvertent compression of the vein during routine scanning (**Table 7**). Symptomatic or hemodynamically significant renal vein stenosis may be treated by venoplasty and stenting, or treatment of the underlying condition.

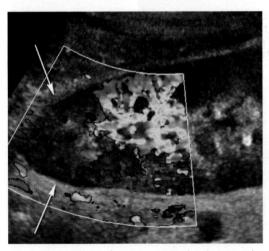

Fig. 4. Segmental infarction. Sagittal color Doppler image shows lack of flow (*arrows*) to upper pole of a transplant kidney owing to ligation of an upper pole accessory renal artery.

Pseudoaneurysm and Arteriovenous Fistula

Percutaneous biopsy may lead to formation of a pseudoaneurysm (PSA) or, more commonly, arteriovenous fistula (AVF). In a recent study, AVF occurred in 7.3% of biopsies.[12] In most cases these complications resolved spontaneously, with self-limiting gross hematuria occurring in 3.5% of biopsies.

A PSA forms when the arterial wall is injured by the biopsy needle, and appears as an anechoic or minimally complex cyst on gray-scale ultrasonography with yin-yang flow on color Doppler (**Fig. 7**). Extrarenal PSAs are rare and usually occur at the anastomosis, and can be precipitated by infection.

The spectral Doppler appearance of PSAs varies depending on presence of communication with a vein. PSAs with a narrow neck and no venous communication will show a classic arterial to-and-fro waveform when the neck is interrogated with spectral Doppler. PSAs that communicate with a vein can show turbulent high-velocity low-resistance flow at the neck and mildly pulsatile high-velocity flow in the draining vein (**Table 8**). Treatment with transcatheter embolization may be necessary if the PSA enlarges or ruptures, and is recommended for extrarenal PSAs.

AVFs typically occur in a single segmental or interlobar artery and paired vein. On color Doppler, they appear as a localized region of turbulent flow or color mosaic extending beyond the confines of a normal vessel (**Table 9**). This appearance is secondary to soft-tissue vibration surrounding the AVF. Spectral Doppler shows a high-velocity low-resistance waveform in the feeding artery and arterialized venous flow in the draining vein (**Fig. 8**). A steal phenomenon may occur with large AVFs, whereby redirection of blood flow to the AVF results in decreased renal perfusion and ischemia of the allograft (**Fig. 9**). In this instance, angiography and embolization may be required.

Compartment Syndrome

The renal allograft is usually placed in a compartment between the anterior abdominal wall and the parietal peritoneum. In the immediate

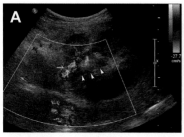
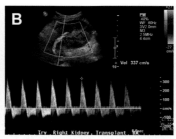
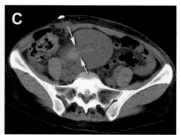

Fig. 5. Renal vein thrombosis. (*A*) Transverse color Doppler of the transplant kidney shows turbulent flow in the main renal artery (*arrows*) and linear decreased echogenicity with no flow in the area of the main renal vein (*arrowheads*). (*B*) Transverse color and spectral Doppler of the main renal artery shows complete diastolic reversal of flow. (*C*) Axial unenhanced computed tomography (CT) of the graft shows hyperdense blood clot (*arrows*) in the area of the main renal vein.

postoperative period, pressures may increase in this extraperitoneal compartment, and this can lead to global compression of the kidney or formation of a kink in the renal artery, resulting in decreased renal perfusion. Renal transplant compartment syndrome (CS) is analogous to abdominal CS whereby elevated intra-abdominal pressures cause organ dysfunction unless the pressure is relieved. CS after renal transplantation is rare, with a reported incidence of between 1.2% and 2%.[13,14] Nonetheless, it is the most common immediate postsurgical complication requiring reoperation. If recognized early, urgent reoperation with placement of the kidney into the peritoneum will salvage the graft. Alternative surgical procedures include retroperitoneal fasciotomy and decompression with closure using an interposition mesh.

Ultrasonography plays a crucial role in this diagnosis. Imaging of the transplant kidney in the immediate postoperative period can detect CS and other major vascular complications so that reoperation may preserve graft function. The typical findings of CS on ultrasonography include poor color Doppler flow, parvus-tardus waveforms in the arcuate arteries, and a patent renal vein (**Fig. 10, Table 10**). Main renal artery velocities may be either very elevated when a renal artery kink occurs, or very low when there is no kink. Isolated

high renal artery velocities with normal color Doppler immediately after transplantation should not be ascribed to CS. A higher than normal renal artery velocity is not uncommon secondary to perivessel edema and high velocities in the ipsilateral external iliac artery resulting from the hemodynamic state of the patient.

Torsion of the Transplant Kidney

Torsion of the allograft is a rare complication of intraperitoneal transplant kidneys. Torsion may occur as early as the first week, but can occur several months following transplant.[15]

Prompt diagnosis is crucial to ensure graft survival. Patients may be asymptomatic and undergoing imaging for routine surveillance, or present with a decline in renal function. Torsion should be suspected when there is a change in renal axis compared with baseline (**Fig. 11, Table 11**). The degree of compromise of vascular flow depends on the degree and duration of torsion, and can result in a high-resistance arterial flow pattern. Additional less specific findings include changes in parenchymal echogenicity, hydronephrosis if the ureter is kinked, and urothelial thickening.

The presence of surgical wounds or dressings may alter the acoustic window and result in a spurious change of renal axis. Images in the

Table 6	
Ultrasonography of transplant renal vein thrombosis	
Timing	Immediate: within the first week posttransplantation
Ultrasonography findings	Enlarged kidney Complete reversal of diastolic flow in the main renal artery and intrarenal arterial branches with absent or diminished flow in main renal vein
Pitfall	Reversal of diastolic flow may be present in acute rejection, severe acute tubular necrosis, Page kidney (compression of parenchyma by subcapsular fluid collection), although the renal vein will remain patent

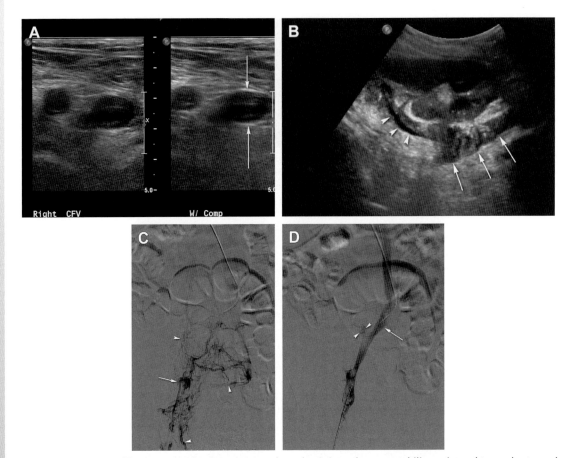

Fig. 6. Propagation of lower extremity deep venous thrombosis into the external iliac vein and transplant renal vein. (*A*) Dual-compression ultrasonography shows noncompressibility of the right common femoral vein (*arrows*) secondary to thrombus. (*B*) Sagittal ultrasonography shows extension of thrombus into the right external iliac vein (*arrows*) and transplant renal vein (*arrowheads*). The thrombus in the transplant renal vein is nonocclusive. (*C*) Venogram with the inferior catheter tip in the external iliac vein (*arrow*) shows thrombosis of the external iliac and common femoral veins with extensive network of collateral flow (*arrowheads*). (*D*) After catheter-directed thrombolysis and venoplasty, there is restoration of flow in the right external iliac vein (*arrow*) and common femoral vein without collateral flow. Note opacification of the proximal renal vein (*arrowheads*).

transverse plane are least operator dependent and should be used as a baseline. Often computed tomography (CT) is helpful in confirming the diagnosis.

UROLOGIC AND COLLECTING SYSTEM COMPLICATIONS

Urologic complications after renal transplantation include urine leaks and urinomas, hydronephrosis, vesicoureteral reflux, and calculi. Large retrospective studies report rates of 6% to 15% for such complications, but often include heterogeneous populations and transplants performed 15 to 20 years ago. With current surgical techniques and ureteral stents, rates of urologic complications are probably between 1% and 8%.[16–18]

Table 7
Ultrasonography of transplant renal vein stenosis

Timing	Late: >1 mo posttransplantation
Ultrasonography findings	Elevated velocity in a narrowed renal vein segment
Pitfall	Inadvertent compression during scanning may falsely narrow the vein and elevate the velocity

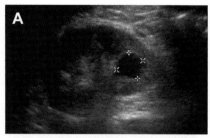 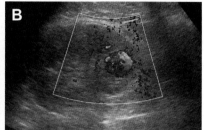

Fig. 7. Pseudoaneurysm presenting as gross hematuria after biopsy. (*A*) Sagittal ultrasonography shows an anechoic cystic structure demarcated by calipers in the lower pole of the transplant kidney. (*B*) Color Doppler shows yin-yang flow in the cystic structure consistent with a postbiopsy pseudoaneurysm, which was subsequently treated with coil embolization.

Most series report urinary leaks, ureteral obstruction, and strictures as the most frequent urologic complications, typically occurring within the first few months after surgery as a result of vascular insufficiency and necrosis at the ureterovesical junction. Most of these complications can be treated percutaneously with a combination of ureteral angioplasty, drainage of collections, ureteral stents, and Foley catheters.[19] Late obstruction may be due to adhesions or fibrosis related to multiple procedures or chronic rejection, and is more likely to require surgical management.

A urine leak manifests sonographically as a simple fluid collection located between the kidney and bladder. Urinary ascites may occur if the transplant is intraperitoneal in location. Percutaneous sampling under ultrasound guidance will yield fluid with a high creatinine level. Cystograms and radionuclide studies can also be used to confirm the suspected leak.

Hydronephrosis can result from a variety of complications including clots, calculi, sloughed papilla, fungus balls, strictures, and extrinsic compression of the ureter by a collection. Dilatation of the collecting system can also occur from vesicoureteral reflux, which is more common in pediatric patients.[20] Patients with acute obstruction will not present with typical ureteral colic because the kidney is denervated; rather, they present with oliguria or anuria, decreased renal function, and occasional gross hematuria. It is noteworthy that mild to moderate dilatation of the collecting system may not be due to obstruction, but commonly results from loss of tone caused by denervation or mild reflux.

The incidence of clinically significant urolithiasis after renal transplant ranges between 1% and 2%.[21] Calculi may originate from the donor or develop de novo at any time, although hypercalcemia as a cause is most common within 1 year of surgery. Elicitation of the color Doppler twinkle artifact is extremely helpful in the detection of renal calculi. Optimal sonographic technique includes a high pulse-repetition frequency to minimize normal color flow and placing the focal zone below the kidney.

Medullary nephrocalcinosis may be more easily appreciated using higher-frequency transducers. Cortical nephrocalcinosis is usually a late process that heralds chronic rejection and failure of the allograft.

PERINEPHRIC FLUID COLLECTIONS

Fluid collections around the kidney are among the most common complications after transplantation. The appearance and timing of presentation help to suggest the nature of the fluid. Ultrasonography is often the first study performed to detect a collection, for which meticulous technique must be used with an extended field of view with varying depths and frequencies, so that complex

Table 8	
Ultrasonography of renal transplant pseudoaneurysm	
Timing	Late: usually occurs as a complication of percutaneous biopsy
Ultrasonography findings	Anechoic or minimally complex cyst on gray-scale ultrasonography with yin-yang flow on color Doppler
	Varying spectral Doppler appearance. May display classic "to and fro" waveform in pseudoaneurysms with no venous communication and narrow neck
	Extrarenal pseudoaneurysms are rare

Table 9 Ultrasonography of renal transplant arteriovenous fistula (AVF)	
Timing	Late: occurs as a complication of percutaneous biopsy
Ultrasonography findings	Localized region of color flow extending beyond confines of a normal vessel with feeding artery and draining vein A steal phenomenon may occur with large AVFs, resulting in decreased parenchymal perfusion and ischemia

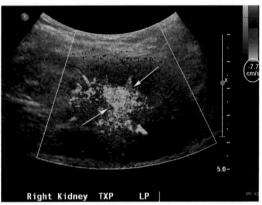

Fig. 9. Large arteriovenous fistula with steal phenomenon. Color Doppler of renal transplant after biopsy shows a large color Doppler bruit (*arrows*) in the lower pole corresponding to an AVF, resulting in poor perfusion of the peripheral renal parenchyma, despite using very sensitive color Doppler settings (*circled*).

collections, and those that extend away from the kidney, are not missed (**Table 12**).

Hematomas are the most common peritransplant collections, usually occurring in the immediate posttransplant period, although they are occasionally a complication of percutaneous biopsy. Acute hematomas are echogenic and are often indistinguishable from surrounding soft tissues; they can be easily overlooked, and can be perinephric or subcapsular in location (**Fig. 12**). Large hematomas may compromise the kidney by compressing vessels or the collecting system, necessitating percutaneous or surgical drainage. Subcapsular hematomas may compress the renal cortex, resulting in increased interstitial pressure and elevation of the RIs because of Page kidney physiology.

Abscesses are rare and usually result from superinfection of hematomas, although any fluid collection may become superinfected in an immunocompromised patient. An abscess should be suspected when there are symptoms of infection and a relatively simple collection becomes more sonographically complex or contains gas (**Fig. 13**).

Lymphoceles are common after renal transplantation, occurring in as many as 20% of cases. Lymphoceles typically present within 1 to 2 months after transplantation, are rounded or ovoid, and relatively anechoic, but may contain thin septations (**Fig. 14**). Various predisposing factors have been reported, including diabetes, various immunosuppressive regimens, and rejection.[22–24] Treatment may be percutaneous with sclerotherapy, or surgical for recurrent collections.

Urinomas are a relatively rare type of peritransplant collection that may occur at any time, but usually in the first few weeks to months after transplantation. The most common location is adjacent to the ureterovesical anastomosis or between the bladder and the kidney (**Fig. 15**). Sonographically

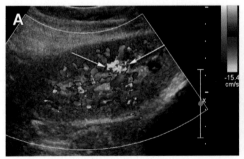
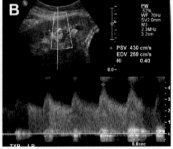

Fig. 8. Arteriovenous fistula (AVF) without steal. (*A*) Color Doppler of a transplant kidney shows a focal color Doppler bruit (*arrows*) representing an AVF with satisfactory perfusion of the peripheral renal parenchyma. Note that the color Doppler settings are sensitive. (*B*) Spectral Doppler shows high-velocity low-resistance arterial flow, characteristic of an AVF.

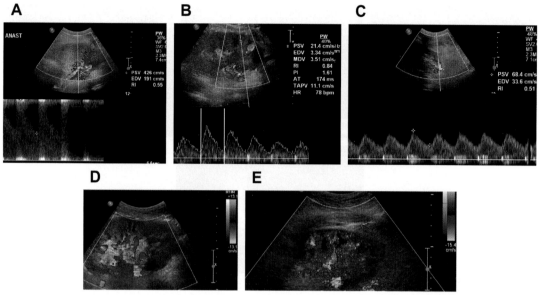

Fig. 10. Compartment syndrome: kink in main renal artery. (A) Color and spectral Doppler shows markedly elevated main renal artery peak systolic velocities at anastomosis. (B, C) Downstream arcuate and hilar renal artery waveforms show delay in upstroke, worrisome for a proximal stenosis. (D) Color Doppler of allograft shows global decreased perfusion. (E) Improved color Doppler flow of the allograft following intraperitoneal placement of transplant kidney.

they are simple in appearance in comparison with hematomas, lymphoceles, and abscesses.

RENAL PARENCHYMAL ABNORMALITIES

Parenchymal abnormalities of the renal transplant include ATN, acute and chronic rejection, medication toxicity, and pyelonephritis. The timing of

Table 10 Ultrasonography of renal transplant compartment syndrome	
Timing	Immediate (<1 wk)
Ultrasonography findings	Decreased renal perfusion on color Doppler, very high or very low main renal artery velocities, parvus-tardus waveforms in the arcuate arteries, patent renal vein
Pitfall	High renal artery velocities secondary to edema at anastomosis with normal parenchymal color Doppler flow may be normal in the immediate posttransplant period

disease presentation is an important factor in diagnosing these causes of diminished renal transplant function. Gray-scale ultrasonography findings are nonspecific and subjective, with negative predictive values ranging from 17% to 50%.[2] These gray-scale findings are listed in **Box 3**.

Evaluation of the arcuate or intralobular artery RIs allows for long-term monitoring of the transplanted kidney and recipient over time, and may be useful in guiding a clinician on whether to proceed with biopsy. An RI cutoff value of 0.80 has been shown to be predictive of recipient mortality, although it may not predict the need for dialysis. Regardless, ATN and antibody-mediated rejection are associated with higher RI values overall than in patients with normal biopsy results.[25] However, ultimately biopsy is necessary for diagnosis in an overwhelming majority of cases.

Acute Tubular Necrosis

Delayed graft function, defined as the need for dialysis in the first week following kidney transplantation, is most commonly caused by ATN. ATN is manifested clinically by a decreased glomerular filtration rate, and is caused by impaired active transport of sodium chloride. The development of ATN is common in the early transplant period and is principally related to the donor kidney, with cold ischemia times of more than 24 to 30 hours resulting in a higher frequency of

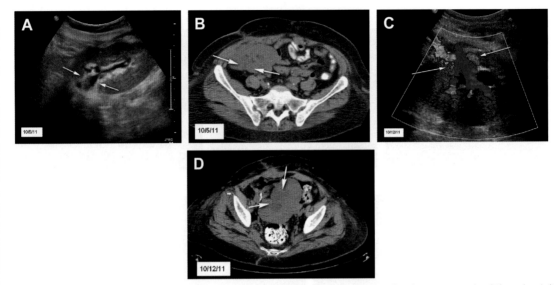

Fig. 11. Torsion of right intraperitoneal transplant kidney. Transverse gray-scale ultrasonography (*A*) and axial unenhanced CT (*B*) of the transplant kidney show a posterolateral oriented hilum (*arrows*) of the transplant kidney. Transverse color Doppler ultrasonography (*C*) and axial unenhanced CT (*D*) one week later show new mild hydronephrosis and a superolateral oriented hilum (*arrows*), secondary to torsion of the intraperitoneal transplant kidney. The patient was taken emergently to the operating room for detorsion and pexy of the transplant.

ATN.[26] As a result, ATN is less commonly seen in patients receiving transplants from living donors. Up to 10% to 30% of patients with ATN require dialysis in the early stages, but most cases resolve spontaneously over the first 2 postoperative weeks.[27] The incidence and severity of ATN after transplantation has increased in recent years as the donation criteria have been expanded to include kidneys that have been subjected to more stress from sicker and older patients.

Gray-scale ultrasonography evaluation of the transplant kidney in patients with ATN is usually normal, but nonspecific findings of renal enlargement, increased or decreased parenchymal echogenicity, loss of corticomedullary differentiation, and elevated RIs may be present (**Table 13**).

Table 11 Ultrasonography of renal transplant torsion	
Timing	Can occur at any time
Ultrasonography findings	Intraperitoneal transplant kidney. Change in renal axis compared with baseline, with variable compromise of vascular and collecting systems
Pitfall	Changes in scanning technique may create the appearance of transplant torsion. Transverse images are least operator dependent

Table 12 Ultrasonography of perinephric collections	
Hematoma	Usually occurs in immediate postoperative period, although may occur after percutaneous biopsy. Hematomas may be perinephric or subcapsular. Acute hematomas are echogenic and may be easily overlooked
Abscess	Abscess should be suspected when a collection becomes more complex or contains gas. Pitfall: Surgicel
Lymphocele	Typically presents within 1–2 mo after transplantation. Relatively anechoic. May contain thin septations
Urinoma	Usually occurs in the first few weeks to months. More simple in appearance than other perinephric collections. Most commonly occurs adjacent to ureterovesical anastomosis

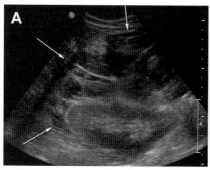
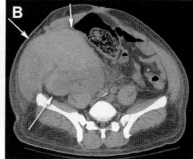

Fig. 12. Perinephric and abdominal wall hematoma. (*A*) Bedside ultrasonography shows a large heterogeneous predominantly hypoechoic perinephric and abdominal wall collection (*arrows*). (*B*) Axial unenhanced CT at the same level better shows the acute perinephric and abdominal wall hematoma (*arrows*).

Acute Rejection

Acute rejection occurs in up to 40% of patients in the early transplant period, peaking at 1 to 3 weeks posttransplant.[27] If promptly recognized, acute rejection can be reversible with high-dose steroid therapy. It can be distinguished from ATN based on time course, with acute rejection rarely occurring in the first few days following transplant. Instead, acute rejection manifests on serial laboratory and ultrasonography evaluations. If acute rejection occurs later than this time period, noncompliance with immunosuppressive therapy should be considered. The occurrence of acute rejection confers a poor long-term prognosis and is a well-recognized predisposing factor to chronic rejection.

The clinical differential diagnosis for acute rejection includes urinary tract obstruction, ATN, pyelonephritis, and medication toxicity. Ultrasonography can be valuable in distinguishing among some of these entities; however, renal biopsy serves as the gold standard for diagnosis. Histologically, acute rejection typically manifests as arteriolar vasculitis and tubular inflammation.[28] Acute rejection may increase renal length to a greater extent than ATN, and can result in a globular appearance.[29] The likelihood of acute rejection increases with higher RIs, with complete absence of diastolic flow, or flow reversal, occurring in more severe cases (**Fig. 16**). In these severe cases, demonstration of a patent renal vein is important in distinguishing rejection from RVT (**Table 14**).

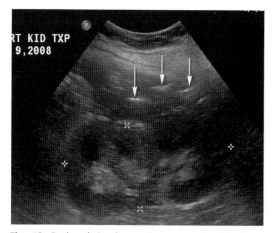

Fig. 13. Perinephric abscess in a patient with fever. Sagittal ultrasonography shows a complex, heterogeneous collection containing echogenic foci (*arrows*) with dirty shadowing corresponding to gas bubbles, anterior to the transplant kidney, representing an abscess. Surgicel in the postoperative bed can have a similar appearance.

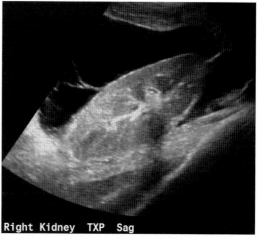

Fig. 14. Lymphocele. Sagittal ultrasonography shows a large perinephric collection containing thin septations and minimal internal echoes.

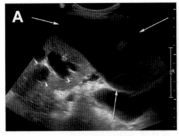
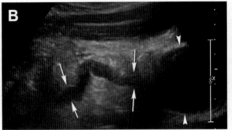
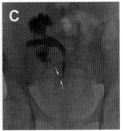

Fig. 15. Urinoma and hydronephrosis secondary to a ureterovesical stricture. (*A*) Sagittal ultrasonography shows a large, predominantly anechoic collection (*arrows*) anterior to the transplant kidney and urinary bladder, which represents a urinoma. Note the moderate hydronephrosis of the transplant kidney (*arrowheads*). (*B*) Sagittal ultrasonography shows moderate hydroureter (*arrows*) extending to the urinary bladder (*arrowheads*), suggesting a stricture at the ureterovesical anastomosis. (*C*) Antegrade nephroureterography confirms hydroureteronephrosis secondary to a ureterovesical junction stricture (*arrows*). This condition was treated with a percutaneous nephrostomy tube, which was converted into a nephroureteral stent.

Hyperacute rejection occurs immediately at the time of vascular anastomosis and, therefore, is rarely imaged; it is due to the presence of preformed antibodies in the recipient.

Chronic Rejection

Chronic rejection is the most common cause of late graft loss, and is characterized by progressive decline and eventual loss of the renal transplant beginning at greater than 3 months following transplantation. Prior episodes of acute rejection are the most consistent predisposing risk factor for the development of chronic rejection. Renal biopsy is required for diagnosis, with sclerosing vasculitis and interstitial infiltration and fibrosis being the predominant histologic features.

Ultrasonography features of chronic rejection include mild hydronephrosis, increased parenchymal echogenicity, cortical thinning, loss of corticomedullary differentiation, urothelial thickening, and reduction of intraparenchymal vascularity (**Table 15**).

Medication Toxicity

Most of the currently used immunosuppressive drugs are nephrotoxic, with cyclosporine conferring the greatest nephrotoxic potential. Dehydration and decreased renal perfusion may accentuate the effects of nephrotoxic drugs, delaying recovery from ATN and leading to irreversible graft dysfunction.[30] Medication toxicity has a variable effect on renal Doppler waveforms. Ultrasonography may be normal, or RIs mildly increased.

Pyelonephritis

Potential ultrasonography findings of pyelonephritis include poor corticomedullary differentiation, increased renal size, and patchy or wedge-shaped areas of increased cortical echogenicity. Doppler imaging shows decreased perfusion in regions of increased echogenicity, with potentially increased RIs (**Fig. 17**). On imaging, pyelonephritis may be indistinguishable from acute rejection, and is occasionally diagnosed on biopsy performed for suspected cases of rejection (**Table 16**).[27]

Neoplasm (Posttransplant Lymphoproliferative Disorder)

Renal transplant patients have a generally increased risk of neoplasm related primarily to

---

Box 3
Possible gray-scale findings of renal transplant dysfunction

- Renal enlargement or atrophy
- Increased cortical thickness or cortical atrophy
- Increased or decreased parenchymal echogenicity
- Loss of corticomedullary differentiation
- Urothelial thickening

Table 13 Ultrasonography of acute tubular necrosis	
Timing	Immediate: occurs in first week posttransplantation
Ultrasonography findings	Usually normal, but renal enlargement, increased or decreased parenchymal echogenicity, loss of corticomedullary differentiation, and elevated intralobular artery resistive indices may be present

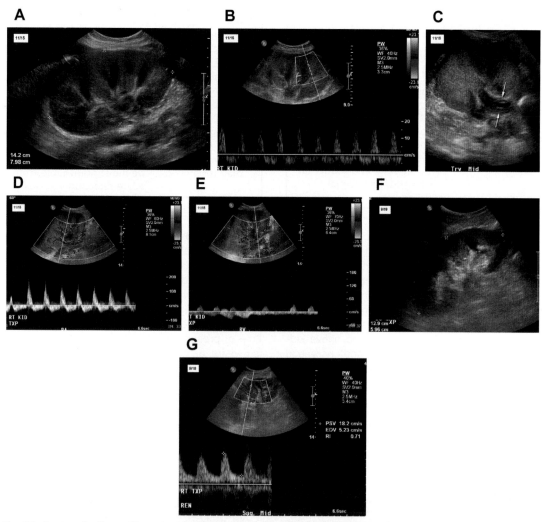

Fig. 16. Acute rejection with reversed diastolic flow. (*A*) Sagittal ultrasonography shows an enlarged, globular-shaped allograft with loss of renal sinus fat. (*B*) Color and spectral Doppler of arcuate artery shows elevated resistive index of 1.0 and complete reversal of diastolic flow. (*C*) Transverse image shows urothelial thickening (*arrows*), a nonspecific finding. (*D*) Spectral Doppler of main renal artery shows complete reversal of diastolic flow. (*E*) Spectral Doppler of main renal vein shows patency with mild phasic flow. (*F, G*) Comparison with ultrasonogram from 2 months earlier confirms the marked change. At that time the transplant was normal in size with normal sinus fat, and showed a normal intrarenal resistive index of 0.71 on spectral Doppler.

Table 14
Ultrasonography of acute renal transplant rejection

Timing	Early: occurs from 1 wk to 1 mo after transplantation
Ultrasonography findings	Increased transplant size with globular appearance Elevated resistive indices with absence of diastolic flow or diastolic flow reversal in severe cases
Pitfall	Demonstration of a patent renal vein is important in cases with reversal of diastolic flow, to distinguish from renal vein thrombosis

Table 15 Ultrasonography of chronic renal transplant rejection	
Timing	Late
Ultrasonography findings	Nonspecific findings of: mild hydronephrosis, increased parenchymal echogenicity, cortical thinning, loss of corticomedullary differentiation, urothelial thickening, and reduction of intraparenchymal vascularity

Table 16 Ultrasonography of pyelonephritis	
Timing	Can occur at any time
Ultrasonography findings	Decreased perfusion in patchy or wedge-shaped regions of increased cortical echogenicity Resistive indices may be increased
Differential diagnosis	Diffuse pyelonephritis may be indistinguishable from acute rejection

chronic immunosuppression. Most neoplasms are skin cancers and lymphomas. Patients are also at increased risk for renal cell carcinoma, although most of these are in the native kidneys in patients with acquired cystic disease from hemodialysis. Ultrasonography may be used to screen for renal neoplasms in both the transplant and native kidneys, although marked atrophy and increased echogenicity in the native kidneys may decrease the ability to detect small tumors with ultrasonography.

Posttransplantation lymphoproliferative disorder (PTLD) is a general term for a variety of lymphoid disorders ranging from lymphoid hyperplasia to frank lymphoma. Most cases of PTLD are B-cell lymphocyte proliferations related to Epstein-Barr virus, although the heterogeneity of these disorders suggests a variety of mechanisms that predispose to lymphoproliferation. PTLD after solid organ transplantation usually occurs within the first year; however, the median time of presentation for renal transplant patients is 5 years, as a result of less aggressive immunosuppressive therapy.[31] The most common site for PTLD in renal transplant patients is the allograft, followed by extranodal involvement, with particular predilection for the gastrointestinal tract and liver. Typical patterns of kidney involvement include a heterogeneous hilar mass and multiple

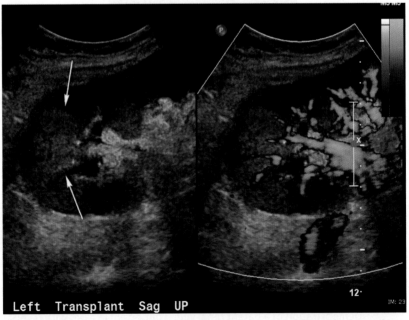

Left   Transplant   Sag   UP

Fig. 17. Pyelonephritis. Sagittal power Doppler-comparison shows a wedge-shaped region of increased echogenicity (*arrows*) in the upper pole of the transplant kidney with corresponding decreased flow on power Doppler.

parenchymal masses. Although one may suspect PTLD based on sonographically detected renal or gastrointestinal abnormalities, the high frequency of multisystem involvement makes positron emission tomography combined with CT the preferred imaging modality.[32]

SUMMARY

Ultrasonography is an excellent tool for evaluation of renal transplantation from the immediate postoperative period through long-term follow up. The combination of gray-scale ultrasonography with color and spectral Doppler is necessary to evaluate complications that may arise in the perinephric space, renal vasculature, renal parenchyma, or collecting system. Further division of complications into immediate, early, and late categories helps formulate an appropriate differential diagnosis.

REFERENCES

1. Nixon JN, Biyyam DR, Stanescu L, et al. Imaging of pediatric renal transplants and their complications: a pictorial review. Radiographics 2013;33:1227–51.
2. Brown ED, Chen MY, Wolfman NT, et al. Complications of renal transplantation: evaluation with US and radionuclide imaging. Radiographics 2000;20:607–22.
3. Gao J, Ng A, Shih G, et al. Intrarenal color duplex ultrasonography. J Ultrasound Med 2007;26:1403–18.
4. De Morais RH, Muglia VF, Mamere AE, et al. Duplex Doppler sonography of transplant renal artery stenosis. J Clin Ultrasound 2003;31:135–41.
5. Dodd GD, Tublin AS, Sajko AB. Imaging of vascular complications associated with renal transplants. AJR Am J Roentgenol 1991;157:449–59.
6. Rees CR, Palmaz JC, Becker GJ, et al. Palmaz stent in artherosclerotic stenosis involving the ostia of the renal arteries: preliminary report of a multicenter study. Radiology 1991;181:507–14.
7. Jordan ML, Cook GT, Cardella CJ. Ten years of experience with vascular complications in renal transplantation. J Urol 1982;128:689–92.
8. Lockhart ME, Wells CG, Morgan DE, et al. Reversed diastolic flow in the renal transplant: perioperative implications versus transplants older than 1 month. AJR Am J Roentgenol 2008;190(3):650–5.
9. Cercuel JP, Chevet D, Mousson C, et al. Acquired vein stenosis of renal allograft-Percutaneous treatment with self-expanding metallic stent. Nephrol Dial Transplant 1997;12:825–6.
10. Olliff S, Negus R, Deane C, et al. Renal transplant vein stenosis: demonstration and percutaneous venoplasty of a new vascular complication in the transplant kidney. Clin Radiol 1991;43:42–6.
11. Obed A, Uihlein DC, Zorger N, et al. Severe renal vein stenosis of a kidney transplant with beneficial clinical course after successful percutaneous stenting. Am J Transplant 2008;8:2173–7.
12. Schwarz A, Gwinner W, Hiss M, et al. Safety and adequacy of renal transplant protocol biopsies. Am J Transplant 2005;5:1992–6.
13. Ball CG, Kirkpatrick AW, Yilmaz S, et al. Renal allograft compartment syndrome: an underappreciated postoperative complication. Am J Surg 2006;191:619–24.
14. Horrow MM, Parsikia A, Zaki R, et al. Immediate postoperative sonography of renal transplants: vascular findings and outcomes. AJR Am J Roentgenol 2013;201:W479–86.
15. Wong-You-Cheong JJ, Grumbach K, Krebs TL, et al. Torsion of intraperitoneal renal transplants: imaging appearances. AJR Am J Roentgenol 1998;171:1355–9.
16. Dinckan A, Tekin A, Turkyilmaz S, et al. Early and late urological complications corrected surgically following renal transplantation. Transpl Int 2007;20:702–7.
17. Nie ZL, Zhang KQ, Li QS, et al. Urological complications in 1,223 kidney transplantations. Urol Int 2009;83:337–41.
18. Zavos G, Pappas P, Karatzas T, et al. Urological complications: analysis and management of 1525 consecutive renal transplantations. Transplant Proc 2008;40:1386–90.
19. Kobayashi K, Censullo ML, Rossman LL, et al. Interventional radiologic management of renal transplant dysfunction: indications, limitations, and technical considerations. Radiographics 2007;27:1009–130.
20. Barrero R, Fijo J, Fernandez-Hurtado M, et al. Vesicoureteral reflux after kidney transplantation in children. Pediatr Transplant 2007;11(5):498–503.
21. Challacombe B, Dasgupta P, Tiptaft R, et al. Multimodal management of urolithiasis in renal transplantation. BJU Int 2005;96(3):385–9.
22. Khauli RB, Stoff JS, Lovewell T, et al. Post-transplant lymphoceles: a critical look into the risk factors, pathophysiology and management. J Urol 1993;150:22–6.
23. Zietek Z, Sulikowski T, Tejchman K, et al. Lymphocele after kidney transplantation. Transplant Proc 2007;39:2744–7.
24. Ulrich F, Niedzwiecki S, Fikatas P, et al. Symptomatic lymphoceles after kidney transplantation - multivariate analysis of risk factors and outcome after laparoscopic fenestration. Clin Transplant 2010;24:273–80.
25. Naesens M, Heylen L, Lerut E, et al. Intrarenal resistive index after renal transplantation. N Engl J Med 2013;369:1797–806.
26. Isoniemi HM, Krogerus L, von Willebrand E, et al. Histopathological findings in well-functioning, long-term renal allografts. Kidney Int 1992;41:155–60.

27. Baxter GM. Ultrasound of renal transplantation. Clin Radiol 2001;56:802–18.

28. Irshad A, Ackerman S, Sosnouski D et al. A review of sonographic evaluation of renal transplant complications. Curr Probl Diagn Radiol. 37(2): 67–79.

29. Pozniak MA, Kelcz F, D'Alessandro A, et al. Sonography of renal transplants in dogs: the effect of acute tubular necrosis, cyclosporine nephrotoxicity and acute rejection on resistive index and renal length. AJR Am J Roentgenol 1992;158:791–7.

30. Myers BD, Sibley R, Newton L, et al. The long term course of cyclosporine associated chronic nephropathy. Kidney Int 1988;33:590–600.

31. Opelz G, Dohler B. Lymphomas after solid organ transplantation: a collaborative transplant study report. Am J Transplant 2004;4:222–30.

32. Borhani AA, Hosseinzadeh K, Almusa O, et al. Imaging of posttransplantation lymphoproliferative disorder after solid organ transplantation. Radiographics 2009;29:981–1002.

The Essentials of Extracranial Carotid Ultrasonographic Imaging

Katherine A. Kaproth-Joslin, MD/PhD[a],*,
Shweta Bhatt, MBBS[a], Leslie M. Scoutt, MD[b],
Deborah J. Rubens, MD[a]

KEYWORDS

- Carotid arteries • Ultrasonography • Sonography • Doppler imaging • Stenosis • Plaque
- Atherosclerosis • Hemodynamics

KEY POINTS

- Sonographic evaluation of the carotid arteries is the imaging modality of choice for screening, diagnosis, and monitoring of atherosclerotic disease of these vessels.
- Accurate and reproducible results come from good standard imaging technique as well as a complete understanding of the normal grayscale, color Doppler, and spectral Doppler imaging of the extracranial carotid arteries.
- Proper assessment of carotid atherosclerosis is dependent on knowledge of plaque characterization as well as an understanding of the sequelae of luminal narrowing, including the common changes identified on grayscale, color Doppler, and spectral Doppler imaging.
- Evaluation of the carotid arteries after intervention is dependent on familiarity with the normal appearance of the carotid arteries after endarterectomy or angioplasty with stenting, as well as an awareness of the complications associated with each procedure.

BACKGROUND

Atherosclerotic stroke is the fourth leading cause of death in the United States, occurring on average every 40 seconds and causing a death every 4 minutes. Approximately 795,000 people per year are projected to suffer from a new or recurrent stroke.[1,2] As one of the most frequent causes of long-term disability, the direct cost of stroke in 2010 was estimated at $36.5 billion, with the total cost of care exceeding $75 billion.[1,2] As the risk factors for stroke (obesity, high cholesterol levels, and diabetes mellitus) increase in the general population, management of atherosclerosis has become a primary focus of preventative care medicine.

Carotid atherosclerosis is a major risk factor for stroke, as a result of stenosis or unstable (vulnerable) plaque with subsequent distal embolization. In at-risk populations, carotid endarterectomy (CEA) and carotid artery angioplasty and stenting (CAS) can reduce or prevent stroke when

No financial support obtained for this project.
Dr L. Scoutt receives honoraria form Philips Healthcare for CME lectures on vascular ultrasonography. The other authors have nothing to disclose.
[a] Department of Imaging Sciences, University of Rochester, 601 Elmwood Avenue, Rochester, NY 14642, USA;
[b] Department of Diagnostic Radiology, Yale School of Medicine, New Haven, CT 06510, USA
* Corresponding author. Department of Imaging Sciences, University of Rochester Medical Center, 601 Elmwood Avenue, Box 648, Rochester, NY 14642.
E-mail address: katherine_kaproth-joslin@urmc.rochester.edu

Radiol Clin N Am 52 (2014) 1325–1342
http://dx.doi.org/10.1016/j.rcl.2014.07.010
0033-8389/14/$ – see front matter © 2014 Elsevier Inc. All rights reserved.

compared with medical therapy alone. Sonographic evaluation of the carotid arteries is the imaging modality of choice for the screening, diagnosis, and monitoring of atherosclerotic disease of these vessels and, occasionally, is the only imaging modality used before intervention.

In this article, the standard ultrasonographic scanning techniques and Doppler settings necessary to produce reliable and reproducible imaging results are discussed. The normal carotid anatomy is reviewed, including grayscale, color Doppler, and spectral Doppler imaging appearances. The vascular abnormalities caused by carotid atherosclerosis are examined, including plaque morphology characterization as well as waveform and velocity changes caused by stenosis. In addition, special situations are explored, such as imaging in the presence of an arrhythmia or cardiac assist devices. Imaging after carotid surgical intervention is discussed, including complications associated with these procedures.

TECHNIQUE
General

Imaging should be performed with the patient supine, arms down by their side, the neck slightly extended, and the head turned away from the side being examined. For patients with a poor imaging window, especially those with short or thick necks, a pillow can be placed under the shoulders of the patient to hyperextend the neck. The sonographer position is variable depending on operator preference; some individuals choose to sit at the patient's head, facing caudally, scanning from the head to the shoulders, and others prefer to sit by the patient's side, facing superiorly, scanning from the shoulders to the head.

The carotid vessels are superficial; therefore, imaging is performed using a high-frequency linear transducer optimized to the near field view. Grayscale images should be obtained using a 5-MHz to 12-MHz transducer and Doppler imaging performed at 3 to 7 MHz, with the frequency choice dependent on patient body habitus and the technical parameters of the ultrasound machine used. The focal zone should be placed at the level of the carotid vasculature to improve fine detail of the vessel. Imaging is preferably from a posterolateral approach, using the sternocleidomastoid muscle as an acoustic window. A direct anterior approach may be used as necessary for tortuous vessels or a poor imaging window laterally.

Grayscale Imaging

Grayscale imaging evaluates the course and caliber of the carotid arteries and should include an estimation of vessel stenosis as well as characterization of intimal-media thickness and plaque, including echotexture, ulceration, and other surface irregularities. Starting in the transverse plane, each carotid artery is scanned in its entirety from the level of the supraclavicular notch to the angle of the mandible. Imaging of the common carotid artery (CCA) origins can be difficult because of depth and position. In particular, the left CCA may require inferior transducer angulation to see the origin. Transverse imaging establishes the orientation of the internal carotid artery (ICA) and external carotid artery (ECA) and identifies areas of luminal narrowing. Longitudinal imaging of the carotids is then performed, with optimal scanning planes and regions of stenosis identified by the previously performed transverse images.

Color/Power Doppler Imaging

Color Doppler imaging permits rapid detection of flow disturbance (ie, those areas that require further evaluation with spectral analysis). It also provides an average blood flow velocity within the vessel, giving a qualitative assessment of stenosis. Each section of the carotid artery requires optimization of scanning parameters to achieve superior imaging results. The first parameter to adjust is the color Doppler gain. Color Doppler gain should be increased until color speckles are identified in the tissues surrounding the lumen of the vessel, and then the gain is decreased until color is seen only within the vessel lumen. Incorrectly high color Doppler gain settings can cause a bleed or bloom artifact where the color signal projects beyond the true lumen of the vessel. This artifact may cause nonvisualization or reduced visualization of plaque or stenosis, hence, the importance of the initial grayscale images. If the color Doppler gain setting is set too low, there is a risk that no or reduced color flow is depicted on the monitor, leading to a misdiagnosis of slow flow or even vessel occlusion. If slow or no flow is detected, power Doppler should be used to reassess the vessel, because this technique is angle independent and more sensitive to slow flow states. The second parameter to adjust is the color velocity scale. As with the color Doppler gain, the color velocity scale should be increased until color is seen in the entire vessel and the direction of flow is clearly established. Improper velocity scale settings may cause the interpreter to miss areas of turbulent flow, stenotic jets or other areas of flow disturbance. Scale settings that are too low cause aliasing throughout the vessel, without true regions of stenosis, and scale settings that are too high reduce the expected aliasing in regions of luminal irregularity or stenosis. If an occlusion is suspected, the wall filter and scale should be reduced as much as possible to detect the presence of slow flow.

Spectral Doppler

Spectral Doppler waveform analysis is the key component of carotid artery imaging. Like color Doppler imaging, optimization of scanning parameters for each segment of the carotid artery is important for accurate measurement of the spectral Doppler signal. The Doppler angle should optimally be between 45° and 60° and should be kept constant on follow-up imaging for reproducible velocity calculations. As the Doppler angle increases higher than 60°, even small shifts in Doppler signal can cause significant variations in Doppler velocity, leading to greater inaccuracy in estimated calculation of velocity. The angle correction cursor should be set parallel to the posterior carotid wall when there is no evidence of stenosis. However, when a region of turbulent flow is encountered, the cursor should be set parallel to the direction of flow observed on color Doppler imaging. The sample gate should be kept as small as possible,

between 1.5 and 2.5 mm, to produce a thin spectral waveform based on a narrow range of red blood cell velocities. The gate should be set in the center of the vessel or the center of a stenotic jet to capture the region of highest velocity flow. The spectral Doppler gain should also be optimized for carotid vessel analysis. When the gain is set too low, the spectral waveform is weak and challenging to evaluate. When the gain setting is too high, noise is introduced into the spectral tracing, which can give the appearance of spectral broadening or turbulent flow. A spectral gain error should be suspected when the grayscale and color Doppler images do not confirm turbulent flow in an area with spectral broadening.

NORMAL CAROTID IMAGING
Anatomy

The first branch off the normal adult aorta is the brachiocephalic artery, also known as the innominate artery, which divides into the right CCA and the right subclavian artery (SCA). The second branch from the aorta is the left CCA, and the third branch is the left SCA (**Fig. 1**). A common

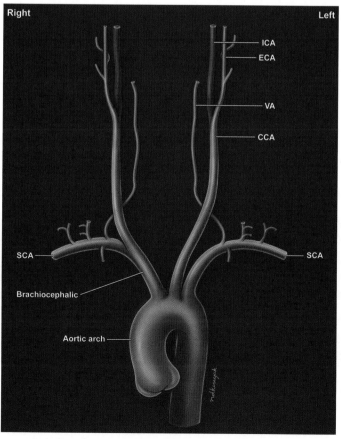

Fig. 1. Branches of the aortic arch and extracranial cerebral arteries. VA, vertebral artery.

anatomic variant is the bovine arch, in which the left CCA arises from the brachiocephalic trunk instead of directly off the aortic arch. The bilateral CCAs are located deep to the jugular veins and sternocleidomastoid muscles and posterolateral to the thyroid gland. Just before the carotid bifurcation, the CCA dilates slightly to form the carotid bulb. The CCA then divides into the ICA and the ECA. The ICA gives off no cervical branches. However, the ECA has multiple cervical branches supplying the musculature of the face and neck. In most patients, the ICA is larger, posterior and lateral to the ECA; however, in a few patients, the ICA is medial to the ECA.[3]

Grayscale Imaging

On longitudinal imaging, the CCA wall is composed of 2 nearly parallel echogenic lines separated by a thin hypoechoic to anechoic layer. Although present in both the near and far walls of the CCA, the anechoic arterial lumen serves as an acoustic window, improving visualization of the double echogenic lines of the far wall compared with the near wall, which may also be degraded by near field artifact. As the vessel caliber narrows, especially at the level of the ICA and ECA, there is decreased visualization of these echogenic lines as 2 separate structures. The echogenic band along the vessel lumen represents the lumen-intima interface, and the second more peripheral echogenic band comprises the media-adventitia interface, with the intima-media layer corresponding to the hypoechoic intervening band. Intima-media thickness (IMT) is defined as the distance between the inner echogenic line and the outer echogenic line, as measured by a caliper placed at the level of the echogenic interface of the intima with the anechoic vessel lumen and a second caliper placed at the echogenic

interface of the adventitia with the hypoechoic media (**Fig. 2**). The normal distance between these 2 echogenic layers is less than 0.9 mm (please see section on plaque characteristics for further details with regards to IMT measurements). The carotid blub can be identified as a mild widening of the CCA just inferior to the bifurcation of the vessel. The ECA can be reliably identified by its branches, whereas the ICA has none (**Fig. 3**A).

Color and Spectral Doppler Imaging

On color Doppler imaging, carotid blood flow is normally directed toward the head, without evidence of turbulent or high-velocity flow. An exception to this rule is seen at the level of the carotid bulb, where there is a normal transient reversal of flow laterally as a result of the widening of the vessel in this location and resultant decreased pressure gradient adjacent to the vessel wall, termed boundary layer separation or helical blood flow. The branches of the ECA are best identified using color or power Doppler (see **Fig. 3**B). Spectral Doppler imaging shows unique waveforms for each of the 3 segments of the carotid artery. The ICA provides the sole blood supply for the brain, which requires oxygenation during both systole and diastole. The ICA waveform, therefore, shows a low-resistance morphology, with a brisk systolic upstroke and a moderate amount of diastolic flow, with antegrade flow throughout the cardiac cycle (**Fig. 4**A). Peak systolic velocity (PSV) in the ICA typically ranges from 60 to 100 cm/s. The ECA supplies the muscles of the face, which do not require blood flow during diastole. The ECA waveform, therefore, shows a high-resistance morphology, with a brisk systolic upstroke followed by a quick return to baseline, with little to no diastolic flow during diastole (see **Fig. 4**B). Although the amount of diastolic flow in the ECA

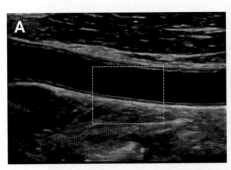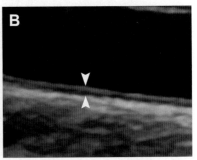

Fig. 2. Normal appearance and size of the IMT. (*A*) Normal appearance of the CCA vessel wall showing 2 nearly parallel echogenic lines separated by a thin hypoechoic to anechoic region. *Dashed box* represents area of magnification shown in image *B*. (*B*) Magnified view of the posterior wall of the CCA shows a normal IMT distance of less the 0.9 mm, as measured by a caliper placed at the level of the echogenic interface of the intima with the anechoic vessel lumen and a second caliper placed at the echogenic interface of the adventitia with the hypoechoic media (*arrowhead* to *arrowhead*).

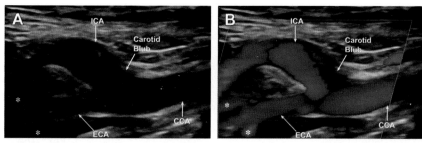

Fig. 3. Grayscale (*A*) and color Doppler (*B*) appearance of the extracranial carotid arteries at the level of the carotid bifurcation. Note that the branches of the ECA (*asterisk*) are best seen on color Doppler imaging.

may be variable patient to patient, diastolic flow in the ECA should be symmetric right to left and less than the amount of diastolic flow in the ICA. When disease is present, it may be difficult to separate the ECA from the ICA based on waveform and location alone. Tapping the superficial temporal artery, which is positioned slightly anterior to the ear, can help to distinguish the ECA from the ICA. As a branch of the ECA, the pulsations produced by tapping the superficial temporal artery transmit preferentially into the ECA and can be visualized as rhythmical saw-tooth deflections of

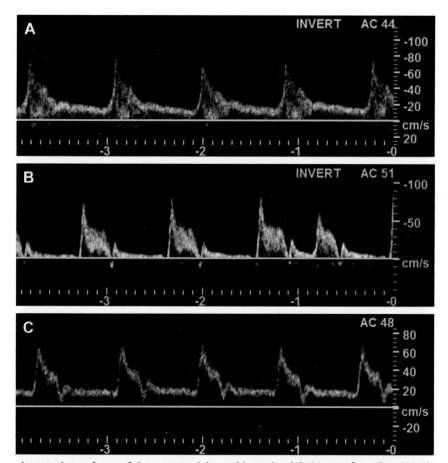

Fig. 4. Normal spectral waveforms of the extracranial carotid arteries. (*A*) ICA waveform showing a low-resistance morphology, with a brisk systolic upstroke and a moderate amount of diastolic flow, with antegrade flow throughout the cardiac cycle. (*B*) ECA waveform showing a high-resistance morphology, with a brisk systolic upstroke followed by a quick return to baseline with little to no diastolic flow during diastole. (*C*) CCA waveform showing a brisk systolic upstroke with forward antegrade flow throughout the cardiac cycle without spectral broadening.

the spectral waveform, best seen in diastole, with limited extension into the ICA and CCA (**Fig. 5**). The CCA waveform shape combines the ECA and ICA waveforms, most similar to the ICA because most of the blood flow goes to supply this vessel (see **Fig. 4**C). Overall the CCA waveform should show a brisk systolic upstroke with forward antegrade flow, without spectral broadening. The CCA, ICA, and ECA waveforms should be symmetric from side to side.

WAVEFORM PATTERN RECOGNITION

Two waveform changes are commonly observed downstream from a severe stenosis: pulsus tardus (delayed upstroke) and pulsus parvus (diminished waveform), together often referred to as a tardus parvus waveform. The waveform reflects decreased systolic propagation distal to a stenosis with prolonged acceleration time (defined as the time from the start of systole to the early systolic peak) and rounding and widening of the systolic portion of the waveform (**Fig. 6**).[4,5] The tardus parvus waveform appears more exaggerated as the vessel is imaged more distal to the stenosis. When the waveform is observed bilaterally, central obstruction should be suspected, such as aortic valve stenosis.[5]

A high-grade stenosis or occlusion distal to the area being sampled may cause a high-resistance waveform, with diminished, absent, or reversed diastolic flow and a reciprocal decrease in PSV, often described as a knocking waveform (**Fig. 7**).[5] The change in diastolic flow and decrease in PSV are more pronounced closer to the region of obstruction that the vessel is sampled. Although typically secondary to atherosclerotic disease, this waveform can also be seen in the setting of vasospasm, carotid dissection, or arteritis. A unilateral knocking waveform

in the CCA typically indicates high-grade ICA stenosis or occlusion. A bilateral pattern suggests increased intracranial pressure, diffuse intracerebral vasospasm, or arteritis.

Internalization of the ECA waveform occurs in the setting of an ipsilateral ICA occlusion or high-grade stenosis, in which case the ECA switches from a high-resistance to a low-resistance waveform pattern as the vessel is recruited to provide cerebral blood flow (**Fig. 8**A).[6] The cause of this increased diastolic flow is believed to be secondary to collateral vessel formation between the distal ICA and the ECA via the ophthalmic bed or through superficial vessels.[7,8] Similarly, occlusion of the CCA can cause low-resistance reversed flow in the ipsilateral ECA, which becomes the primary blood supply for the ipsilateral ICA (see **Fig. 8**B).[8]

Pulsus bisferiens (Latin *bis* meaning "twice" and *ferire* meaning "to beat") has 2 systolic beats per cardiac cycle, creating 2 sharp systolic peaks with an interposed midsystolic dip on the spectral waveform (**Fig. 9**). The most common pathologic cause of this waveform is moderate to severe aortic regurgitation, identified in 50% of patients with aortic valvular disease. However, this waveform can also be seen in athletic younger individuals or older adults with no known aortic disease and may represent a normal variant in these individuals.[5,9] The waveform abnormality becomes exaggerated when aortic stenosis is also present in patients with aortic regurgitation.[5]

Pulsus alternans describes a waveform showing alternating strong and weak peak systolic velocities in the setting of a regular cardiac rhythm. It is often caused by left ventricular systolic impairment, and other causes have been postulated to include intrinsic myocardial disease, such as ischemic cardiomyopathy and valvular heart disease, hypocalcemia, or impaired venous return (**Fig. 10**).[5,10]

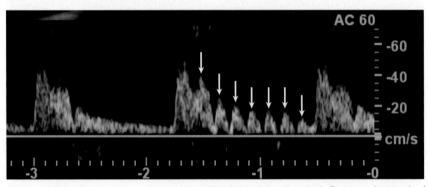

Fig. 5. Identification of the ECA using a temporal tap. Rhythmical saw-tooth deflections (*arrows*) of the spectral waveform are transmitted preferentially into the ECA, best seen in diastole, secondary to the tapping of the superficial temporal artery by the sonographer, helping to distinguish the ECA from the ICA.

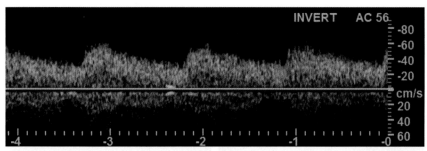

Fig. 6. Tardus parvus waveform after stenosis. Pulsus tardus (delayed upstroke) and pulsus parvus (diminished waveform), reflecting decreased systolic propagation after stenosis, causing a prolonged acceleration time (as defined by the start of systole to the time to reach the early systolic peak) and rounding and widening of the systolic portion of the waveform.

Cardiac arrhythmias are common causes of abnormal carotid waveform and changes in PSV. Bradycardia causes artificial increase of PSV and reduction of end-diastolic velocity (EDV), mimicking a high-resistance waveform, whereas the reverse is typically true in tachycardia, except when tachycardia occurs in the setting of an increased cardiac output, in which the PSV is also increased. Consequently, PSV is falsely low after a premature ventricular contraction (mimicking tachycardia) and subsequently, high after the compensatory pause (mimicking bradycardia) (**Fig. 11**A).[11] Atrial fibrillation, one of the most commonly encountered cardiac arrhythmias, causes irregular waveform morphology with varying PSV amplitudes, making velocity measurements difficult to perform (see **Fig. 11**B). Overall, when a cardiac arrhythmia is present, PSV should be calculated from the most normal appearing waveform and use of the PSV ICA/PSV CCA ratio may be more reliable in the setting of bradycardia and tachycardia then PSV alone for the evaluation of stenosis.

Waveform analysis is difficult in patients with cardiac assistance, such as an intra-aortic balloon pump (IABP) or a left ventricular assist device (LVAD). IABPs create a characteristic waveform with 2 peaks followed by flow reversal at end diastole. The first peak represents the natural systolic upstroke. The second wave of antegrade flow occurs as the balloon inflates during early diastole, increasing flow both to the coronary arteries (the intended effect) and to the carotid arteries (**Fig. 12**A). Flow reversal at the end of diastole corresponds to deflation of the balloon. IABPs can be adjusted to inflate with each cardiac cycle, with a 1:1 ratio, or cycle less frequently, such as a 1:2 ratio, in which the balloon is inflated every other cardiac cycle. This overall increase in antegrade flow in systole decreases the PSV. This situation limits the role of PSV in the evaluation of a carotid stenosis, making grayscale imaging and color Doppler evaluation as well as velocity ratio the more important for assessment of carotid stenosis in these patients.[12] Most LVADs produce monophasic antegrade flow, with a slow systolic upstroke and a rounded systolic peak of decreased velocity, mimicking a tardus parvus waveform (see **Fig. 12**B). In some cases, the waveform is nonpulsatile, without a clear systolic peak. As with the IABP, grayscale and color Doppler evaluation provide the most reliable assessment

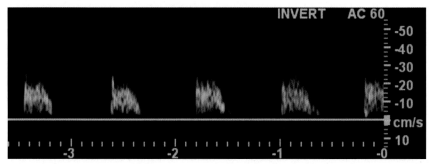

Fig. 7. Knocking waveform proximal to high-grade stenosis or occlusion showing a high-resistance waveform with absent diastolic flow and decreased PSV.

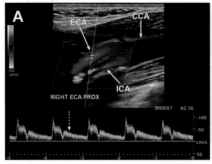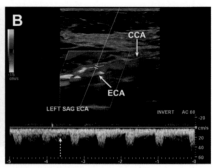

Fig. 8. Internalization of the ECA. (*A*) High-grade stenosis of the ipsilateral ICA (*asterisk*), causing a change in the ECA waveform to a low-resistance pattern, with increased diastolic flow (*dashed arrow*). (*B*) In a different patient with occlusion of the ipsilateral CCA, the ECA shows reversed flow, with a low-resistance waveform pattern (*dashed arrow*), characterized by increased diastolic flow, because the ECA now provides the blood supply for the ipsilateral ICA.

for stenosis in these patients. For patients with either IABP or LVAD, abnormal waveforms should be present bilaterally in the carotid vessels and are often seen throughout the systemic arterial vasculature.

ESTIMATION OF STENOSIS

The goal of carotid ultrasonographic imaging is to identify regions of atherosclerotic plaque formation and estimate the severity of luminal stenosis. NASCET (the North American Symptomatic Carotid Endarterectomy Trial) found that symptomatic patients benefited from endarterectomy in the setting of 70% to 99% ICA stenosis.[13,14] The Asymptomatic Carotid Atherosclerosis Study found that asymptomatic patients with luminal stenosis 60% or greater had a reduced risk of stroke after endarterectomy.[15]

Before the NASCET study, luminal narrowing was traditionally calculated based on a ratio comparing the smallest diameter of the residual lumen with the estimated diameter of the outer wall to the outer wall of the ICA at the same level (**Fig. 13**). However, interobserver error could be high with this methodology, especially in the

setting of dense atherosclerotic calcification, because it is difficult angiographically to be certain as to the exact location of the outer wall, although the residual lumen is well visualized. The NASCET study introduced a new method of calculating an ICA stenosis, which compares the smallest residual luminal diameter with the normal ICA diameter as measured distally past any area of poststenotic dilatation (see **Fig. 13**). For a given residual lumen, the percent stenosis is generally calculated to be higher when using the traditional technique for calculating an ICA stenosis when compared with the NASCET method. The NASCET method is considered the standard by which patient management decisions are made in North America.[16]

Estimating luminal stenosis via ultrasonography can be a demanding task. Imaging of the carotid artery in the longitudinal plane can greatly exaggerate or minimize the degree of luminal narrowing when plaque is eccentrically located within the vessel lumen (**Fig. 14**). Viewing the vessel in the transverse plane reduces this potential error; however, hypoechoic to anechoic plaque can be difficult to perceive on grayscale imaging alone, and heavily calcified plaque can be difficult to penetrate secondary to posterior acoustic shadowing.

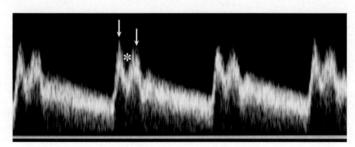

Fig. 9. Pulsus bisferiens waveform secondary to aortic regurgitation showing 2 sharp systolic peaks (*arrows*) with an interposed midsystolic dip (*asterisk*).

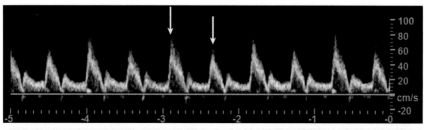

Fig. 10. Pulsus alterans waveform secondary to left ventricular systolic impairment showing alternating strong and weak systolic upstrokes (*arrows*) in the setting of a regular cardiac rhythm.

However, color/power Doppler imaging is prone to color bleeding or blooming artifact, often overestimating the size of the residual lumen. Because of these limitations, direct measurement of luminal narrowing on ultrasonographic imaging may be helpful in assessing the degree of carotid stenosis, but spectral Doppler analysis is considered the primary method to determine stenosis.

Spectral Doppler imaging provides a more reliable measurement of carotid stenosis through the investigation of velocity and waveform changes. The 3 most reliable Doppler parameters include PSV, EDV, and the ratio of PSV in the ICA at the site of stenosis to the PSV in the ipsilateral CCA as measured 2 cm proximal to the carotid bifurcation (PSV ICA/PSV CCA). The Society of Radiologists in Ultrasound (SRU) established criteria for estimating ICA stenosis based on these variables, as well as the presence of plaque, in a consensus panel convened in 2002. These criteria are commonly used as the reference standard across the United States (Table 1), but techniques and

protocols should be independently validated if possible in individual laboratories, because patient populations and equipment may vary.[17]

PSV is the most generally accepted criterion for grading an ICA stenosis until the stenosis is greater than approximately 95%. For luminal narrowing less than 50%, there is generally no significant change in PSV or spectral waveform; however, as the stenosis becomes more severe, the PSV and EDV increase incrementally. Turbulent flow is often seen in the region of stenosis, with broadening of the spectral envelope and fill-in of the spectral window, as well as reversal of flow lower than the baseline (Fig. 15). As the degree of stenosis exceeds 95%, PSV begins to decrease from its point of maximal velocity and can be normal or low, although spectral broadening and turbulent flow in the setting of extensive plaque formation should raise the suspicion for high-grade stenosis. Many factors can cause variation in PSV independent of stenosis. As described earlier, cardiac arrhythmia or heart

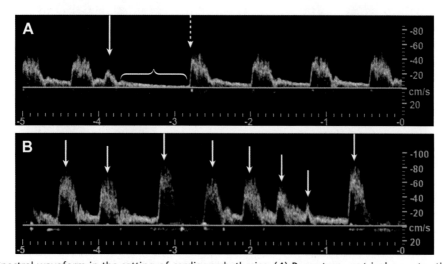

Fig. 11. Spectral waveform in the setting of cardiac arrhythmias. (*A*) Premature ventricular contraction causing an artificially low PSV (*solid arrow*) followed by a compensatory pause (*bracket*) and a subsequently high PSV (*dashed arrow*). (*B*) Atrial fibrillation causing irregular waveform morphology with varying PSV amplitudes (*arrows*). Note as the rhythm becomes tachycardic, the PSV begins to decrease.

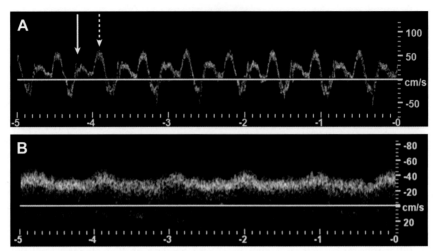

Fig. 12. Spectral waveform in the setting of cardiac assist devices. (A) IABP creating a characteristic waveform with 2 peaks followed by flow reversal at end diastole. The first peak represents the natural systolic upstroke (*solid arrow*). The second wave of antegrade flow occurs as the balloon inflates during early diastole (*dashed arrow*). Flow reversal at the end of diastole corresponds to deflation of the balloon. (B) LVAD creating a monophasic antegrade waveform pattern with a slow systolic upstroke and a rounded systolic peak, mimicking a tardus parvus waveform. On occasion, waveforms in patients with LVADs may look almost venous in configuration.

rate can dramatically affect PSV, as can high or low cardiac output. The presence of a second non-visualized stenosis, such as at the origin of the CCA or brachiocephalic artery, may decrease the velocity of the distal common carotid artery and cause underestimation of an ICA stenosis based on PSV alone. In addition, the presence of a high-grade ICA stenosis on 1 side can lead to

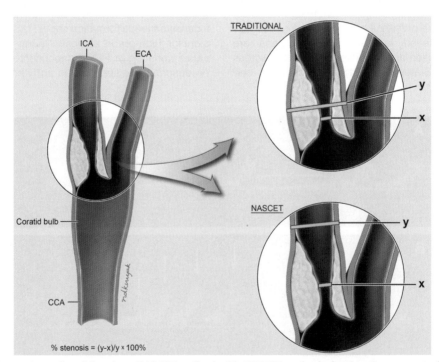

% stenosis = (y-x)/y x 100%

Fig. 13. Comparison of traditional pre-NASCET method with NASCET method of estimating percent of ICA stenosis. Traditional method compares the diameter of the residual lumen (x) with the distance between outer walls of the ICA (y) at the level of stenosis. The NASCET method compares the diameter of the residual lumen (x) with the distance between the outer walls of the ICA (y) at a level of the distal to the stenosis.

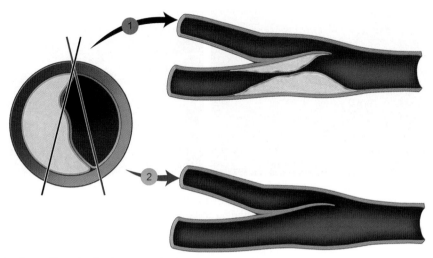

Fig. 14. Limitations of longitudinal imaging in the estimation of stenosis in the setting of eccentric plaque. When the transducer is angled toward the plaque in the longitudinal plane (1), the lumen appears to be significantly narrowed; however, when the transducer is angled away from the plaque at the same level (2), the vessel appears to be widely patent. This inconsistency is secondary to the eccentric location of the plaque and highlights the problems with using longitudinal plane imaging to calculate luminal stenosis.

compensatory increased flow in the contralateral carotid artery, artificially increasing the contralateral PSV, with or without a hemodynamically significant stenosis.[18,19] ICA tortuosity can increase PSV without a hemodynamically significant stenosis, especially when the Doppler correction angle is greater than 60°.

Comparison of PSV in the ICA at the level of stenosis with the PSV ipsilateral CCA can overcome some of these limitations that are observed with isolated PSV values, especially when there is incongruity between the grayscale and color/spectral Doppler images. This ratio creates an internal control for factors altering the baseline velocity involving the entire ipsilateral carotid vessel, such as high or low cardiac output or compensatory increase of velocity secondary to contralateral high-grade carotid stenosis. However, because measurement variability is inherent in the independent calculations of PSV at both the ICA and CCA levels, measurement error is compounded in a ratio calculation. Therefore, the PSV ICA/PSV

Table 1
SRU consensus panel grayscale and spectral Doppler ultrasonography criteria for the diagnosis of ICA stenosis

| Degree of Stenosis (%) | Primary Parameters | | Secondary Parameters | |
	ICA PSV (cm/s)	Plaque Estimate (%)[a]	PSV ICA/PSV CCA Ratio	ICA EDV (cm/s)
Normal	<125	None	<2.0	<40
<50	<125	<50	<2.0	<40
50–69	125–230	≥50	2.0–4.0	40–100
≥70 but less than near occlusion	>230	≥50	>4.0	>100
Near occlusion	High, low, undetectable	Visible	Variable	Variable
Total occlusion	Undetectable	Visible, no detectable lumen	Not applicable	Not applicable

[a] Plaque estimate (diameter reduction) with grayscale and color Doppler ultrasonography.
From Grant EG, Benson CB, Moneta GL, et al. Carotid artery stenosis: Gray-scale and Doppler US diagnosis-Society of Radiologists in Ultrasound consensus conference. Radiology 2003;229:344; with permission.

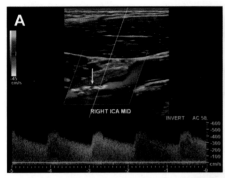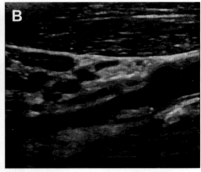

Fig. 15. High-grade stenosis of the ICA. (A) Color and spectral Doppler imaging of the ICA at the level of high-grade stenosis shows turbulent flow (arrow), increase of the PSV, a broad spectral envelope, and filling of the spectral window. Based on SRU guidelines, this finding indicates a hemodynamically significant stenosis with 70% or greater diameter reduction. (B) Grayscale image shows narrowing secondary to calcified and noncalcified plaque.

CCA ratio is less reliable than ICA PSV as an isolated measure.

Like ICA PSV, EDV increases as luminal narrowing becomes greater than 50%. This finding is most useful when the PSV becomes too high to accurately calculate, depicted as aliasing on color Doppler imaging, whereas the EDV continues to be present as an increased but measurable value. An EDV greater than 100 cm/s is a relatively specific, although not a sensitive, criterion for an ICA stenosis greater than 70%.[17]

PLAQUE CHARACTERIZATION

IMT has been proposed as a noninvasive surrogate marker for the presence of coronary atherosclerosis, with each increase of 0.03 mm causing a 2.2 increase in relative risk of nonfatal myocardial infarction (MI) or coronary death.[20] Normal IMT is considered to be less than 0.9 mm as measured at the level of the distal CCA on grayscale imaging, although normal values are related to age, race, and gender. Each interval increase in IMT thickness by 0.1 mm higher than normal is associated with a 13% to 18% higher risk of future stroke and 10% to 15% higher risk of future MI.[21] Furthermore, in patients older than 65 years, an IMT of 0.9 mm has been reported to be associated with single-vessel coronary artery disease, an IMT of 1.2 mm associated with 2-vessel disease, and an IMT of 1.3 mm is associated with 3-vessel disease (**Fig. 16**).[22]

A key component of the carotid ultrasonographic examination is evaluation of atherosclerotic plaque, identifying the location, echotexture, and surface characteristics of the lesion. The most common cause of transient ischemic attack is embolus, often from unstable or vulnerable plaque in the carotid system and not from hemodynamically significant carotid artery stenosis

(so-called watershed infarcts). Plaque should be evaluated in both the longitudinal and transverse planes on grayscale imaging. Use of color or power Doppler imaging has a limited role in evaluating plaque, because the projected color map can obstruct visualization of the plaque surface contour, possibly obscuring regions of ulceration or intraplaque hemorrhage. However, color or power Doppler can be helpful in identifying extremely hypoechoic or anechoic plaque, which may not be apparent on grayscale imaging alone. The most common site for plaque formation is in the ICA, within 2 cm of the bifurcation, an area readily imaged on ultrasonography.

Plaque echotexture is described as homogeneous or heterogeneous. Homogeneous plaques are the most common form of atherosclerosis and are believed to represent stable lesions.[11] These plaques show a uniform echo pattern, with a smooth external contour, and comprise primarily dense fibrous connective tissue (**Fig. 17A**). Small regions of sonolucency may be present but

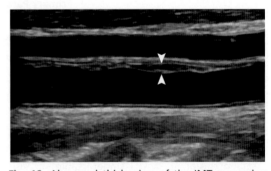

Fig. 16. Abnormal thickening of the IMT measuring 1.5 mm thick as measured from arrowhead to arrowhead in a patient who underwent radiation therapy to the neck. Such patients often develop accelerated atherosclerosis.

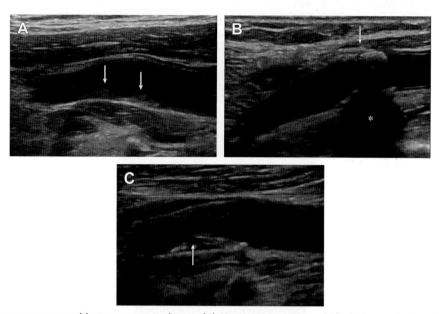

Fig. 17. Homogeneous and heterogeneous plaque. (*A*) Homogeneous noncalcified plaques (*arrows*) showing a uniform echo pattern with a smooth external contour, likely comprising primarily dense fibrous connective tissue, although diffusely hemorrhagic or lipid-laden plaque may have a similar appearance. (*B*) Calcified plaque is highly echogenic (*arrow*), producing strong posterior acoustic shadowing (*asterisk*), often limiting evaluation of the vessel lumen. (*C*) Heterogeneous plaque is more complex in echotexture, containing 1 or more regions of focal sonolucency, which make up more than 50% of the total plaque volume (*arrow*).

compromise less than 50% of the total plaque volume. Calcified plaque is often found in asymptomatic individuals and is highly echogenic, producing strong posterior acoustic shadowing, often limiting evaluation of the vessel lumen (see **Fig. 17**B). Heterogeneous plaque is more complex in echotexture, containing 1 or more regions of focal sonolucency, which make up more than 50% of the total plaque volume (see **Fig. 17**C). These hypoechoic regions often represent foci of intraplaque hemorrhage, lipid, cholesterol, or proteinaceous material.[23,24] This form of atherosclerosis is considered unstable and has a high embolic potential with subsequent neurologic symptoms.[11] Plaque ulceration is another source of emboli; however, it can be difficult to identify on grayscale and color Doppler imaging. Sonographically, plaque ulceration appears as a focal depression or defect on the surface of a plaque or as an anechoic area extending from within the plaque to the lumen of the vessel without a separating region of echogenicity (**Fig. 18**). On color Doppler examination, an eddy of slow flow or turbulent flow may be visualized within the anechoic defect, assisting in the detection of this lesion.

POSTOPERATIVE CAROTID IMAGING

CEA is a commonly performed procedure to treat hemodynamically significant carotid artery stenosis.

Ultrasonographic examination after CEA shows disruption of the normal intima-media layer at the level of the endarterectomy site, with occasional visualization of echogenic suture material or synthetic patch material (**Fig. 19**A). A small percentage of patients may also have persistent postoperative abnormalities, including residual moderate to severe stenosis, occluded ECAs, or carotid flaps.[25]

Percutaneous transluminal CAS is gaining popularity as an alternative to CEA for significant carotid artery disease. Carotid stents are easily visualized on ultrasonography as an echogenic structure adjacent to the carotid wall, and detailed assessment of the proximal vessel, the intrastent portion, and the vessel distal to the stent should be performed (see **Fig. 19**B, C). Velocities within the stent are usually increased compared with the normal carotid artery, with PSVs of 125 to 140 cm/s and higher commonly seen in widely patent stents. In addition, the velocity of the nonstenotic ICA beyond the level of the stent is often increased. Hence, the SRU velocity criteria for grading an ICA stenosis in a native vessel cannot be applied to stented carotid arteries, and alternative systems have been proposed. In a study published by Setacci and colleagues,[26] PSV of 104 cm/s or less was shown to be associated with less than 30% stenosis, PSV of 105 to 174 cm/s is associated with 30% to 50% stenosis, PSV of 175 to 299 cm/s is associated with 50% to

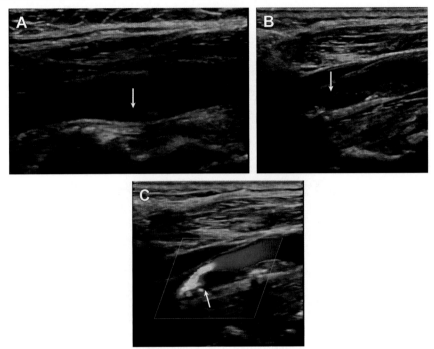

Fig. 18. Plaque ulceration. (*A*) Shallow ulcer appearing as a focal depression or defect on the surface of a plaque (*arrow*). (*B*) Grayscale imaging of a deep ulcer appearing as an anechoic cleft (*arrow*) extending from within the plaque to the lumen of the vessel without a separating border of echogenicity. (*C*) Color Doppler imaging of the deep cleft showing turbulent color flow within the anechoic defect (*arrow*), assisting in the detection of this lesion.

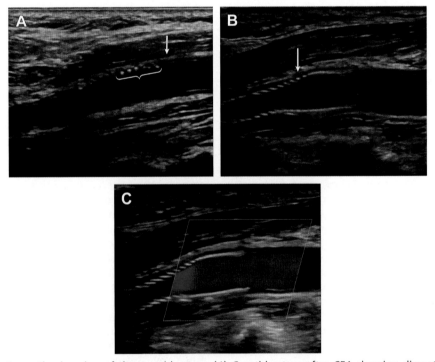

Fig. 19. Postoperative imaging of the carotid artery. (*A*) Carotid artery after CEA showing disruption of the normal intima-media layer (*arrow*) at the level of the endarterectomy site, with visualization of echogenic synthetic patch material (*bracket*). (*B*) Grayscale images of the carotid artery after CAS showing the echogenic metallic stent (*arrow*) in normal position directly opposed to the carotid wall. (*C*) Color Doppler imaging after CAS shows nonturbulent flow through the stent.

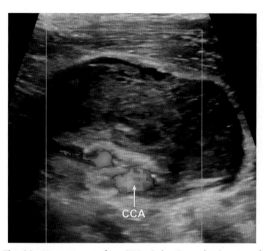

Fig. 20. Hematoma after CEA. Color Doppler image of the cervical soft tissues showing a large heterogeneous fluid collection surrounding the CCA after CEA. No color flow is identified within this collection.

70% stenosis, and PSV of 330 cm/s or greater is associated with 70% stenosis or greater. Depending on the length, width, and type of the stent used, each patient has a different baseline nonstenotic velocity. Therefore, following changes in PSV over time, using ICA/CCA ratio criteria, and detailed evaluation of the grayscale/color Doppler findings are valuable when screening for stenosis after CAS.

Restenosis is one of the most common complications encountered after carotid intervention, with a complication rate of approximately 6% within 2 years after the procedure for both CEA and CAS placement.[27] Hematoma is another common postoperative complication of carotid intervention, typically occurring at the site of vessel puncture, with approximately 5% of patients developing cervical hematomas after CEA.[28] The sonographic appearance of hematoma varies with age. An acute hematoma appears well defined and hypoechic; however, as the

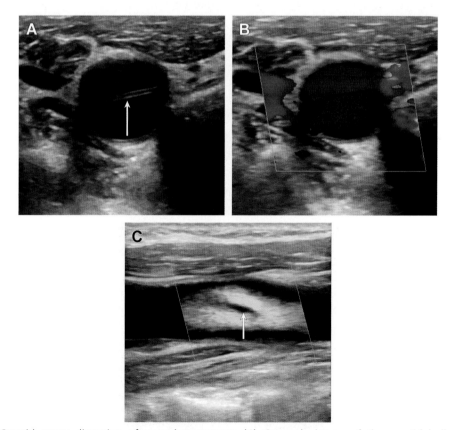

Fig. 21. Carotid artery dissection after endarterectomy. (*A*) Grayscale image of the carotid bulb showing an echogenic flap (*arrow*) dividing the vessel into 2 separate lumens. (*B*) Color Doppler image of the carotid bulb showing a dual pattern of flow within the vessel secondary to the presence of a intimal flap. (*C*) Longitudinal B-flow image of the carotid bulb showing a linear flap (*arrow*) protruding into the vessel lumen.

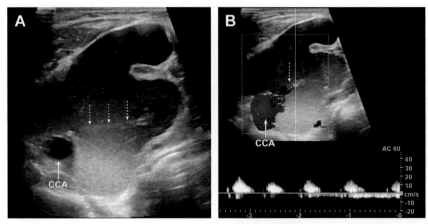

Fig. 22. Pseudoaneurysm after carotid artery intervention. (*A*) Grayscale image of a large pseudoaneurysm sac surrounding the CCA (*solid arrow*). Note the jet of blood flow entering the pseudoaneurysm (*dashed arrows*), which was shown to have pulsatile flow (*dashed arrow*) on color and spectral Doppler imaging (*B*).

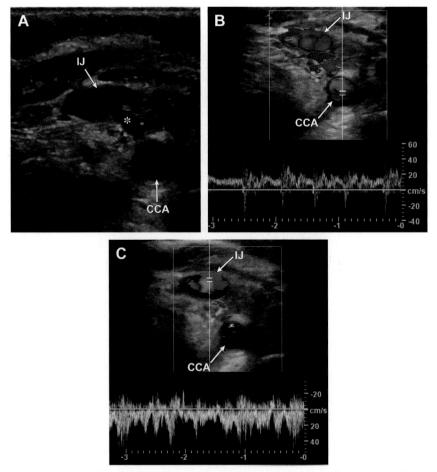

Fig. 23. Arteriovenous fistula after carotid intervention. (*A*) Grayscale image of a fistulous tract (*asterisk*) connecting the CCA to the jugular vein (IJ). Spectral Doppler imaging shows altered flow pattern in the CCA (*B*) and IJ (*C*), consistent with mixing of arterialized and venous flow.

hematoma ages and coagulation occurs, the hematoma appears more echogenic and heterogeneous. No blood flow should be seen within the fluid collection, and the collection should regress over time (**Fig. 20**).[29] Carotid artery dissections may also be visualized after carotid intervention, occurring in less than 1% of patients undergoing CEA.[30] Ultrasonographic imaging shows an echogenic intimal flap or double lumen within the vessel, which is often associated with an abnormal pattern of flow (**Fig. 21**).

Two rare complications of CEA and CAS include pseudoaneurysm and arterial venous fistula formation.[31,32] Pseudoaneurysms can occur after any penetrating trauma, including postsurgical intervention. These lesions represent false aneurysms, because they do not contain all 3 layers of the normal vessel wall, often occurring secondary to intimal dissection and subsequent vessel rupture, with the pseudoaneurysm sac contained by the adjacent soft tissues and thrombus. The patient may complain of a palpable mass, with or without pulsation; however, pseudoaneurysms may be asymptomatic in some individuals. Sonographically, a direct communication should be detectable between the pseudoaneurysm and the arterial lumen on color Doppler imaging. Spectral Doppler often shows a high-velocity to-and-fro waveform at the level of the pseudoaneurysm neck, with a characteristic yin-yang pattern of color flow within the pseudoaneurysm sac (**Fig. 22**).

Another uncommon complication of carotid intervention is the development of a fistulous communication between the carotid artery and an adjacent vessel, often a neck vein or the cavernous sinus, occurring secondary to direct puncture after operative intervention. Turbulent flow should be seen on color Doppler imaging in the affected vein with arterialization of the spectral Doppler waveform. In addition, an anechoic tract may also be seen on grayscale imaging connecting the 2 vessels, which may fill in with flow on Doppler imaging (**Fig. 23**). If the cavernous sinus is involved, ultrasonography can show dilatation and reversal of flow from intracranial to extracranial in the superior ophthalmic vein.

SUMMARY

Ultrasonographic imaging of the carotid arteries plays a key noninvasive role in the clinical evaluation for hemodynamically significant ICA stenosis, estimating the degree of luminal narrowing as well as identifying and characterizing atherosclerotic plaque associated with these regions. High-quality imaging is dependent on a systematic and reproducible approach, following the measurement guidelines established by NASCET and the velocity recommendations established by the SRU consensus panel or other criteria validated within individual laboratories. Image interpretation is based on a complete understanding of the normal carotid hemodynamics, as well as how alterations to the luminal diameter lead to changes in grayscale, color Doppler, and spectral Doppler imaging patterns.

ACKNOWLEDGMENTS

Illustrations were created by N.D. Kiriyak and G. Mack, Medical Imagers, Department of Imaging Sciences, University of Rochester, Rochester, NY. Figures were created by M. Kowaluk, Graphic Designer, Department of Imaging Sciences, University of Rochester, Rochester, NY.

REFERENCES

1. Fonarow GC, Alberts MJ, Broderick JP, et al. Stroke outcomes measures must be appropriately risk adjusted to ensure quality care of patients: a presidential advisory from the American Heart Associate/American Stroke Association. Stroke 2014;45: 1589–601.
2. Go AS, Mozaffarian D, Roger VL, et al. Executive summary: heart disease and stroke statistics–2014 update: a report from the American Heart Association. Circulation 2014;129:399–410.
3. Bailey MA, Scott DJ, Turnstall RG, et al. Lateral external carotid artery: implications for the vascular surgeon. Eur J Vasc Endovasc Surg 2007;14:22–4.
4. Bude RO, Rubin JM, Platt JF, et al. The effect of poststenotic vessel wall compliance upon the pulsus tardus phenomenon. Angiology 1994;45:605–11.
5. Rohren EM, Kliewer MA, Carroll BA, et al. A spectrum of Doppler waveforms in the carotid and vertebral arteries. Am J Roentgenol 2003;181: 1695–704.
6. AbuRahma AF, Pollack JA, Robinson PA, et al. The reliability of color duplex ultrasound in diagnosing total carotid artery occlusion. Am J Surg 1997;174: 185–7.
7. Macchi C, Catini C. The anatomy and clinical significance of the collateral circulation between the internal and external carotid arteries through the ophthalmic artery. Ital J Anat Embryol 1993;98(1): 23–9.
8. Verbeeck NY, Vazquez-Rodriguez C. Patent internal and external carotid arteries beyond an occluded common carotid artery: report of a case diagnosed by color Doppler. JBR-BTR 1999;82(5):219–21.
9. Kallman CE, Gosink BB, Gardner DJ. Carotid duplex sonography: bisferious pulse contour in patients

with aortic valvular disease. Am J Roentgenol 1991; 157:403–7.

10. Sipido KR. Understanding cardiac alternans: the answer lies in the Ca^{2+} store. Circ Res 2004;94: 570–2.

11. Tahmasebpour HR, Buckley AR, Cooperberg PL, et al. Sonographic examination of the carotid arteries. Radiographics 2005;25:1561–75.

12. Scoutt LM, Kirsch JD, Hamper UM. Ultrasound evaluation of the carotid arteries. In: Ho VB, Reddy GP, editors. Cardiovascular imaging. St Louis (MO): Elsevier; 2011. p. 1227–50. Chapter 90.

13. North American Symptomatic Carotid Endarterectomy Trial Collaborators. Beneficial effect of carotid endarterectomy in symptomatic patients with high-grade carotid stenosis. N Engl J Med 1991;325: 445–53.

14. Barnett HJ, Taylor DW, Eliasziw M, et al, North American Symptomatic Carotid Endarterectomy Trial Collaborators. Benefit of carotid endarterectomy in patients with symptomatic moderate or severe stenosis. N Engl J Med 1998;339(20):1415–25.

15. Endarterectomy for asymptomatic carotid artery stenosis. Executive Committee for the asymptomatic carotid atherosclerosis study. JAMA 1995;273: 1421–8.

16. Scoutt LM, Grant EG. Carotid ultrasound. In: Practical sonography for the radiologists: categorical course syllabus. Leesburg (VA): ARRS; 2009. p. 99–111.

17. Grant EG, Benson CB, Moneta GL, et al. Carotid artery stenosis: gray-scale and Doppler US diagnosis-Society of Radiologists in Ultrasound consensus conference. Radiology 2003;229:340–6.

18. AbuRahma AF, Richmond BK, Robinson PA, et al. Effect of contralateral severe stenosis or carotid occlusion on duplex criteria of ipsilateral stenosis: comparative study of various duplex parameters. J Vasc Surg 1995;22:751–62.

19. Busuttil SJ, Franklin DP, Youkey JR, et al. Carotid duplex overestimation of stenosis due to severe contralateral disease. Am J Surg 1996;172(2):144–7.

20. Hodis HN, Mack WJ, LaBree L, et al. The role of carotid arterial intima-media thickness in predicting clinical coronary events. Ann Intern Med 1998;128: 262–9.

21. Lorenz MW, Markus HS, Bots ML, et al. Prediction of clinical cardiovascular events with carotid intima-media thickness. Circulation 2007;115:459–67.

22. Mattace Raso F, van Popele NM, Schalekamp M, et al. Intima-media thickness of the common carotid arteries is related to coronary atherosclerosis and left ventricular hypertrophy in older adults. Angiology 2002;53:569–74.

23. Bluth EI, Kay D, Merritt CR, et al. Sonographic characterization of carotid plaque: detection or hemorrhage. Am J Roentgenol 1986;146:1061–5.

24. ten Kate GL, Sijbrands EJ, Staub D, et al. Noninvasive imaging of the vulnerable atherosclerotic plaque. Curr Probl Cardiol 2010;35:556–91.

25. Jackson MR, D'Addio VJ, Gillespie DL, et al. The fate of residual defects following carotid endarterectomy detected by early postoperative duplex ultrasound. Am J Surg 1996;172(2):184–7.

26. Setacci C, Chisci E, Setacci F, et al. Grading carotid intrastent restenosis, A 6-year follow-up study. Stroke 2008;39:1189–96.

27. Lal BK, Beach KW, Roubin GS, et al. Restenosis after carotid artery stenting and endarterectomy: a secondary analysis of CREST, a randomized controlled trial. Lancet Neurol 2012;11:755–63.

28. Greenstein AJ, Chassin MR, Wang J, et al. Association between minor and major surgical complications after carotid endarterectomy: results of the New York carotid artery surgery study. J Vasc Surg 2007;46:1138–46.

29. Carra BJ, Bui-Mansfield LT, O'Brien SD, et al. Sonography of musculoskeletal soft-tissue masses: techniques, pearls, and pitfalls. Am J Roentgenol 2014; 202:1281–90.

30. Radak D, Tanaskovic S, Sagic D, et al. Carotid angioplasty and stenting is safe and effective for treatment of recurrent stenosis after endarterectomy. J Vasc Surg 2014;60(3):645–51.

31. Abdelhamid MF, Wall ML, Vohra RK. Carotid artery pseudoaneurysm after carotid endarterectomy: case series and a review of the literature. Vasc Endovascular Surg 2009;43(6):571–7.

32. Bakar B, Cekirge S, Tekkok IH. External carotid-internal jugular fistula as a late complication after carotid endarterectomy: a rare case. Cardiovasc Intervent Radiol 2011;2(34 Suppl):S53–6.

A Practical Approach to Interpreting Lower Extremity Noninvasive Physiologic Studies

Thomas E. McCann, MD, Leslie M. Scoutt, MD,
Gowthaman Gunabushanam, MD*

KEYWORDS

- Peripheral arterial disease • Vascular laboratory • Ankle brachial index
- Segmental pressure measurements • Pulse volume recording

KEY POINTS

- Resting ankle brachial index (ABI) less than 0.90 is abnormal. Exercise ABI should be done in symptomatic patients with normal ABIs at rest.
- When rest and postexercise ABIs are normal, there is a low likelihood of an abnormal segmental pressure measurement or pulse volume recording (PVR).
- Toe brachial index (TBI) is especially helpful in patients in whom an ABI cannot be reliably obtained because of incompressibility of the calf arteries, often due to arteriolosclerotic mural calcifications. A TBI value less than 0.70 is abnormal.
- Segmental pressure measurements and pulse volume recording (PVR) studies help determine the level of obstruction. A pressure gradient more than 20 mm Hg between different levels, or between the 2 sides at the same level, is considered significant.
- PVR waveforms distal to a site of significant stenosis are characterized by loss of the dicrotic notch, smaller amplitude of the pulse wave, increased time-to-peak, a more rounded peak, and a downslope that is convex away from the baseline.

INTRODUCTION

Peripheral arterial disease (PAD) is an important manifestation of atherosclerosis, with an estimated age-adjusted prevalence of approximately 13% in people older than 50.[1] PAD affects men and women equally and is associated with an increased relative risk of death from cardiovascular causes that is approximately the same as in patients with a history of cardiovascular disease.[2] The major risk factors for PAD include age older than 40 years, smoking, diabetes, hyperlipidemia, hypertension, and hyperhomocysteinemia.[3–6]

Because even asymptomatic individuals with PAD have an increased relative risk of death, screening of the at-risk population should be considered to identify the disease and begin treatment.[2] Early intervention with lipid-lowering therapy and antiplatelet drugs may delay disease progression and prevent premature death from cardiovascular causes.[7]

Ten percent to 30% of patients with PAD have symptoms of claudication.[8] Typical claudication is defined as pain in one or both legs on walking, primarily affecting the calves, that does not go

---

Department of Diagnostic Radiology, Yale University School of Medicine, 333 Cedar Street, PO Box 208042, New Haven, CT 06520, USA
* Corresponding author.
E-mail address: gowthaman.gunabushanam@yale.edu

Radiol Clin N Am 52 (2014) 1343–1357
http://dx.doi.org/10.1016/j.rcl.2014.07.006
0033-8389/14/$ – see front matter Published by Elsevier Inc.

away with continued walking and is relieved by rest. However, more than 50% of patients found to have PAD by ankle brachial index screening (ABI) do not have typical claudication or evidence of limb ischemia at rest.[9] Initial evaluation of a patient suspected of having PAD should include a careful history to determine whether the patient has a history of walking impairment or if the patient experiences discomfort at rest. In patients with a history of walking impairment, it is important to quantify the degree of impairment by documenting the degree of exertion (eg, the distance walked) before the development of symptoms. A thorough physical examination is also performed to assess for abnormal pulses, skin discoloration, skin integrity, and ulcerations.[2] PAD can be further classified using the Rutherford Classification Index or the Fontaine classification system.[10,11] The Rutherford Classification Index classifies patients according to the degree of sensory loss, muscle weakness, and arterial and venous measurements in acute and chronic PAD. The Fontaine classification index classifies patients into 1 of 4 disease states, ranging from asymptomatic (stage 1) to tissue necrosis, death, and gangrene (stage 4).

In this review, we focus on the physiologic noninvasive vascular laboratory methods for screening and follow-up of patients with PAD, such as ABI (without or with exercise), toe brachial index (TBI), segmental pressure measurements, and pulse volume recordings (PVRs), which are considered the mainstays for identifying and quantifying the degree of PAD. Noninvasive imaging of PAD with ultrasound, computed tomography angiography (CTA), or magnetic resonance angiography (MRA) is not included in this review.[12–14]

ABI

The ABI is an objective test that can be used as a screening tool in the initial evaluation of PAD and in differentiating vascular etiology from neurologic and musculoskeletal causes of lower extremity pain, such as nerve root compression (for example by a herniated disc), spinal stenosis, or hip arthritis.[8] ABIs are also helpful in the evaluation of patients with PAD after medical or interventional treatment. Furthermore, ABIs have been validated with angiography and have been shown to provide prognostic information regarding limb survival, wound healing, and even all-cause patient survival.[15–17]

Technique

The patient should rest in the supine position for at least 10 minutes before obtaining the ABI. Blood pressure cuffs that are appropriately sized to the limb circumference are placed on both arms and lower calves. Systolic blood pressure (BP_S) is obtained with the aid of a handheld 5-MHz to 10 MHz continuous wave Doppler scanning probe. BP_S from the brachial arteries in the right and left upper extremities and the dorsalis pedis and posterior tibial arteries in the bilateral lower extremities are obtained. The ABI on each side is then calculated to 2 decimal places by dividing the higher of the dorsalis pedis and posterior tibial artery BP_S on that side by the higher of the BP_S in the arms (left or right arm).

Interpretation

A difference in BP_S in the brachial arteries by more than 20 mm Hg may be observed in patients with aortic dissection or stenosis in the subclavian or axillary arteries, and further workup for this should be considered (**Fig. 1**). Pulse wave reflection in healthy individuals causes the ankle systolic pressure to be approximately 10 to 15 mm Hg (10%) higher than the brachial arterial systolic pressure, causing the ABI to be normally greater than 1.00. An ABI less than 0.90 is considered abnormal. Patients with claudication typically have ABIs ranging from 0.41 to 0.89, and patients with critical leg ischemia have ABI values of 0.40 or less (**Table 1**). Patients with heavily calcified arteries, including arteriolosclerotic calcifications in the tunica media (often found in patients with diabetes and chronic renal failure and elderly individuals), may demonstrate falsely elevated systolic pressure measurements or inability to completely occlude the arterial flow (ie, noncompressible vessels). An ABI value of greater than 1.30 or a systolic pressure measurement higher than 250 mm Hg (some use 200 mm Hg) is an indeterminate result, usually secondary to a noncompressible, calcified vessel that prevents measurement of true arterial pressure. Although vessel wall calcification limits ABI and segmental pressure measurements and interpretation, it usually does not affect pulse volume recording waveforms.[18]

With serial ABI measurements following medical, surgical, or percutaneous interventional treatment, a decrease in ABI of 0.10 or greater when associated with a change in clinical status or an isolated decrease in ABI of 0.15 or greater is considered significant.[19]

Pitfalls and Limitations

An abnormal ABI in itself is not a reliable predictor of symptom magnitude, extent, or location of disease, and should be used primarily to identify patients with PAD, and interpreted in conjunction with segmental pressure measurements and PVR

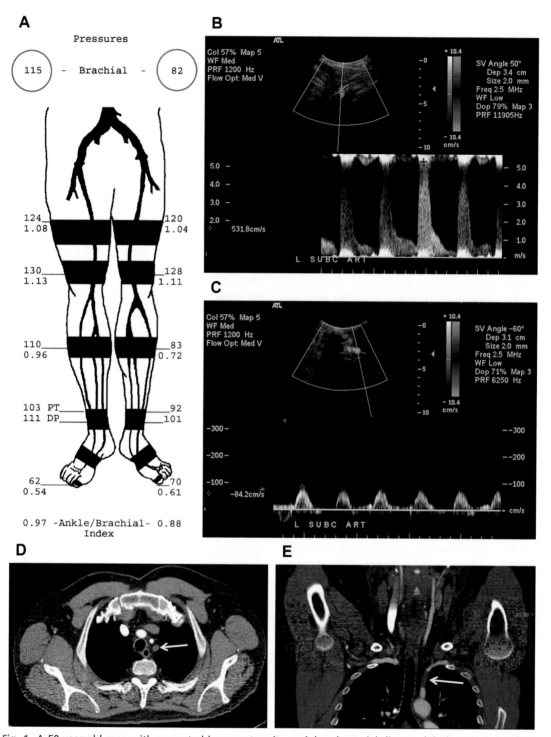

Fig. 1. A 50-year-old man with suspected lower extremity peripheral arterial disease. (*A*) There is a significant pressure difference of 33 mm Hg between the right (115) and left (82) brachial arteries. (*B*) Doppler ultrasound examination shows a markedly increased peak systolic velocity of 532 cm/s in the medial left subclavian artery. (*C*) Doppler ultrasound within the mid left subclavian artery shows tardus parvus waveforms and a relatively low peak systolic velocity of 84 cm/s. These findings are consistent with a high-grade left subclavian artery stenosis. (*D*, *E*) Axial and coronal reformatted CTA scan of the chest in a different patient shows complete occlusion of the left subclavian artery (*arrows*, *D*, *E*) with reconstitution of the distal artery from collaterals.

Table 1
Interpretation of resting ABI

ABI Value	
>1.30	Indeterminate result due to noncompressible artery
0.90–1.30	Normal
0.41–0.89	Mild to moderate peripheral arterial disease
<0.41	Severe peripheral arterial disease

Abbreviation: ABI, Ankle Brachial Index.

to further quantify and localize the extent of PAD.[10] Noninvasive localization of the level of obstruction can be attempted with segmental-limb pressures and PVR (see later in this article). In addition, in patients with severely stenotic or completely occluded iliofemoral arteries, the ABI may be normal at rest if sufficient collaterals are present. In symptomatic individuals with suspected PAD and normal resting ABIs, exercise (stress) ABI should be performed.[2]

It is important to carefully position the patient in the supine position at the time the blood pressures are taken. For each inch the ankle is positioned below the heart, there is a 1 mm Hg increase in systolic ankle blood pressure.[10]

EXERCISE ABI

In symptomatic patients who have a normal ABI at rest, an exercise ABI should be performed. Ideally, the patient is made to walk on a treadmill at 2 mph (3.2 km/h), at a 10% to 12% grade for 5 minutes or until the patient develops symptoms of claudication. If a treadmill is not available, the patient is asked to perform active pedal plantar flexion for approximately 5 minutes. A decrease in the post-exercise ABI by 0.15 to 0.20 (15%–20%) of the resting ABI is concerning for significant PAD.

Contraindications to performing exercise ABI include uncontrolled hypertension, severe aortic stenosis, congestive heart failure, chronic obstructive pulmonary disease, or other comorbidities that prevent the patient from performing exercise. An alternative in nonambulatory patients is to inflate the thigh cuff above the BP_S for 3 to 5 minutes, and then deflate the cuff to cause reactive hyperemia. The ankle pressure 30 seconds after cuff deflation is approximately equivalent to the pressure obtained 1 minute after walking to the point of claudication.

If the rest ABI is indeterminate (>1.30) due to vascular calcifications, exercise ABI is unlikely to be helpful. Also, it is important to have a formally

structured exercise protocol and not simply request that the patient "walk around" the vascular laboratory to elicit the symptoms of claudication, because those measurements tend to be less reliable.

TBI

The digital arteries are much less likely to be affected by the tunica media arteriolosclerotic calcifications that involve the calf arteries. Therefore, the TBI is especially helpful in cases of suspected false elevation of ankle pressures secondary to medial calcification or when PAD is suspected within the foot. A small pneumatic cuff is placed directly on the first or second digit. A photo electrode is then placed on the end of the digit and a photoplethysmographic waveform is recorded. The cuff is inflated until the arterial waveform is no longer seen and then deflated. The systolic pressure is recorded at the time of return of the arterial waveform. The normal toe pressure is 80% to 90% of the brachial artery pressure, so a normal TBI is 0.80 to 0.90. A TBI less than 0.70 is considered abnormal (**Fig. 2**). Patients with claudication typically have a TBI of 0.35 ± 0.15 (mean ± SD), and patients with ischemic rest pain typically have a TBI of 0.11 ± 0.10 (mean ± SD).[20]

SEGMENTAL PRESSURE MEASUREMENTS

Segmental pressure measurements and PVRs are used to attempt to localize the level of stenosis.

Technique

Similar to measuring the ABI, segmental pressure measurements are done with the patient in the supine position. A small cushion is placed under the patient's feet to elevate the ankles to approximately the same level as the heart. Blood pressures are obtained from the bilateral brachial arteries. Appropriately sized pneumatic cuffs are then placed around both lower extremities at the thigh, calf, and ankle levels. Both a 4-cuff technique (upper thigh, lower thigh, calf and ankle levels) as well as a 3-cuff technique (thigh, calf, and ankle) have been described. The ankle cuff is placed just above the malleoli. The calf cuff is placed around the widest portion of the calf. If 2 cuffs are placed in the thigh (4-cuff technique), the upper thigh cuff is positioned such that the upper edge of the cuff is at the highest possible level of the patient's inner thigh. The lower thigh cuff is positioned such that the lower edge of the cuff is just above the patella. Typical cuff bladder widths for an average adult in the upper thigh, lower thigh,

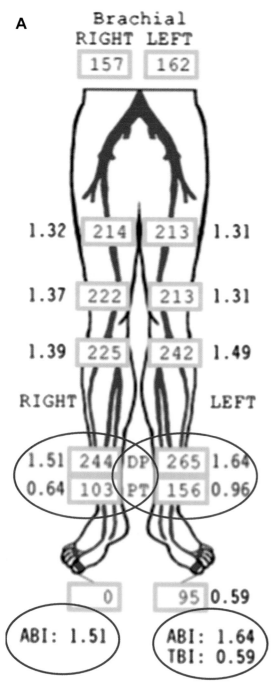

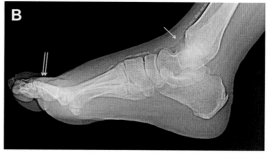

Fig. 2. A 67-year-old woman with diabetes and right great toe gangrene. (*A*) ABIs are indeterminate (>1.3) in bilateral dorsalis pedis arteries: 1.51 on right and 1.64 on left, likely due to arteriosclerotic calcifications associated with diabetes. The ABIs in the posterior tibial artery, 0.64 on right and 0.96, on left appear to be a more reliable indicator of the underlying arterial pressures. TBI is abnormal on left side (0.59) and could not be obtained on right side because of digital gangrene. (*B*) Radiograph of the right foot shows "tram-tracking" type of arterial tunica media calcifications in the anterior tibial (*single arrow*) and dorsalis pedis arteries. Note the lack of calcifications in the digital arteries (*double arrows*).

calf, and ankle are 11, 19, 12, and 10 to 12 cm respectively. The advantage of the 4-cuff method is better localization of the level of disease. Disadvantages include potentially longer time to complete the study, and additionally, in some patients with large thighs, it can be challenging to get a reliable pressure measurement or place the cuff high in the thigh.

Pressure measurements are taken sequentially starting at the ankle, followed by the calf and thighs. The cuff is inflated to well above the systolic BP and then slowly deflated at a rate of approximately 2 to 4 mm Hg per second while using a continuous-wave Doppler device to detect resumption of blood flow distally within the posterior tibial or dorsalis pedis arteries. Segmental pressure indices analogous to the ABI are computed at each level by dividing the pressure at that level by the higher of the right and left brachial artery pressures.

Interpretation

In a healthy individual, blood pressures increase slightly as one proceeds distally within a limb. The presence of a hemodynamically significant arterial stenosis or occlusion will result in a decrease in the segmental pressure measurements distally within that limb.

The normal pressure variation between limb segments should be no more than 20 to 30 mm Hg. To improve sensitivity, at our institution, we use a gradient between adjacent limb segments greater than 20 mm Hg as significant for a hemodynamically significant stenosis in the artery between the 2 segments. In cases of complete arterial occlusion, a gradient of 40 mm Hg or greater is expected. It is also useful to compare measurements in the right and left leg: a pressure difference greater than 20 mm Hg at the same level in the opposite limb is concerning for hemodynamically significant disease.[21]

Pitfalls and Limitations

The accuracy of segmental pressure measurements is significantly affected by the size of the blood pressure cuff that is used. If the cuff is too narrow, the pressure reading will be falsely elevated, and if the cuff is too wide, the pressure reading will be falsely low. For instance, inappropriate cuff sizing during the measurement of brachial artery blood pressures have been shown to produce an average error of 8.5 mm Hg.[22] The American Heart Association recommends that the width of the bladder (inflatable portion) of the pressure cuff be 40% of the circumference of the limb or 20% wider than the limb diameter.[23] Similar to the ABI, assessment of segmental pressure measurements is limited in arteries that are incompressible due to the presence of heavily calcified plaque or medial arteriosclerotic calcifications. A segmental pressure index greater than 1.30 or pressure greater than 250 mm Hg suggests that the pressure measurements are unreliable at that level. Segmental pressure measurements should not be attempted at the level of a previously placed stent or arterial bypass graft because of the risk of stent fracture or trauma to the underlying graft. Also, patients with wounds or cellulitis, or

patients with critical limb ischemia may not be able to tolerate cuff inflation because of severe pain, leading to an incomplete study. Another contraindication is the presence of acute deep venous thrombosis.

PULSE VOLUME RECORDING (PLETHYSMOGRAPHY)

The volume of an extremity changes with each incoming arterial pulse and/or in response to temporary obstruction of the venous system. The commonly used air plethysmogram records the volume changes of an examined body part using a pulse volume recorder. PVR uses pneumatic cuffs placed at multiple levels along an extremity, which are inflated until the underlying veins (but not the arteries) are occluded. By standardizing the volume of air and pressure within the cuff, the subtle volume changes that occur in a limb lead to measurable pulsatile pressure changes within the cuff, which may be used to derive intra-arterial pressures and arterial flow. The contour and amplitude of the PVR waveforms provide a qualitative assessment of the degree of PAD.

Technique

Similar to segmental pressure measurements, pressure cuffs are placed around the limb and attached to the plethysmograph. Most modern plethysmography machines inject a known fixed quantity of air into the cuffs to achieve a preset pressure, after which PVR tracings are recorded over several cardiac cycles. It is important to avoid adjusting the amplitude gain and other settings on the plethysmography machine so as to achieve accurate and reproducible results and enable reliability in comparison between the different levels and follow-up studies on the same patient.

Interpretation

A normal pulse wave is characterized by a steep upslope, a narrow peak, the presence of a dicrotic notch in the downslope, and a downslope that is concave toward the baseline. Normally, the pulse wave amplitude should increase between the thigh and calf. This occurs because of differences in muscle mass, cuff volumes, and decrease in vessel diameter from the thigh to the calf.[24] Pulse wave contour and amplitude should be symmetric when comparing both limbs at the same level. In the presence of a proximal arterial stenosis or occlusion, loss of the dicrotic notch is usually the first observed sign. With increasing severity of atherosclerotic disease, the amplitude of the pulse wave diminishes progressively (**Figs. 3** and **4**). In addition to dampening of the pulse wave contour, the upslope becomes more gradual, the peak appears broader and more rounded, and the downslope becomes convex away from the baseline. If this continues to progress, the pulse wave contour will eventually flat line (**Figs. 5–8**). Note that the presence of a dicrotic notch in the waveforms at the ankle level makes significant proximal arterial occlusive disease unlikely.

Pitfalls and Limitations

The systolic pressure wave created by left ventricular contraction is modified by a number of variables, including stroke volume, vasoconstriction or vasodilation of small-caliber arteries and arterioles, vessel wall elasticity, arterial branching patterns, vascular stenosis or occlusion, presence of collateral vascular beds, arteriovenous shunts, and size and position of the limb.[25] Any of these variables may act as confounding factors, and limit the accuracy of PVR measurements. Specifically, the presence of aortic valvular stenosis, hypotension, tachycardia, patient motion, or a significant proximal arterial stenosis may mask the presence of distal disease due to decreased intra-arterial pressure.

SUMMARY

Noninvasive vascular laboratory physiologic studies are used in screening asymptomatic

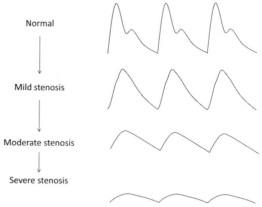

Fig. 4. Schematic diagram showing the changes in PVR waveforms with increasing severity of stenosis. Loss of the dicrotic notch is often the first observed sign. With further increase in stenosis severity, there is a progressive flattening of the waveforms, an increase in the time to peak, and the downslope becomes bowed away from the baseline.

individuals with risk factors for PAD, helping establish an arterial etiology of a patient's symptoms, localizing the level of disease, determining prognosis, and performing surveillance after invasive therapy.

An algorithm that summarizes the noninvasive workup of patients with suspected PAD is provided in **Fig. 9**. In a new patient with suspected PAD, resting ABI is first done. If this is normal, an exercise ABI is done. If resting and exercise ABI are

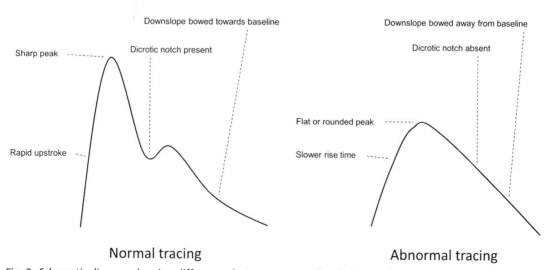

Fig. 3. Schematic diagram showing differences between a normal and abnormal PVR tracing. A normal tracing is characterized by a rapid upstroke, sharp peak, presence of a dicrotic notch, and a downslope that is bowed toward the baseline. An abnormal tracing demonstrates a slower rise time, a flat or rounded peak, absence of the dicrotic notch, and a downslope that is bowed away from the baseline.

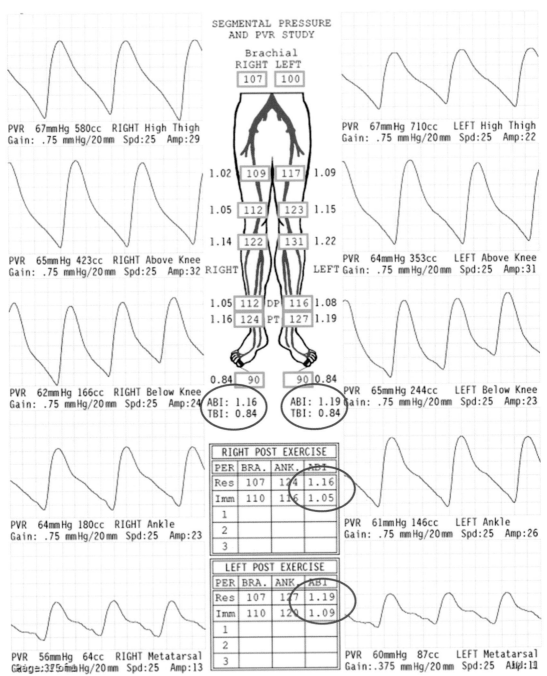

Fig. 5. A 51-year-old woman with bilateral lower extremity claudication. ABIs are normal bilaterally: 1.16 on right and 1.19 on left. TBIs are also normal bilaterally: 0.84 on right and 0.84 on left. Immediately after exercise, ABIs decreased slightly to 1.05 from 1.16 (–0.11) on the right side and decreased slightly to 1.09 from 1.19 (–0.10) on the left side, which are not significant. Therefore, this is a normal study, and there is likely a nonvascular cause of the patient's symptoms. With a normal rest and exercise ABI, there is a very low likelihood of an abnormal PVR study. Note that there are no significant segmental pressure gradients, and the PVR waveforms are symmetric throughout, with a preserved dicrotic notch through the level of the metatarsals.

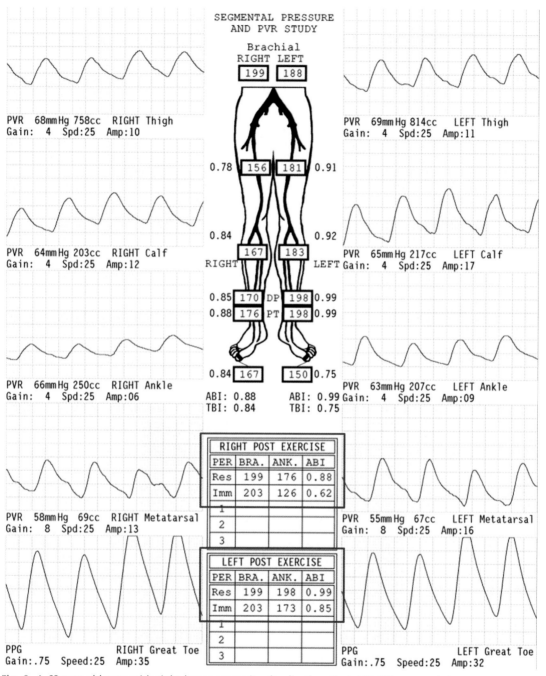

Fig. 6. A 62-year-old man with right lower extremity claudication. Rest ABI, TBI, segmental pressure measurements, and PVR are normal except for a slightly decreased right-sided ABI (0.88). After exercise, the ABI on the right decreased to 0.62, consistent with significant PAD. The patient underwent angiography, which demonstrated stenosis of the right external iliac artery that was treated with a stent (not shown). This case shows the utility of obtaining post exercise ABI.

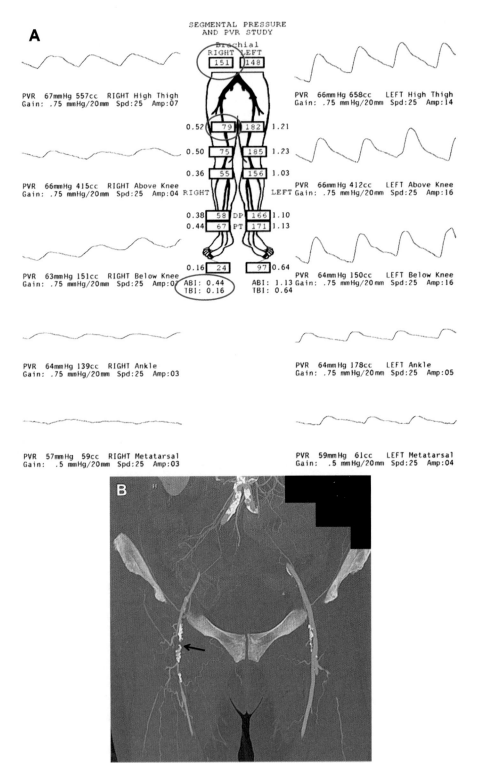

Fig. 7. A 61-year-old woman with right lower extremity claudication. (*A*) Note the markedly decreased ABI (0.44) and TBI (0.16) on the right side. Segmental pressure measurements show a significant gradient of 72 mm Hg between the right brachial artery (151 mm Hg) and right high thigh (79 mm Hg), but no other significant pressure gradients are observed. PVR demonstrates loss of dicrotic notch and dampened waveforms throughout the right lower extremity compared with the left side. These findings are consistent with right iliofemoral (inflow) disease. (*B*) Coronal maximum-intensity projection (MIP) reconstruction of a CT angiogram shows focal occlusion of the right common femoral artery (*arrow*) with reconstitution of the superficial femoral and profunda femoris arteries from collaterals. The patient underwent a right common femoral endarterectomy (not shown). (*C*) Postoperative study shows normal right ABI (1.02) and TBI (0.88). Note the marked improvement in the amplitude and appearance of the PVR waveforms on the right side, which are now very similar to the left.

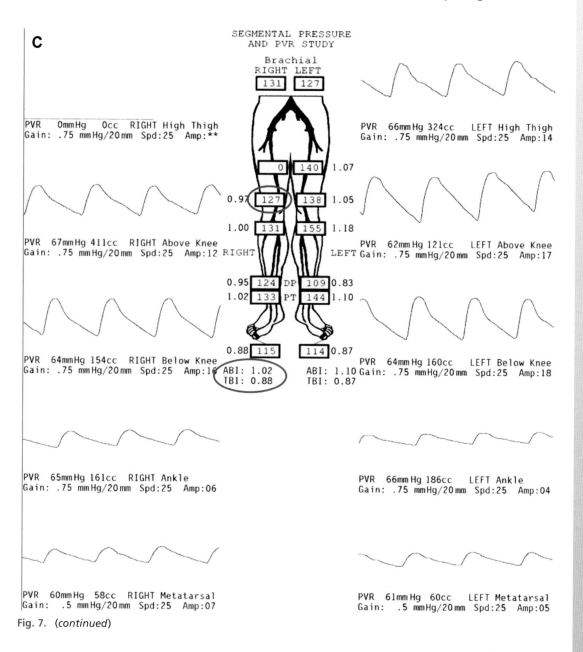

C

SEGMENTAL PRESSURE
AND PVR STUDY

Brachial
RIGHT LEFT
131 127

PVR   0mmHg   0cc   RIGHT High Thigh
Gain: .75 mmHg/20mm Spd:25 Amp:**

PVR   66mmHg 324cc   LEFT High Thigh
Gain: .75 mmHg/20mm Spd:25 Amp:14

0 140 1.07

0.97 127   138 1.05

1.00 131   155 1.18

PVR 67mmHg 411cc RIGHT Above Knee
Gain: .75 mmHg/20mm Spd:25 Amp:12   RIGHT

LEFT PVR 62mmHg 121cc   LEFT Above Knee
Gain: .75 mmHg/20mm Spd:25 Amp:17

0.95 124 DP 109 0.83
1.02 133 PT 144 1.10

0.88 115   114 0.87

PVR 64mmHg 154cc RIGHT Below Knee
Gain: .75 mmHg/20mm Spd:25 Amp:16 ABI: 1.02

ABI: 1.10 PVR 64mmHg 160cc   LEFT Below Knee
TBI: 0.88   TBI: 0.87 Gain: .75 mmHg/20mm Spd:25 Amp:18

PVR 65mmHg 161cc RIGHT Ankle
Gain: .75 mmHg/20mm Spd:25 Amp:06

PVR 66mmHg 186cc   LEFT Ankle
Gain: .75 mmHg/20mm Spd:25 Amp:04

PVR 60mmHg 58cc RIGHT Metatarsal
Gain: .5 mmHg/20mm Spd:25 Amp:07

PVR 61mmHg 60cc   LEFT Metatarsal
Gain: .5 mmHg/20mm Spd:25 Amp:05

Fig. 7. (*continued*)

both normal, it is unlikely that PAD is the cause of patient's symptoms, and alternate (musculoskeletal or neurologic causes) should be considered. If the resting and/or exercise ABI is abnormal, segmental pressure measurements and PVR are done to localize the disease. If these studies are abnormal as well, further evaluation with Doppler ultrasound, CTA, MRA, or angiography should be done as appropriate. If the resting ABI is indeterminate (>1.30), TBI may be helpful. Please note, however, that because of differences in subspecialist versus primary care physician referral patterns and preferences, it is common in many practices,

including our own, to initially perform resting ABI, TBI, segmental pressure measurements, and PVR in all patients with suspected PAD.

A practical approach to the interpretation of vascular laboratory physiologic studies is summarized in **Box 1**. After angiographic or surgical intervention, surveillance is done using review of symptoms, physical examination, noninvasive vascular studies, and/or Duplex ultrasound at regular intervals.[2]

Medical therapy is initially recommended in patients without critical limb ischemia (rest pain, skin changes, or tissue loss) who have abnormal

A

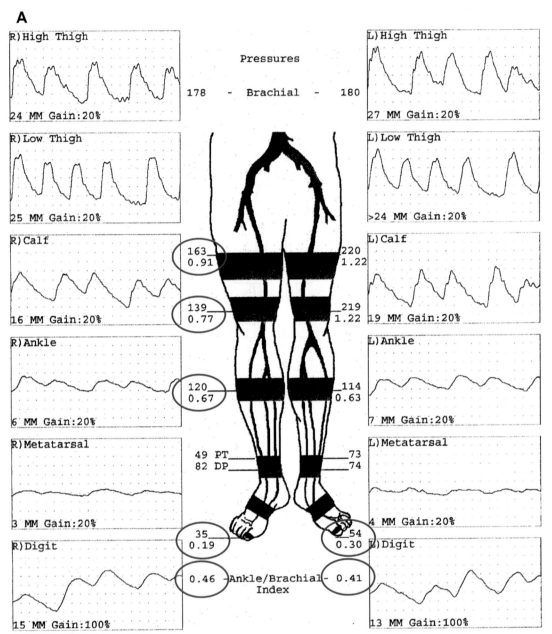

Fig. 8. A 75-year-old man with right leg rest pain. (*A*) The ABIs are decreased bilaterally (0.46 on right and 0.41 on left). There is a 24 mm Hg significant pressure gradient between the right upper thigh (163 mm Hg) and the lower thigh (139 mm Hg) and borderline 19 mm Hg gradient to the upper calf (120 mm Hg). Also note the dampening of waveforms between the right lower thigh to calf, and calf to ankle levels. The values 0.91, 0.77, and 0.67 represent the segmental pressure indices, which are analogous to the ABI. (*B*) CTA shows complete occlusion of the right distal superficial femoral and popliteal arteries (*arrows*). (*C*) Angiogram confirms the above CTA findings (*arrows*). (*D*) Note the complete occlusion of the right posterior tibial and distal peroneal arteries (*double arrows*). The anterior tibial artery (*arrow*) is widely patent to the level of the ankle joint.

vascular laboratory physiologic studies.[7] The patient may also undergo a treadmill test to define maximum walking distance and pain-free walking distance. Patients who have critical limb ischemia or have failed medical therapy will need to be further

evaluated using ultrasound, CTA or MRA, and digital subtraction angiography. Ultrasound has the advantage of being inexpensive, widely available, and does not use contrast media or ionizing radiation; however, it may be limited in individuals with

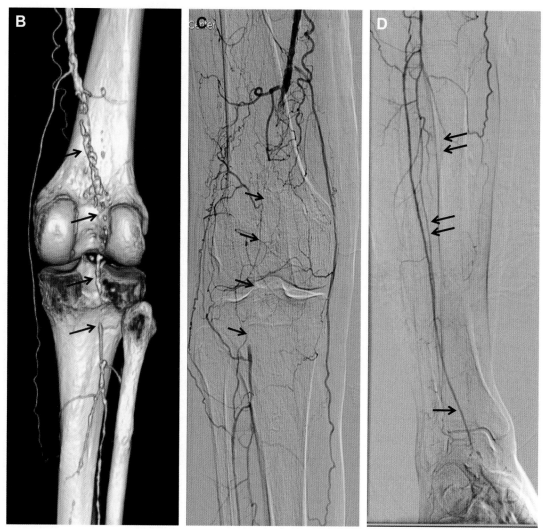

Fig. 8. (*continued*)

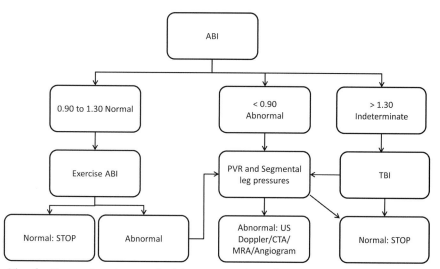

Fig. 9. Algorithm for the noninvasive vascular laboratory workup of patients with suspected peripheral arterial disease. Please note that because of variations in physician preferences, it is common to perform rest ABI, TBI, segmental pressure measurements, and PVR in all patients with suspected PAD. US, ultrasound.

> **Box 1**
> **Checklist for interpreting ankle brachial index/pulse volume recording (ABI/PVR) studies**
>
> 1. Brachial artery systolic blood pressures
>   - If there is a systolic blood pressure difference between right and left brachial arteries greater than 20 mm Hg, consider possibility of thoracic aortic dissection or significant subclavian/axillary artery stenosis
> 2. ABI
>   - Rest ABI less than 0.90: Abnormal
>   - Rest ABI greater than 1.30: Indeterminate
>   - Rest ABI ranging from 0.90 to 1.30: Normal
>   - Exercise ABI (only done if rest ABI is normal): Decrease of 0.15 compared with the rest ABI is abnormal
>   - Follow-up studies: Decrease in ABI by ≥0.15; (or) Decrease in ABI by ≥0.10 accompanied by change in clinical symptoms/signs is significant
> 3. Toe Brachial Index (TBI)
>   - TBI less than 0.70: Abnormal
> 4. Segmental Pressure Measurements
>   - More than 20 mm Hg difference in pressure between the 2 sides or between different levels on the same side is significant
> 5. PVRs
>   - Compare amplitude of waveforms at the same level on both sides
>   - Assess for abnormal features in waveforms, including
>   - Loss of dicrotic notch
>   - Increased time to peak
>   - Smooth or rounded peak
>   - Downslope bowed away from baseline

a large body habitus, those with extensive atherosclerotic or arteriosclerotic calcifications, and in the iliac and below-knee arteries. CTA provides excellent spatial resolution but has the disadvantages of being relatively expensive and using ionizing radiation and potentially nephrotoxic iodinated contrast media. Digital subtraction angiography is an invasive procedure, and with the exception of carbon dioxide angiography in patients with renal failure, is mostly done when there is a high likelihood of performing an intervention at the same time.

REFERENCES

1. Hirsch AT, Criqui MH, Treat-Jacobson D, et al. Peripheral arterial disease detection, awareness, and treatment in primary care. JAMA 2001;286(11): 1317–24.
2. American College of Cardiology Foundation, American College of Radiology, American Institute of Ultrasound in Medicine, et al. ACCF/ACR/AIUM/ASE/ASN/ICAVL/SCAI/SCCT/SIR/SVM/SVS/SVU [corrected] 2012 appropriate use criteria for peripheral vascular ultrasound and physiological testing part I: arterial ultrasound and physiological testing: a report of the American College of Cardiology Foundation appropriate use criteria task force, American College of Radiology, American Institute of Ultrasound in Medicine, American Society of Echocardiography, American Society of Nephrology, Intersocietal Commission for the Accreditation of Vascular Laboratories, Society for Cardiovascular Angiography and Interventions, Society of Cardiovascular Computed Tomography, Society for Interventional Radiology, Society for Vascular Medicine, Society for Vascular Surgery, [corrected] and Society for Vascular Ultrasound. [corrected]. Journal of the American College of Cardiology 2012;60(3): 242–76.
3. Norgren L, Hiatt WR, Dormandy JA, et al. Inter-Society Consensus for the Management of Peripheral

Arterial Disease (TASC II). Journal of Vascular Surgery 2007;45(Suppl S):S5–67.

4. Newman AB, Siscovick DS, Manolio TA, et al. Ankle-arm index as a marker of atherosclerosis in the Cardiovascular Health Study. Cardiovascular Heart Study (CHS) Collaborative Research Group. Circulation 1993;88(3):837–45.

5. Hiatt WR, Hoag S, Hamman RF. Effect of diagnostic criteria on the prevalence of peripheral arterial disease. The San Luis Valley Diabetes Study. Circulation 1995;91(5):1472–9.

6. Graham IM, Daly LE, Refsum HM, et al. Plasma homocysteine as a risk factor for vascular disease. The European Concerted Action Project. JAMA 1997; 277(22):1775–81.

7. Hiatt WR. Medical treatment of peripheral arterial disease and claudication. New England Journal of Medicine 2001;344(21):1608–21.

8. Lau JF, Weinberg MD, Olin JW. Peripheral artery disease. Part 1: clinical evaluation and noninvasive diagnosis. Nature Reviews Cardiology 2011;8(7): 405–18.

9. McDermott MM, Mehta S, Liu K, et al. Leg symptoms, the ankle-brachial index, and walking ability in patients with peripheral arterial disease. Journal of General Internal Medicine 1999;14(3): 173–81.

10. Crawford F, Chappell FM, Welch K, et al. Ankle brachial index for the diagnosis of symptomatic peripheral arterial disease. Cochrane Database of Systematic Reviews 2013;(8):CD010680. Available at: http://onlinelibrary.wiley.com/doi/10.1002/14651858. CD010680/abstract.

11. Khan NA, Rahim SA, Anand SS, et al. Does the clinical examination predict lower extremity peripheral arterial disease? JAMA 2006;295(5):536–46.

12. Foley WD, Stonely T. CT angiography of the lower extremities. Radiologic Clinics of North America 2010; 48(2):367–96, ix.

13. Goyen M, Ruehm SG, Debatin JF. MR angiography for assessment of peripheral vascular disease. Radiologic Clinics of North America 2002;40(4): 835–46.

14. Pellerito JS. Current approach to peripheral arterial sonography. Radiologic Clinics of North America 2001;39(3):553–67.

15. Resnick HE, Lindsay RS, McDermott MM, et al. Relationship of high and low ankle brachial index to all-cause and cardiovascular disease mortality: the Strong Heart Study. Circulation 2004;109(6):733–9.

16. Ankle Brachial Index Collaboration, Fowkes FG, Murray GD, et al. Ankle brachial index combined with Framingham Risk Score to predict cardiovascular events and mortality: a meta-analysis. JAMA 2008;300(2):197–208.

17. Caruana MF, Bradbury AW, Adam DJ. The validity, reliability, reproducibility and extended utility of ankle to brachial pressure index in current vascular surgical practice. European Journal of Vascular and Endovascular Surgery 2005;29(5):443–51.

18. Stein R, Hriljac I, Halperin JL, et al. Limitation of the resting ankle-brachial index in symptomatic patients with peripheral arterial disease. Vascular Medicine 2006;11(1):29–33.

19. Green RM, McNamara J, Ouriel K, et al. Comparison of infrainguinal graft surveillance techniques. Journal of Vascular Surgery 1990;11(2):207–14 [discussion: 214–5].

20. Ramsey DE, Manke DA, Sumner DS. Toe blood pressure. A valuable adjunct to ankle pressure measurement for assessing peripheral arterial disease. Journal of Cardiovascular Surgery 1983;24(1):43–8.

21. Fronek A, Johansen KH, Dilley RB, et al. Noninvasive physiologic tests in the diagnosis and characterization of peripheral arterial occlusive disease. American Journal of Surgery 1973;126(2):205–14.

22. Manning DM, Kuchirka C, Kaminski J. Miscuffing: inappropriate blood pressure cuff application. Circulation 1983;68(4):763–6.

23. Kirkendall WM, Feinleib M, Freis ED, et al. Recommendations for human blood pressure determination by sphygmomanometers. Subcommittee of the AHA Postgraduate Education Committee. Circulation 1980;62(5):1146A–55A.

24. Kupinski AM. Segmental pressure measurement and plethysmography. Journal of Vascular Technology 2002;26(1):32–8.

25. Rose SC. Noninvasive Vascular Laboratory for evaluation of peripheral arterial occlusive disease: part I—hemodynamic principles and tools of the trade. Journal of Vascular and Interventional Radiology 2000; 11(9):1107–14.

Update on the Lower Extremity Venous Ultrasonography Examination

Laurence Needleman, MD

KEYWORDS

- Thrombosis • Ultrasonography • Veins • Diagnosis • Clinical prediction rules

KEY POINTS

- A standard lower extremity venous ultrasonography protocol includes gray scale, color, and spectral Doppler. Normal veins coapt completely with probe compression; a noncompressible vein is either acute deep venous thrombosis (DVT), residual venous thrombosis, or incompletely compressed.
- Ultrasonography is an accurate method to diagnose acute DVT and to differentiate it from residual venous thrombosis (chronic scarring). Recurrent DVT, acute DVT after a prior episode, is often difficult diagnosis.
- The decision to order ultrasonography can be based on pretest risk assessment in order to reduce the number of normal tests. In several guidelines, patients with intermediate or high risk go straight to ultrasonography; patients with low risk get D-dimer blood tests and only go on to ultrasonography if the D-dimer test is positive.
- If the ultrasonography study is negative, the report may recommend follow-up for patients whose clinical condition changes or for patients with specific risks.
- Lower extremity venous ultrasonography is the gold standard for diagnosis of DVT. It is accurate and objective, and because the clinical assessment of patients is limited and its potential complication, pulmonary embolism, is significant, the impact of a positive and negative test is high.

NATURAL HISTORY OF VENOUS THROMBOSIS

The Virchow triad identifies the 3 most important factors that may lead to venous thrombosis: stasis, vessel wall injury, and hypercoagulable states.[1] The function of the venous endothelium is to resist thrombosis but also to create a clot when the vein is disrupted. Therefore, clot formation and thrombolysis occur together. Deep venous thrombosis (DVT) forms when the normal balance is altered.

The earliest location for most venous thrombosis is in the muscular veins of the calf, particularly the soleal sinuses and behind valve leaflets. A fibrin-rich thrombus forms and extends into the vein. Clot can extend from the initial thrombus but commonly independent sites of thrombosis are formed. It is common for more than one site of DVT to be separated by normal veins.[2]

Thrombus formation and propagation occur at the same time as fibrinolysis is breaking it down. Inflammation is part of the body's response to thrombin. Thrombus is lysed by recanalization and retraction. Recanalization creates channels in the clot and retraction affects the edges of the thrombus. Over time, thrombi may completely dissolve or healing may leave residual fibrotic thickening or occlusion.[3] In some patients, DVT may extend even on adequate therapy.[4–6] Residual scars are found in approximately 50% of patients at 1 year after DVT.[7]

Several terms have been used to describe the material that remains in the vein following

Sidney Kimmel Medical College of Thomas Jefferson University, 763 Main Building, 132 South 10th Street, Philadelphia, PA 19107-5244, USA
E-mail address: laurence.needleman@jefferson.edu

Radiol Clin N Am 52 (2014) 1359–1374
http://dx.doi.org/10.1016/j.rcl.2014.08.001
0033-8389/14/$ – see front matter © 2014 Elsevier Inc. All rights reserved.

thrombolysis and anticoagulation therapy. The internal medical literature favors residual venous thrombosis.[8] This term is not used universally and terms such as chronic venous thrombosis and scarring are often used in ultrasonography reports.

ALTERNATIVES TO ULTRASONOGRAPHY: CLINICAL DECISION RULES AND D-DIMER TEST

The risk of anticoagulation requires that a definitive diagnosis be made before treatment is initiated. Only 20% of patients clinically suspected to have DVT are found to have it[9] and several organizations have developed guidelines to exclude the diagnosis and to reduce inefficient imaging. Clinical decision rules to establish pretest probability are recommended by, among others, the American College of Physicians and the American Academy of Family Physicians.[10]

The most common rule set is the Wells criteria (Table 1).[11] A score is given for certain physical examination findings and pertinent history. Each criterion increases the score, except a likely alternative diagnosis, which decreases the final value. The Wells score groups risk of DVT into low, intermediate, or high. A recent modification of the

score creates 2 groups: DVT unlikely or DVT likely.[12]

Approximately 50% of symptomatic patients have a low Wells score. For DVT unlikely, the prevalence of DVT is 5.5% (95% confidence interval [CI], 3.8%–7.6%) and for a low risk, 8%.[12,13] These rates are not low enough to stop the work-up for DVT. Guidelines therefore recommend a D-dimer test for those with low risk.[10,14] The D-dimer test is a degradation product of fibrin. The test is sensitive for DVT, but not specific. Thus, a negative D-dimer test in the setting of a low pretest probability Wells score safely excludes DVT. If the D-dimer test is positive, the patient should go on to ultrasonography. This group includes true-positives but also a substantial number of false-positives.

If the patient is DVT likely, the prevalence of DVT is 27.9% (95% CI, 23.9%–31.8%).[12] The risk of DVT is 27% for intermediate scores and 66% for high scores.[13] These scores are not high enough to recommend treatment without imaging. Therefore, the recommendation for those categories is to go straight to ultrasonography.

A negative D-dimer test paired with intermediate or high risk of DVT scores is not adequate to exclude DVT, and the test is not recommended for these risk categories.[9]

In practice, many patients do not undergo this work-up.[15] Pretest probability requires a physical examination and history taking, and the D-dimer assay requires that the patient receive a blood test and wait for the results. Going straight to sonography is frequently faster than the alternative work-up and, even if the ultrasonography examination is negative for DVT, an alternative diagnosis may be discovered.

ANATOMIC PRINCIPLES AND NOMENCLATURE

The deep veins (Figs. 1A, B and 2) are below the muscular fascia, whereas the superficial veins are in the subcutaneous space above the muscular fascia. The major superficial veins are the great and small saphenous veins. Connections between the superficial and deep systems occur at the saphenofemoral and saphenopopliteal junctions and via perforating veins.

The American College of Radiology-American Institute of Ultrasound in Medicine-Society of Radiologists in Ultrasound (ACR-AIUM-SRU) guidelines[16] recommend using the terms proximal and distal with respect to the hip joint; proximal is closer to the hip and distal further from it. Calf veins are distal veins.

Valves control the flow of blood distal to proximal toward the heart and valves in the superficial

Table 1 Wells criteria for assessing pretest probability of DVT	
Active cancer (treatment ongoing or within previous 6 months or palliative)	1
Paralysis, paresis, or recent plaster immobilization of the lower extremities	1
Recently bedridden for 3 d or more, or major surgery within the previous 12 wk requiring general or regional anesthesia	1
Localized tenderness along the distribution of the deep venous system	1
Entire leg swelling	1
Calf swelling at least 3 cm larger than that on the asymptomatic leg (measured 10 cm below the tibial tuberosity)	1
Pitting edema confined to the symptomatic leg	1
Collateral superficial veins (non-varicose)	1
Previously documented DVT	1
Alternative diagnosis at least as likely as DVT	−2

Risk category: low risk, ≤0 points; intermediate risk, 1 or 2 points; high risk, ≥3 points.

Data from Wells PS. Integrated strategies for the diagnosis of venous thromboembolism. J Thromb Haemost 2007;5:41–50. http://dx.doi.org/10.1111/j.1538-7836.2007.02493.x.

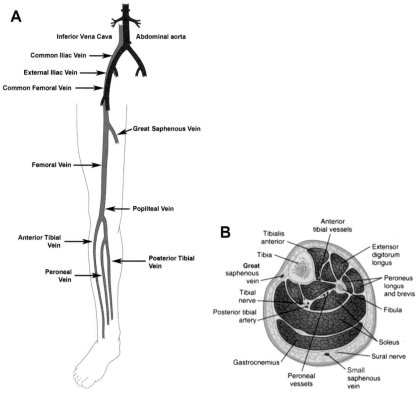

Fig. 1. (*A*) Anatomy of the deep veins of the leg. The peroneal veins and posterior tibial veins join to create the tibioperoneal trunk; caudal to this the anterior tibial vein joins the trunk to create the popliteal vein. (*B*) Cross-sectional anatomy of the midcalf. The paired veins (posterior tibial, peroneal, and anterior tibial) are between calf muscles. The gastrocnemius muscle (larger in the upper calf) and soleus muscle (larger in the midcalf) have intramuscular veins that are frequently the earliest veins to be affected by DVT. (*From* [*A*] Lin EP, Bhatt S, Dogra VS. Lower extremity venous doppler. Ultrasound Clin 2008;3(4):147–58, with permission; and [*B*] Khatri VP, Asensio JA. Operative surgery manual. Philadelphia: Saunders; 2003, with permission.)

veins control flow from superficial to deep. The energy to return blood to the heart comes from contraction of the calf muscle pump, which creates sufficient pressures in the deep muscles of the calf to overcome gravity.

The proximal deep veins are the common femoral, femoral, deep femoral, and popliteal veins. The femoral vein, formerly termed the superficial femoral vein, was renamed in order to avoid confusion because it is a deep vein.[17,18]

Calf veins are anatomically deep veins.[18] Confusion can arise because natural history and treatment of distal DVT is different than those of proximal DVT. Three sets of veins are located

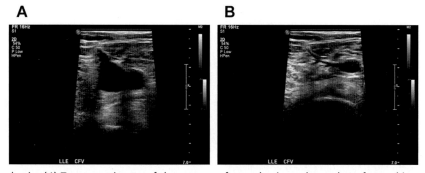

Fig. 2. Normal vein. (*A*) Transverse image of the common femoral vein at the saphenofemoral junction without compression shows the great saphenous vein joining the vein anteriorly at 11 o'clock. (*B*) Compression of the vein collapses it and no residual lumen is observed. A sliver of thin, normal hypoechoic wall can be seen. The compressed vein is frequently no longer visualized with compression.

between the muscles of the calf: the posterior tibial, peroneal, and anterior tibial veins (see **Fig. 1B**). The peroneal veins, also called fibular veins, are located medial to the fibula. The posterior tibial veins are dorsal to the tibia. The anterior tibial veins cross the interosseous membrane and are located in the anterior compartment.

The tibioperoneal trunk is formed from the junction of the posterior tibial and peroneal veins. The standard ultrasonography examination ends at the tibioperoneal trunk. The popliteal vein is formed where the anterior tibial vein meets the tibioperoneal trunk. Because this confluence is not visualized when scanning posteriorly in the popliteal fossa, the distal end of the scan is typically identified when separate peroneal and posterior tibial veins are identified in the upper calf.

There are also calf deep veins that are located within the muscle of the calf: the soleal and gastrocnemius veins. These veins are frequently the first site of DVT formation.[2] The soleal veins drain into the posterior tibial and peroneal veins. The gastrocnemius veins drain into the popliteal vein via lateral and medial stem veins at the popliteal fossa.

PROTOCOL

The ACR-AIUM-SRU guidelines describe the lower extremity duplex venous ultrasonography examination in detail (**Tables 2** and **3**).[16] Gray-scale

Table 2
ACR-AIUM-SRU scanning guidelines for peripheral venous ultrasonography

	Scanning
Thigh: fullest extent of common femoral and femoral veins	√
Knee: fullest extent of popliteal distally to tibioperoneal trunk	√
Symptomatic areas if symptoms not elucidated by the standard examination	Focal symptoms generally require evaluation of those areas This may include the calf for patients with calf symptoms
More can be performed if it is the protocol of the laboratory	—

Data from American Institute of Ultrasound in Medicine, American College of Radiology, Society of Radiologists in Ultrasound. Practice guideline for the performance of peripheral venous ultrasound examinations. J Ultrasound Med 2011;30(1):143–50.

ultrasonography is optimized and all accessible veins are compressed in real time. Compression is performed in the transverse plane, perpendicular to the long axis of the vessel. A normal vein collapses completely with probe pressure. If there is material in the vein or if compression is inadequate, a residual lumen will be present.

The study typically begins at the inguinal crease at the common femoral vein and ends at the tibioperoneal trunk (see **Table 2**). During scanning, compressions are performed every 2 cm or less. A representative subset of the scan is recorded, including images of the common femoral, saphenofemoral junction, proximal deep femoral, proximal and distal femoral, as well as the popliteal veins (see **Table 3**). Additional images may be acquired to characterize an abnormality or to document other areas that are scanned. Long-axis views of thrombus may be helpful to characterize or assess the age of thrombus.

Images must be recorded without and with compression. There are 3 general ways this is done: a cine clip, a side-by-side split-screen image, or separate images without and with compression. Our laboratory prefers separate images. By going back and forth on a picture archiving and communication system, a video effect can be created with only 2 images. Because the eye sees motion well, the vein stands out.

Color and spectral Doppler are performed at the common femoral or external iliac level on both sides, even when the examination is otherwise unilateral. A spectral Doppler waveform is also recorded from the popliteal vein Doppler on the side of interest or in both veins for a bilateral study.

DIFFERENTIATING ACUTE DEEP VENOUS THROMBOSIS FROM RESIDUAL VENOUS THROMBOSIS

The differential diagnosis for a noncompressible vein is acute venous thrombosis, scarring, and inadequate compression of the vein.

SONOGRAPHIC FINDINGS OF ACUTE DEEP VENOUS THROMBOSIS

Fresh thrombus has layers of red blood cells alternating with platelets and fibrin. Although the site of origin is attached to the vessel wall, the propagating portion may be poorly attached or free floating in the lumen.

There are 4 findings of acute venous thrombosis that are specific (one or more may be present): (1) intraluminal material that is deformable during compression, (2) dilatation of the vein, (3) smooth intraluminal material, (4) a free tail floating

Table 3
ACR-AIUM-SRU recording guidelines for peripheral venous ultrasonography

Recording Guidelines	Gray Scale (Transverse Without and With Compression)	Duplex (Color and Spectral Doppler)
Common femoral vein	√	Both common femoral (or iliac veins) even if the study is otherwise unilateral
Saphenofemoral junction	√	—
Proximal deep femoral vein	√	—
Proximal femoral vein	√	—
Distal femoral vein	√	—
Popliteal vein	√	On symptomatic side, both if bilateral study
Symptomatic areas	Symptomatic areas require additional evaluation and images	
Abnormal veins and/or nonvascular abnormalities	In general require additional images. Long-axis views of abnormal vein may help characterization	

Data from American Institute of Ultrasound in Medicine, American College of Radiology, Society of Radiologists in Ultrasound. Practice guideline for the performance of peripheral venous ultrasound examinations. J Ultrasound Med 2011;30(1):143–50.

proximally from the attachment of the clot on the vein wall (**Figs. 3–6**).[19] Long-axis images are frequently helpful to see floating clot and determine whether the clot distends the vein and/or whether it is smooth (see **Fig. 5**).

Acute clot changes shape from circular to elliptical during compression (see **Fig. 4**). Compression must be adequate to confirm a noncompressible vein. Although it is not usually necessary to press this hard, if there is distortion of the adjacent artery, sufficient pressure has been applied. There is an insignificant risk of embolization from normal compression and fear of this should not hinder performing a compression maneuver to obtain the correct diagnosis.

In a normal vein, a thin wall may be seen or the vein may disappear. The technologist should record the vein in the completely collapsed state. Taking an image with some residual lumen (so the vein can be identified) is incorrect and has led to misdiagnoses.

Acute clots may have limited attachments to the wall and color Doppler may show flow around the clot. Color Doppler is usually not necessary because characteristic gray-scale findings indicating acute thrombus are usually present. Moreover, small thrombi may be overwritten by faulty color settings or color blooming (see **Fig. 3C**) and color should not be used as a substitution for gray-scale compression. In small veins, or in

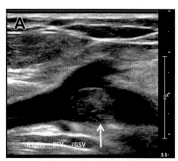 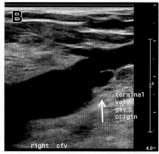 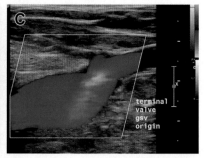

Fig. 3. Acute DVT evolving into residual venous thrombosis. (*A*) Long-axis view of DVT in the common femoral vein at the saphenofemoral junction. The thrombus is heterogeneous and smooth. It has a short attachment to the vein wall (*arrow*). At least 50% of the cephalic portion of the thrombus is unattached to the wall. (*B*) Four weeks after the DVT was detected, a follow-up longitudinal scan showed a small amount of residual venous thrombosis. This irregular material is now incorporated into the wall (*arrow*). The scar is isoechoic to surrounding tissue. A valve at the junction distal to the scar is unaffected and retains its normal thickness. (*C*) A color image taken at the same time as image *B*, showing that the color has falsely overwritten the wall irregularity. Color does not substitute for gray scale evaluation.

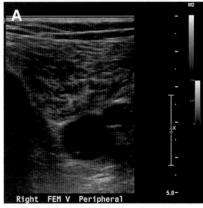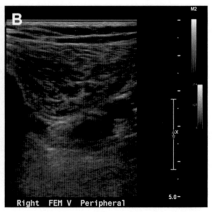

Fig. 4. Acute DVT. (*A*) Short-axis view of the peripheral femoral vein shows the vein to be dilated compared with the superficial femoral artery. Almost no echoes are in the vein. (*B*) Compression image shows that the vein is noncompressible. The vein and the nearly anechoic material in it change shape, indicating that it is soft acute DVT.

those patients with difficult body habitus, color Doppler can be used as a pathfinder but should be turned off when obtaining the gray-scale images. In areas where gray scale is inadequate, demonstration of filling of the vein with color is helpful to determine whether the vein is patent, excluding occlusive thrombus. Nonetheless, if compression is difficult or impossible to see, the report should state that it is limited and that thrombus cannot be excluded.

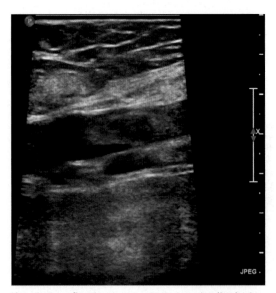

Fig. 5. Free-floating acute DVT. Longitudinal view showing material in the vein that was mobile in real time. There is a short attachment point and the propagating free-floating proximal portion is longer. The thrombus shows variable echogenicity, from nearly anechoic to hypoechoic internally to having a slightly more echogenic surface.

SONOGRAPHIC FINDINGS OF RESIDUAL VENOUS THROMBOSIS

The fibrotic material that persists in the vein following acute DVT has certain characteristic features. The vein is either completely occluded or partially compressible or preferred. As the thrombus heals, it loses bulk. The vein returns to normal size or may scar down to a smaller than normal caliber (Fig. 7). The residual venous thrombosis is firmly adherent and broadly incorporated into the wall (Fig. 8).

The intraluminal soft tissue has a different consistency; scarring is stiff and does not change shape during venous compression (see Fig. 7). An irregular surface may be present (see Fig. 3B).

If lysis occurs via retraction from both edges, a more weblike scar in the vein may result. This material can be wispy and ultrasonography may only pick up the edges of the web where it is specular to the sound beam (see Fig. 8; Fig. 9A). The residual thrombosis may alternatively be thicker and bandlike (see Fig. 9B). Webs, bands, and wall thickening frequently coexist.

If recanalization is the predominant feature of healing, there may only be thickening of the vein wall. This thickening can be uniform or irregular, circumferential in all or part of the wall (Fig. 10).

Color Doppler can be helpful in some cases to determine occlusion, sites of recanalization, or to outline the wall thickening (see Fig. 10; Figs. 11 and 12A). However, for detail of material inside a vein, optimized gray scale without color gives the highest resolution. Color may overwrite some of this detail.

Although echogenicity has been cited by a variety of investigators to help differentiate acute venous

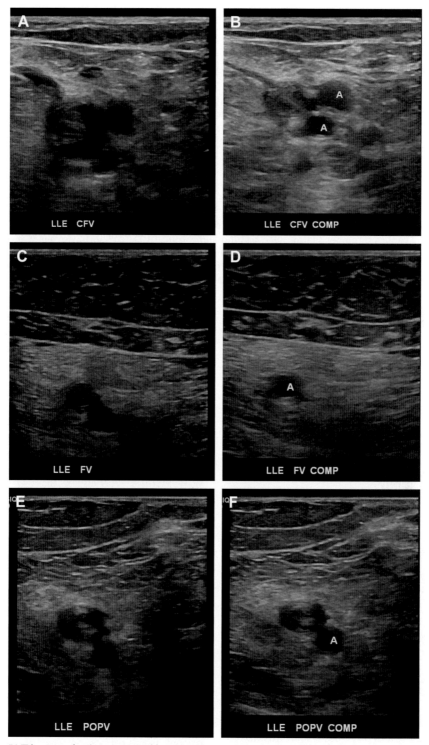

Fig. 6. Acute DVT in several veins separated by normal vein. Independent sites of DVT can develop. DVT does not usually grow in one continuous column. (*A*) Short-axis view of the common femoral vein at the level of the superficial femoral artery–deep femoral artery bifurcation shows a heterogeneous acute DVT that involves about half of the lumen. (*B*) Common femoral vein acute DVT is deformable with compression. (*C, D*) Femoral vein without and with compression. The femoral vein was compressible through its course. (*E*) Short-axis view of the popliteal vein shows heterogeneous acute DVT in a dilated popliteal vein. (*F*) Popliteal vein DVT with compression has a more elliptical shape, indicating that it is soft. A, artery.

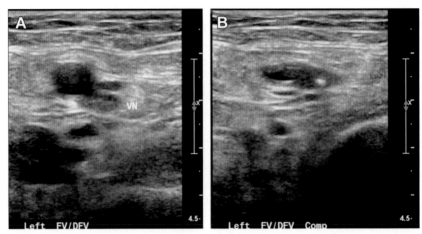

Fig. 7. Residual venous thrombosis (also called scarring and chronic DVT). (*A*) Short-axis vein of the femoral vein shows heterogeneous material in the vein. The material is wider than it is tall and the vein is small compared with its corresponding artery. (*B*) With compression the vein maintains its flattened shape, indicating that it is stiff. An echogenic focus is seen in the vein, which is likely a small calcified phlebolith.

thrombosis from residual venous thrombosis, it is too variable to be helpful (see **Fig. 5**; **Fig. 13**). This variability has been documented in several articles.[20,21] Echogenicity is subjective and can be altered based on the ultrasound angle and the degree of compression. In most cases, acute clot is heterogeneous and shows internal echoes (see **Fig. 6**). Chronic changes similarly can have a wide variety of echogenicity and can be nearly anechoic if the fibrotic material is homogeneous (see **Fig. 13**).

DOPPLER FINDINGS

The examination is a duplex study and selected spectral Doppler waveforms and their

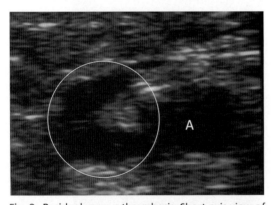

Fig. 8. Residual venous thrombosis. Short-axis view of femoral vein (in the *circle*) next to its artery. The vein at the 2 o'clock to 3 o'clock axis shows a small, triangular-shaped scar with irregular borders. It has a broad attachment to the wall compared with the narrower portion projecting into the lumen. A few fine webs, also called synechiae, are seen at 9 o'clock as well as inferior to the scar.

corresponding color Doppler images are recorded (separately or as 1 image). Spectral Doppler waveforms are taken from the center of the vessel and are performed in the longitudinal plane (along the long axis of the vessel) (**Fig. 14**).

Color should fill the normal vein.[19] Thrombosis is identified as a filling defect in the color column (see **Figs. 11** and **12A**); however, it should be confirmed with compression ultrasonography. Adjustment of settings during the study may be necessary because the color signal can vary between veins of different sizes because of different velocities and blood volumes. Too much gain may overwrite a thrombus, whereas too little gain may produce a false filling defect.

Spectral Doppler waveforms of normal veins show mild variation that corresponds with inspiration and expiration (see **Fig. 14**). This variation is referred to as phasicity. When the vein is obstructed, phasicity is attenuated or absent (continuous, flat waveform). Subtle changes may require comparison with the contralateral vessel scanned in the same position (**Fig. 15**). An occluded vessel shows no spectral Doppler signal and no flow by color Doppler.

In cases of increased right heart pressure or tricuspid regurgitation the cardiac pulse may be observed in the waveform (a pulsatile waveform), producing a longer than normal retrograde component. Some retrograde flow can be seen in the normal common femoral veins. Therefore, abnormal pulsatility should be suggested when the changes are seen more distally in the leg. This condition can be evaluated on the popliteal venous waveform because this is part of the protocol in all patients (see **Fig. 15A**).

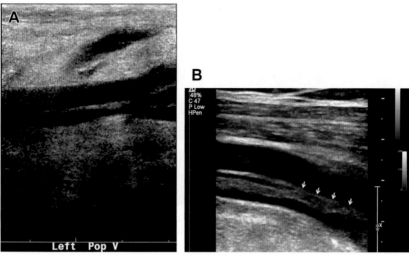

Fig. 9. Residual venous thrombosis. (*A*) Web. Longitudinal view of the popliteal vein shows a fixed, slightly irregular linear filling defect. As retraction occurs, the material in the vein loses bulk and can become a thin fibrotic web of tissue. It is distinguished from free-floating DVT because this material is stiff, immobile, and flat or wispy. Even though these webs are not bulky, they can produce venous obstruction. (*B*) Band. Longitudinal view of the popliteal vein in a different patient shows an irregularly thickened immobile band of material. The surface is irregular rather than smooth, which is another difference from a free-floating acute DVT. There is a long attachment to the vein wall (*arrows*).

An obstructive waveform indicates that the obstruction is proximal to the site of the sample (see **Fig. 12**). There is a differential diagnosis for a blunted signal that includes acute venous thrombosis, vein scarring, and extrinsic compression on the vein. Extrinsic compression may be seen from pathologic processes such as pelvic adenopathy or tumors but can also be seen in more benign circumstances such as a pregnant uterus or overfilled bladder. In those cases, emptying the bladder or turning the patient slightly up may return the waveform to normal.

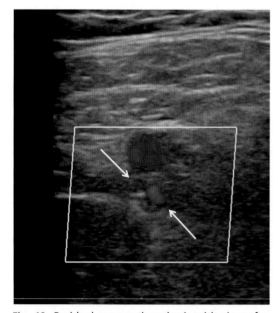

Fig. 10. Residual venous thrombosis with circumferential wall thickening. Short-axis power Doppler image. After recanalization, the vein may return to normal or be left with a narrowed residual lumen and a thickened wall (*arrows*).

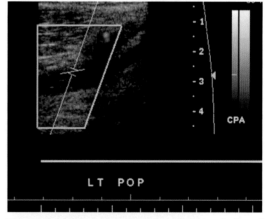

Fig. 11. Residual venous thrombosis with occlusion of the vein. Long-axis view of the popliteal vein shows very hypoechoic material in the vein months after the original DVT. The lack of echoes is likely caused by homogeneous fibrosis of the residual material. There is no flow in the occluded vein by power Doppler and no signal with spectral Doppler.

A   **B**

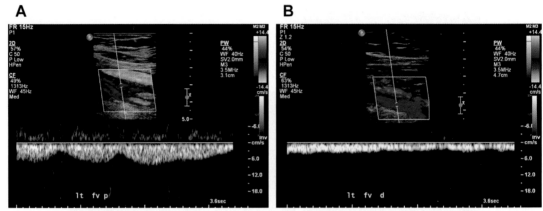

Fig. 12. Residual venous thrombosis with irregular recanalization and venous obstruction. (*A*) Color spectral Doppler of the proximal femoral vein has a normal phasic waveform. However, the color image is abnormal. There are multiple flow channels (*blue lines*) separated by elongated residual material. (Red corresponds with flow in the femoral artery above and deep femoral artery below the vein). (*B*) Color spectral Doppler in the distal femoral vein below the area of scarring has a flattened, near-continuous waveform (compared with the normal phasic waveform proximally), which indicates obstruction above the site of the Doppler signal from the scarred proximal vein.

Because the pelvic veins are generally not evaluated as part of this examination, the protocol calls for duplex of the right and left common femoral or iliac veins to get indirect evidence of pelvic or central obstruction. A unilateral obstructive waveform may indicate ipsilateral pelvic disease or pelvic DVT. Bilateral abnormalities may indicate caval, bi-iliac, or bilateral pelvic disease. Because Doppler waveforms are indirect evidence of obstruction to flow, further evaluation with pelvic imaging should be considered when 1 or both proximal waveforms are blunted and the cause is not determined.

Some centers use distal augmentation to help determine whether the Doppler signal is normal. A rapid increase with distal compression is normal, whereas an attenuated response is abnormal. Because of the subjectivity of this finding, it is not mandated in the guidelines.

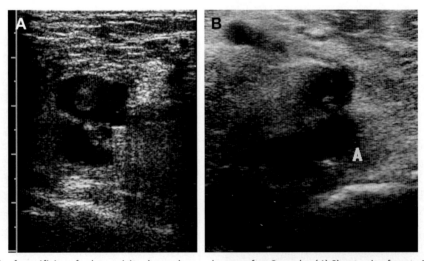

Fig. 13. Lack of specificity of echogenicity shown by no change after 8 weeks. (*A*) Short axis of acute DVT. There is heterogeneous material in the vein at the time the patient presented with DVT after surgery. The material was deformable with compression (not shown). (*B*) Short axis of the vein after 8 weeks. The vein is now irregularly shaped. The few echoes remain in the vein adjacent to the artery (*A*). At compression (not shown) much of the vein was noncompressible and filled with anechoic residual venous thrombosis. The scar has become less echogenic during healing.

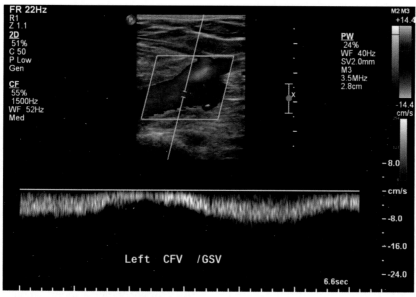

Fig. 14. Long-axis color spectral Doppler of the common femoral vein. All spectral waveforms are performed in long axis. This image shows normal phasicity, and mild variation of the waveform from respiration. Color fills the normal vein.

RECURRENT DEEP VENOUS THROMBOSIS

Acute DVT occurring after a prior episode of DVT is called recurrent DVT. It is a frequent complication of proximal DVT, occurring in 16% to 41% of patients at 5 years following the DVT.[22]

Ultrasonography has 2 potential roles to play in recurrent disease: (1) to determine risk of recurrence near or after therapy, and (2) to detect recurrent disease when the patient returns with symptoms.

RISK FOR RECURRENT DEEP VENOUS THROMBOSIS

The identification of residual venous occlusion (RVO) to determine risk for recurrent DVT is controversial.[23] Tan and colleagues[8] reviewed

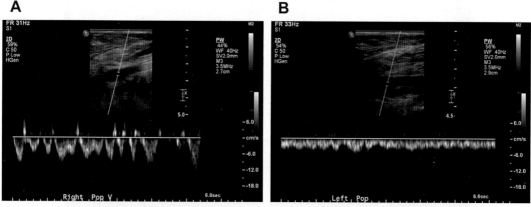

Fig. 15. Bilateral abnormal spectral Doppler with asymmetry of spectral Doppler waveforms. (*A*) Spectral Doppler of the right popliteal vein shows excessive variation of the waveform with an abnormally large retrograde component (above the baseline, toward the transducer). This waveform is pulsatile and should not be present in the popliteal vein. It is caused by increased right heart pressure or tricuspid regurgitation. There is no Doppler sign of obstruction. (*B*) Spectral Doppler of the left popliteal vein is blunted compared with the right, which indicates obstruction of flow above the signal. If the ipsilateral common femoral vein waveform is symmetric, the obstruction is in the leg between the two sites. If the common vein is abnormal (as it was in this case [not shown]) the obstruction is above the leg. This finding may be caused by iliac DVT, scarring, or pelvic obstruction. It is not at the caval level because the other side shows no obstruction.

the limitations of these studies, but reported a positive relationship between residual thrombosis and recurrent DVT. Two different methods of determining RVO were reviewed. In some studies the criterion was more than 2 mm of residual venous thrombosis. In others, the criterion was a ratio of the size of the residual material at compression; more than 40% of the size of the uncompressed vein. The latter criterion had a far higher odds ratio to predict recurrent DVT. How RVO is to be used clinically is still evolving. Other tests at the end of therapy are also being researched. For instance, an increased D-dimer level identifies a 2.4-fold increased risk. However, the D-dimer test must be done after finishing anticoagulation therapy, whereas the ultrasonography can be performed before anticoagulation is stopped.[8]

SONOGRAPHIC FINDINGS OF RECURRENT DEEP VENOUS THROMBOSIS

Recurrent DVT is a difficult diagnosis.[9] The definitive way to diagnose recurrent DVT is to find an acute thrombus in a previously uninvolved segment of vein. This segment can be ipsilateral or contralateral to the prior clot and a bilateral study is recommended in those patients with a prior history of DVT.

Identifying acute findings in a previously involved vein is also diagnostic (**Fig. 16**), but

may be difficult because the vein may be scarred and noncompressible or may be small.[24] An acute DVT may not be able to expand a scarred vein.

Some investigators have evaluated an increase in the size of the residual material in the vein from baseline to indicate recurrent DVT.[25] An increase of 4 mm between studies has been proposed.[9] Other investigators think that the measurement errors of residual venous thrombosis can limit the usefulness of this approach.[21]

Identification of changes from study to study is easiest when there is a baseline ultrasonography scan after treatment. For this reason, some authorities recommend baseline ultrasonography at the end of treatment. However, this is infrequently obtained.

INDETERMINATE RESULTS

The ultrasonography report should attempt to distinguish between residual scarring in the vein from acute venous changes because treatment varies between the two. However, only a small number of abnormal patients show equivocal results. In the absence of a baseline study, the differential diagnosis in these indeterminate cases is residual venous thrombus with incomplete resolution or recurrent DVT. Determining dilatation or retraction of a vein may be difficult if there is a

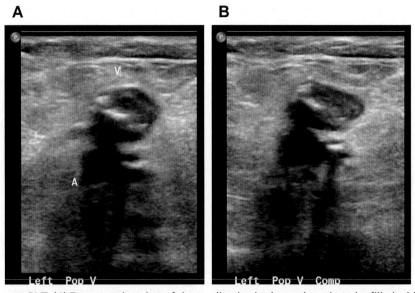

Fig. 16. Recurrent DVT. (*A*) Transverse imaging of the popliteal vein shows the vein to be filled with hypoechoic material in the upper portion of the vein (V) and bright irregular hyperechoic material in the midplane. A smaller vein to the right of the artery (A) at 3 o'clock is small and contains a calcification with shadowing (phlebolith). The calcification and echogenic material are scars from prior DVT. (*B*) Compression of the popliteal vein shows that the vein is partially compressible and the anterior hypoechoic area is deformable. The anechoic area posteriorly does not compress or change shape. This finding indicates acute DVT superimposed on residual venous thrombosis, which is one finding of recurrent DVT.

duplicated vein, which is a common anatomic variation (**Fig. 17**).

Indeterminate findings should be interpreted along with clinical findings, perhaps using D-dimer test or serial ultrasonography examinations for further clarification. There may be value in magnetic resonance venography in some cases.[26,27]

CALF VEINS

Proximal DVT usually presents with swelling. In contrast, calf DVT may result in focal tenderness over the thrombus. For that reason, the ACR-AIUM-SRU guidelines recommend evaluating symptomatic areas in the calf if the proximal examination has not elucidated the source of the symptoms (**Fig. 18**). Scanning the area of pain has other value. Patients may be confused if they come in for calf pain and the test ends above their area of concern. Alternative diagnosis can sometimes be found or suspected. The most common alternative diagnosis other than DVT is a musculoskeletal abnormality; popliteal cysts, joint effusions, muscle trauma, and other findings may be present. Ultrasonography readers may recognize an abnormal finding even if they cannot render a definitive diagnosis. All such findings should be reported, and can be described in a general way with the patient referred for a definitive test.

Calf imaging is becoming more common and calf imaging is required for accreditation by the Intersocietal Accreditation Commission[28] but the role of calf imaging is still evolving. The exact protocol to study calf veins is not established. The Intersocietal Accreditation Commission recommends scans of the posterior tibial and peroneal veins. Some groups also take images of the soleal and/or gastrocnemius veins.

In the American College of Chest Physicians guidelines for antithrombotic therapy routine ultrasonography of the calf is not favored.[29] Serial evaluation to detect proximal DVT, and not the

detection of calf DVT, is favored rather than a complete compression ultrasonography from thigh to ankle.

The rate at which calf DVT becomes proximal DVT is extremely variable, from 0% to 44%.[30] Calf DVT is rarely associated with symptomatic pulmonary embolism. The risk for recurrent venous thrombosis is less dangerous; half that of those with proximal DVT.[22] This more benign natural history favors managing patients with serial examination of proximal veins and treating only if proximal DVT appears. This management avoids overtreating a frequently self-limited process.[30]

If calf DVT is detected, the patient may or may not be treated. If treated, no further imaging is needed. If treatment is not initiated, repeat examinations up to 10 to 14 days is warranted to determine whether there is propagation.[29] At 1 week, if there is no propagation, a second test at 2 weeks should be performed. If the DVT has resolved, no imaging is needed. If proximal DVT or significant progression of disease occurs, treatment is instituted.[29]

The person interpreting the ultrasonography may not know whether a patient with calf DVT will be treated. A general statement should be included: "If this calf DVT is not treated, a follow-up in 1 week is recommended to evaluate for progression."

COMPLETE VENOUS ULTRASONOGRAPHY VERSUS MORE LIMITED EXAMINATIONS

Some clinicians recommend a complete compression ultrasonography examination from the thigh to the ankle. The rationale is to attempt to detect any DVT that may be present in the leg. This strategy is generally safe, with less than 1% venous thromboembolic disease at 3-month follow-up in most analyses.[31,32] This approach has the advantage of diagnosing proximal and calf DVT, but may result in overtreatment of calf DVT.

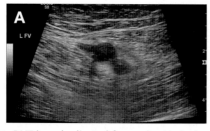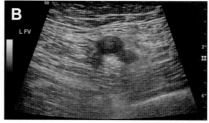

Fig. 17. Acute DVT in a duplicated femoral vein. Each vein is smaller than a single (nonduplicated) femoral vein and it is difficult to determine if material in the vein enlarges it without a baseline. (*A*) Transverse view of the femoral veins shows duplicated veins at 10 o'clock and 4 o'clock on the accompanying artery. (*B*) With compression, the vein at 4 o'clock does not compress but does change shape, indicating acute DVT. The vein at 10 o'clock compresses completely.

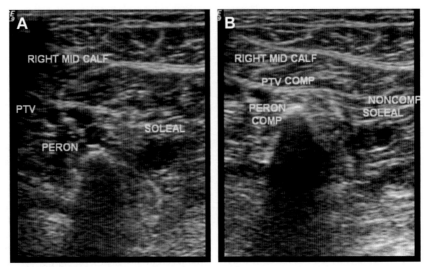

Fig. 18. Acute soleal calf (muscular branch) DVT. (*A*) Noncompression short-axis views of the midcalf show paired posterior tibial veins (PTV) and peroneal veins (PERON) and a single soleal branch, which is enlarged and shows intraluminal echoes consistent with thrombus. (*B*) Compression images show normal compression (COMP) in the posterior tibial and peroneal veins. The soleal vein does not compress (NONCOMP) but is deformable, consistent with acute thrombus.

More limited examinations are also being proposed. With the advent of point-of-care ultrasonography a variety of specialties are performing this examination in office settings, intensive care units, and emergency departments. These examinations frequently are less detailed than the standard examination.

The 2-point ultrasonography examination of the common femoral vein and the popliteal vein has been widely evaluated in the medical literature.[33,34] The test consists of compression of the common femoral vein from the inguinal crease to its bifurcation into the femoral and deep femoral veins and the popliteal vein from the proximal popliteal fossa to a point 10 cm distal from the midpatella. Most, but not all, proximal DVT is detected with this approach. This approach requires a serial evaluation in 1 week to detect proximal DVT that propagated from the calf, formed in the interim, or was undetected at baseline. Two studies, 1 week apart, predict a low likelihood of venous thromboembolism in the months following the tests.[32]

Two-point ultrasonography has a 2% to 5.7% chance of detecting DVT at a repeat ultrasonography at 1 week.[7,32,33] If a D-dimer test is performed at the time of the first ultrasonography and it is positive, 5.5% of patients have a positive study at 1 week.[34]

SAFE STRATEGIES

The sensitivity and specificity of ultrasonography for proximal DVT is 89% to 96% sensitive and 94% to 99% specific.[14] Ultrasonography is less sensitive for calf DVT (73%–75%), but with 99% specificity.[14]

In those with low pretest probability, either a negative D-dimer test or normal ultrasonography (standard, 2 point, or complete) is a safe strategy. Likewise a single complete compression ultrasonography or serial testing of proximal veins are also safe,[31] with low subsequent venous thromboembolic disease at follow-up after several months.

RECOMMENDATIONS FOR FOLLOW-UP

If the patient's examination is negative and the patient's clinical condition worsens, follow-up ultrasonography is warranted.

In patients with documented DVT on treatment, a repeat examination during treatment is rarely warranted. Repeat scans should not be ordered unless there is a clinical change.[35]

In patients with isolated calf DVT, a follow-up at 1 week is warranted if the patient is not treated.

Reevaluating patients near the anticipated end of anticoagulation should be encouraged to determine whether there is scarring and to establish a new baseline for patients who return for new symptoms.

Most studies have evaluated patients during their initial presentation of DVT. The accuracy of a single ultrasonography scan with other patient history is not established. Risk factors, D-dimer results, and relevant history may not be known by the imaging facility. Therefore, in some patients with normal examinations, it may be prudent to recommend follow-up in 1 week. This follow-up could include patients with a prior history of DVT, patients in whom scarring is identified, pregnant women, patients in whom the scan is technically limited, or patients in whom there is calf pain and DVT is not identified. This approach is inferred because it is established that 2 more limited studies, 1 week apart, is a safe strategy.[33]

In general, a comment in the otherwise normal report that "If there remains suspicion of DVT or the clinical condition worsens, a follow-up should be considered" may be a helpful reminder to the referrer.

REFERENCES

1. Esmon CT. Basic mechanisms and pathogenesis of venous thrombosis. Blood Rev 2009;23(5):225–9. http://dx.doi.org/10.1016/j.blre.2009.07.002.
2. Thomas DP. Overview of venous thrombogenesis. Semin Thromb Hemost 1988;14(1):1–8. http://dx.doi.org/10.1055/s-2007-1002749.
3. Patel K. Deep venous thrombosis. Medscape Reference; 2014. p. 1–33. Available at: http://emedicine.medscape.com/article/1911303-overview#aw2aab6b2b4.
4. Killewich LA, Bedford GR, Beach KW, et al. Spontaneous lysis of deep venous thrombi: rate and outcome. J Vasc Surg 1989;9(1):89–97.
5. Meissner MH, Caps MT, Bergelin RO, et al. Propagation, rethrombosis and new thrombus formation after acute deep venous thrombosis. J Vasc Surg 1995;22(5):558–67. http://dx.doi.org/10.1016/S0741-5214(95)70038-2.
6. van Ramshorst B, van Bemmelen PS, Hoeneveld H, et al. Thrombus regression in deep venous thrombosis. Quantification of spontaneous thrombolysis with duplex scanning. Circulation 1992;86(2):414–9. http://dx.doi.org/10.1161/01.CIR.86.2.414.
7. Kearon C, Julian JA, Newman TE, et al. Noninvasive diagnosis of deep venous thrombosis. McMaster Diagnostic Imaging Practice Guidelines Initiative. Ann Intern Med 1998;128(8):663–77.
8. Tan M, Mos IC, Klok FA, et al. Residual venous thrombosis as predictive factor for recurrent venous thromboembolism in patients with proximal deep vein thrombosis: a systematic review. Br J Haematol 2011;153(2):168–78. http://dx.doi.org/10.1111/j.1365-2141.2011.08578.x.
9. Tan M, van Rooden CJ, Westerbeek RE, et al. Diagnostic management of clinically suspected acute deep vein thrombosis. Br J Haematol 2009;146(4):347–60. http://dx.doi.org/10.1111/j.1365-2141.2009.07732.x.
10. Qaseem A, Snow V, Barry P, et al. Current diagnosis of venous thromboembolism in primary care: a clinical practice guideline from the American Academy of Family Physicians and the American College of Physicians. Ann Fam Med 2007;5(1):57–62. http://dx.doi.org/10.1370/afm.667.
11. Wells PS. Integrated strategies for the diagnosis of venous thromboembolism. J Thromb Haemost 2007;5:41–50. http://dx.doi.org/10.1111/j.1538-7836.2007.02493.x.
12. Le Gal G, Carrier M, Rodger M. Clinical decision rules in venous thromboembolism. Best Pract Res Clin Haematol 2012;25(3):303–17. http://dx.doi.org/10.1016/j.beha.2012.06.001.
13. Kraaijenhagen RA, Piovella F, Bernardi E, et al. Simplification of the diagnostic management of suspected deep vein thrombosis. Arch Intern Med 2002;162(8):907–11.
14. Segal JB, Eng J, Tamariz LJ, et al. Review of the evidence on diagnosis of deep venous thrombosis and pulmonary embolism. Ann Fam Med 2007;5(1):63–73. http://dx.doi.org/10.1370/afm.648.
15. Squizzato A, Micieli E, Galli M, et al. Diagnosis and management of venous thromboembolism: Results of a survey on current clinical practice. Thromb Res 2010;125(2):134–6. http://dx.doi.org/10.1016/j.thromres.2009.05.008.
16. American Institute of Ultrasound in Medicine, American College of Radiology, Society of Radiologists in Ultrasound. Practice guideline for the performance of peripheral venous ultrasound examinations. J Ultrasound Med 2011;30(1):143–50.
17. Bundens WP, Bergan JJ, Halasz NA, et al. The superficial femoral vein. A potentially lethal misnomer. JAMA 1995;274(16):1296–8.
18. Caggiati A, Bergan JJ, Gloviczki P, et al. Nomenclature of the veins of the lower limbs: an international interdisciplinary consensus statement. J Vasc Surg 2002;36:416–22.
19. Hamper UM, DeJong MR, Scoutt LM. Ultrasound evaluation of the lower extremity veins. Radiol Clin North Am 2007;45(3):525–47. http://dx.doi.org/10.1016/j.rcl.2007.04.013.
20. Murphy TP, Cronan JJ. Evolution of deep venous thrombosis: a prospective evaluation with US. Radiology 1990;177(2):543–8.
21. Linkins LA, Stretton R, Probyn L, et al. Interobserver agreement on ultrasound measurements of residual vein diameter, thrombus echogenicity and Doppler venous flow in patients with previous venous thrombosis. Thromb Res 2006;117(3):241–7. http://dx.doi.org/10.1016/j.thromres.2005.02.011.
22. Galioto NJ, Danley DL, Van Maanen RJ. Recurrent venous thromboembolism. Am Fam Physician 2011;83(3):293–300.
23. Watson HG. RVO–real value obscure. J Thromb Haemost 2011;9(6):1116–8. http://dx.doi.org/10.1111/j.1538-7836.2011.04296.x.

24. Cronan JJ, Leen V. Recurrent deep venous thrombosis: limitations of US. Radiology 1989;170(3 Pt 1):739–42.

25. Prandoni P, Lensing AW, Bernardi E, et al. The diagnostic value of compression ultrasonography in patients with suspected recurrent deep vein thrombosis. Thromb Haemost 2002;88(3):402–6. http://dx.doi.org/10.1267/THRO88030402.

26. Spritzer CE. Progress in MR imaging of the venous system. Perspect Vasc Surg Endovasc Ther 2009; 21(2):105–16. http://dx.doi.org/10.1177/153100350 9337259.

27. Westerbeek RE, Van Rooden CJ, Tan M, et al. Magnetic resonance direct thrombus imaging of the evolution of acute deep vein thrombosis of the leg. J Thromb Haemost 2008;6(7):1087–92. http://dx. doi.org/10.1111/j.1538-7836.2008.02986.x.

28. IAC standards and guidelines for vascular testing accreditation. 2014:1–67. Available at: http://www. intersocietal.org/vascular/main/vascular_standards. htm. Accessed April 14, 2014.

29. Guyatt GH, Akl EA, Crowther M, et al. Executive summary: antithrombotic therapy and prevention of thrombosis, 9th ed: American College of Chest Physicians evidence-based clinical practice guidelines. Chest 2012;141(Suppl 2):7S–47S. http://dx.doi.org/ 10.1378/chest.1412S3.

30. Palareti G, Schellong S. Isolated distal deep vein thrombosis: what we know and what we are doing. J Thromb Haemost 2012;10(1):11–9. http://dx.doi. org/10.1111/j.1538-7836.2011.04564.x.

31. Johnson SA, Stevens SM, Woller SC, et al. Risk of deep vein thrombosis following a single negative whole-leg compression ultrasound: a systematic review and meta-analysis. JAMA 2010;303(5):438–45. http://dx.doi.org/10.1001/jama.2010.43.

32. Guanella R, Righini M. Serial limited versus single complete compression ultrasonography for the diagnosis of lower extremity deep vein thrombosis. Semin Respir Crit Care Med 2012;33(2):144–50. http://dx.doi.org/10.1055/s-0032-1311793.

33. Birdwell BG, Raskob GE, Whitsett TL, et al. The clinical validity of normal compression ultrasonography in outpatients suspected of having deep venous thrombosis. Ann Intern Med 1998;128(1): 1–7.

34. Bernardi E, Camporese G, Büller HR, et al. Serial 2-point ultrasonography plus D-dimer vs whole-leg color-coded Doppler ultrasonography for diagnosing suspected symptomatic deep vein thrombosis: a randomized controlled trial. JAMA 2008; 300(14):1653–9. http://dx.doi.org/10.1001/jama.300. 14.1653.

35. Society for Vascular Medicine. Five things physicians and patients should question. Choosing wisely; 2014. p. 1–2. Available at: http://www.choosing-wisely.org/doctor-patient-lists/society-for-vascular-medicine/. Accessed April 14, 2014.

Index

Note: Page numbers of article titles are in **boldface** type.

Radiol Clin N Am 52 (2014) 1375–1383
http://dx.doi.org/10.1016/S0033-8389(14)00161-4
0033-8389/14/$ – see front matter © 2014 Elsevier Inc. All rights reserved.

radiologic.theclinics.com

United States Postal Service

Statement of Ownership, Management, and Circulation
(All Periodicals Publications Except Requestor Publications)

1. Publication Title	2. Publication Number	3. Filing Date
Radiologic Clinics of North America	5 9 6 - 5 1 0	9/14/14

4. Issue Frequency	5. Number of Issues Published Annually	6. Annual Subscription Price
Jan, Mar, May, Jul, Sep, Nov	6	$460.00

7. Complete Mailing Address of Known Office of Publication (Not printer) (Street, city, county, state, and ZIP+4®)

Elsevier Inc.
360 Park Avenue South
New York, NY 10010-1710

Contact Person
Stephen R. Bushing

Telephone (Include area code)
215-239-3688

8. Complete Mailing Address of Headquarters or General Business Office of Publisher (Not printer)

Elsevier Inc., 360 Park Avenue South, New York, NY 10010-1710

9. Full Names and Complete Mailing Addresses of Publisher, Editor, and Managing Editor (Do not leave blank)

Publisher (Name and complete mailing address)

Linda Belfus, Elsevier, Inc., 1600 John F. Kennedy Blvd. Suite 1800, Philadelphia, PA 19103-2899

Editor (Name and complete mailing address)

John Vassallo, Elsevier, Inc., 1600 John F. Kennedy Blvd. Suite 1800, Philadelphia, PA 19103-2899

Managing Editor (Name and complete mailing address)

Adrianne Brigido, Elsevier, Inc., 1600 John F. Kennedy Blvd. Suite 1800, Philadelphia, PA 19103-2899

10. Owner (Do not leave blank. If the publication is owned by a corporation, give the name and address of the corporation immediately followed by the names and addresses of all stockholders owning or holding 1 percent or more of the total amount of stock. If not owned by a corporation, give the names and addresses of the individual owners. If owned by a partnership or other unincorporated firm, give its name and address as well as those of each individual owner. If the publication is published by a nonprofit organization, give its name and address.)

Full Name	Complete Mailing Address
Wholly owned subsidiary of	1600 John F. Kennedy Blvd, Ste. 1800
Reed/Elsevier, US holdings	Philadelphia, PA 19103-2899

11. Known Bondholders, Mortgagees, and Other Security Holders Owning or Holding 1 Percent or More of Total Amount of Bonds, Mortgages, or Other Securities. If none, check box ☐ None

Full Name	Complete Mailing Address
N/A	

12. Tax Status (For completion by nonprofit organizations authorized to mail at nonprofit rates) (Check one)
The purpose, function, and nonprofit status of this organization and the exempt status for federal income tax purposes:
☐ Has Not Changed During Preceding 12 Months
☐ Has Changed During Preceding 12 Months (Publisher must submit explanation of change with this statement)

PS Form 3526, August 2012 (Page 1 of 3 (Instructions Page 3)) PSN 7530-01-000-9931 PRIVACY NOTICE: See our Privacy policy in www.usps.com

---

13. Publication Title	14. Issue Date for Circulation Data Below
Radiologic Clinics of North America	July 2014

15. Extent and Nature of Circulation			Average No. Copies Each Issue During Preceding 12 Months	No. Copies of Single Issue Published Nearest to Filing Date
a. Total Number of Copies (Net press run)			2,830	2,776
b. Paid Circulation (By Mail and Outside the Mail)	(1)	Mailed Outside-County Paid Subscriptions Stated on PS Form 3541. (Include paid distribution above nominal rate, advertiser's proof copies, and exchange copies)	1,764	1,719
	(2)	Mailed In-County Paid Subscriptions Stated on PS Form 3541 (Include paid distribution above nominal rate, advertiser's proof copies, and exchange copies)		
	(3)	Paid Distribution Outside the Mails Including Sales Through Dealers and Carriers, Street Vendors, Counter Sales, and Other Paid Distribution Outside USPS®	522	539
	(4)	Paid Distribution by Other Classes Mailed Through the USPS (e.g. First-Class Mail®)		
c. Total Paid Distribution (Sum of 15b (1), (2), (3), and (4))			2,286	2,258
d. Free or Nominal Rate Distribution (By Mail and Outside the Mail)	(1)	Free or Nominal Rate Outside-County Copies Included on PS Form 3541	50	43
	(2)	Free or Nominal Rate In-County Copies Included on PS Form 3541		
	(3)	Free or Nominal Rate Copies Mailed at Other Classes Through the USPS (e.g. First-Class Mail)		
	(4)	Free or Nominal Rate Distribution Outside the Mail (Carriers or other means)		
e. Total Free or Nominal Rate Distribution (Sum of 15d (1), (2), (3) and (4))			50	43
f. Total Distribution (Sum of 15c and 15e)			2,336	2,301
g. Copies not Distributed (See instructions to publishers #4 (page #3))			494	475
h. Total (Sum of 15f and g)			2,830	2,776
i. Percent Paid (15c divided by 15f times 100)			97.86%	98.13%

16. Total circulation includes electronic copies. Report circulation on PS Form 3526-X worksheet.

17. Publication of Statement of Ownership
If the publication is a general publication, publication of this statement is required. Will be printed in the November 2014 issue of this publication.

18. Signature and Title of Editor, Publisher, Business Manager or Owner

Stephen R. Bushing – Inventory Distribution Coordinator

Date: September 14, 2014

I certify that all information furnished on this form is true and complete. I understand that anyone who furnishes false or misleading information on this form or who omits material or information requested on the form may be subject to criminal sanctions (including fines and imprisonment) and/or civil sanctions (including civil penalties).

PS Form 3526, August 2012 (Page 2 of 3)

Moving?

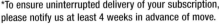

Make sure your subscription moves with you!

To notify us of your new address, find your **Clinics Account Number** (located on your mailing label above your name), and contact customer service at:

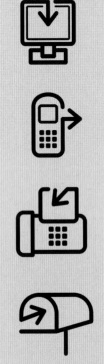

Email: journalscustomerservice-usa@elsevier.com

800-654-2452 (subscribers in the U.S. & Canada)
314-447-8871 (subscribers outside of the U.S. & Canada)

Fax number: 314-447-8029

Elsevier Health Sciences Division
Subscription Customer Service
3251 Riverport Lane
Maryland Heights, MO 63043

ELSEVIER